Textbook for the Veterinary Assistant

Textbook for the Veterinary Assistant

Second Edition

Kara M. Burns, MS, MEd, LVT, VTS (Nutrition)
Independent Consultant
Lafayette, IN, USA

Lori Renda-Francis, LVT, BBA, M.Ed, PhD
Macomb Community College
Clinton Township, MI, USA

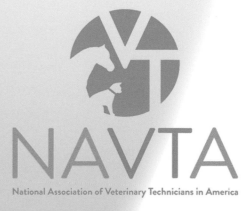

WILEY Blackwell

NAVTA
National Association of Veterinary Technicians in America

Registered Office
John Wiley & Sons, Inc., 111 River Street, Hoboken, NJ 07030, USA

Editorial Office
111 River Street, Hoboken, NJ 07030, USA

For details of our global editorial offices, customer services, and more information about Wiley products visit us at www.wiley.com.

Wiley also publishes its books in a variety of electronic formats and by print-on-demand. Some content that appears in standard print versions of this book may not be available in other formats.

Library of Congress Cataloging-in-Publication Data Applied for:

ISBN: 9781119565314

Cover Design: Wiley
Cover Images: Courtesy of Lori Renda-Francis; Courtesy of Lynn Roland, LVT

Set in 10/12pt Minion by Straive, Pondicherry, India

Printed in Singapore
M095433_031121

Dedication

The editors wish to thank the contributors from the first edition.

Your contributions aided in the success of the first edition and allowed for the expansion of topics in this second edition.

Contents

Acknowledgments

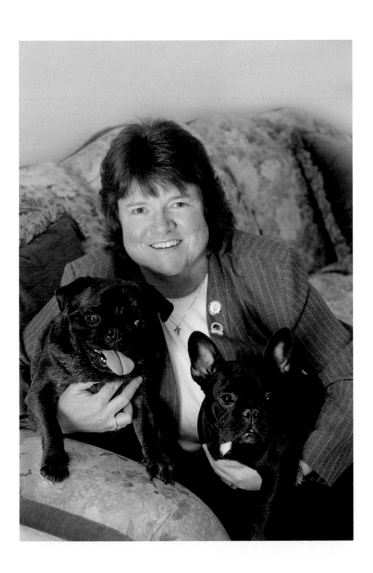

Writing a book is no small feat. Developing this second edition has truly been an honor. This would not have been possible without the support of several individuals who have helped me throughout this journey.

First and foremost, I want to thank my wife Ellen Lowery, DVM, PhD, MBA. You make my life complete and give me the courage to pursue all of my dreams. Thank you for your encouragement and support in this endeavor and for inspiring me to always follow my dreams! Thank you for being the love of my life!

I would like to thank my co-author Lori Renda-Francis, LVT, PhD for her friendship and support as our second edition came to fruition. May God continue to watch over you and your family – two and four legged!

Thank you to our colleagues at Wiley Blackwell. Specifically, our managing editor Merryl Le Roux and our executive editor Erica Judisch. We are truly grateful for your support and guidance on this journey.

Thank you to the National Association of Veterinary Technicians in America (NAVTA) for the support given to Lori and myself to write this book and for the support NAVTA gives to the entire veterinary profession and all healthcare team members.

Finally, thank you to all the pets, past and present, which have gifted our lives with your presence. To name them all would be a book in itself, but each of you have touched my life and brought infinite joy.

Kara M. Burns

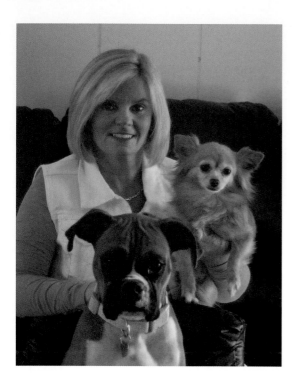

It has been an honor and a privilege to have the opportunity to write a textbook for veterinary assistants. I can only hope that this second edition continues to teach and inspire students to become loving and caring professionals.

I have been very fortunate to have the support of friends, family, and colleagues throughout the writing of this textbook. These individuals have provided the assistance and encouragement necessary for me to successfully complete this book. To all of them, I express my sincere thanks.

I would like to thank my parents, Marilyn and Joe Renda, for always believing in me, encouraging me, and supporting my love for animals, and for allowing me to keep all the little critters that I snuck into the house. Mom's heartfelt encouraging words and Dad's strong work ethic and persistence taught me that working hard for things you want will be worth it in the end.

I would also like to thank my sisters Wendy and Shelly, my son Brad and daughter-in-law Jen for being by my side encouraging me. Most of all, I would like to thank my husband Steve for the incredible sacrifices he has made to ensure I was successful in this endeavor. Steve, you are a great husband and wonderful father. Thank you for your love, dedication, support, and encouragement and for believing in me even when I did not believe in myself.

Thank you to all of the contributors of this book. Most importantly, thank you to my wonderful staff members, who always support me through all of my endeavors, and to my students, who continue to teach me as much as I teach them.

In addition, I would like to thank Merryl LeRoux and Erica Judisch at Wiley Blackwell for their patience and guidance, and a very special thank you to my co-author and good friend Kara Burns. It has been a true honor working on the second edition with someone I admire and respect so much. The idea for this book came about because of the love that we share for veterinary technicians and veterinary assistants. I pray that we can inspire students to reach their goals.

Finally, I am grateful to God for His gracious blessings and guiding hands.

Lori Renda-Francis

About the Companion Website

This book is accompanied by a companion website:

www.wiley.com/go/burns/textbookvetassistant2

The website includes:

An Instructor Site:

- Textbook Fill in Blank Questions Key
- Homework Assignments Key
- Power Points for teaching

A Student Site:

- Student Study Guide Notes
- Textbook Fill in Blank Questions
- Homework Assignments
- Multiple Choice Questions
- Figures from the book in Power Point per chapter

Chapter 1 Introduction to the Veterinary (or Assistant) Profession

Welcome to veterinary medicine! Congratulations on choosing one of the most rewarding and enriching professions! Veterinary medicine is a profession that involves medicine, compassion, technical skills, and teamwork. It provides care for species that cannot speak for themselves. As in human medicine, the veterinary health-care team is composed of many members, each with an important role in the proper care of patients and functioning of a veterinary hospital.

The goal of the veterinary practice should be excellent patient care and exceptional customer service. This textbook will look at the veterinary assistant's role in making this goal a reality. Veterinary practices should also provide team members with a friendly, well-organized, and safe workplace. Every veterinary health-care team member is responsible for the success of the practice.

The veterinary health-care team works together in the best interest of the patient. All team members, regardless of their role in the veterinary hospital, have the responsibility to ensure the safety and comfort of all patients. Each member of the health-care team has specific roles and responsibilities, and often times these responsibilities are shared. Whatever the hierarchy in the practice, all members must provide the best care to all patients at all times. The American Veterinary Medical Association (AVMA) likewise recognizes the value of the various health-care team members: "The veterinary profession is enhanced through efficient utilization of each member of the veterinary healthcare team by appropriate delegation of tasks and responsibilities to support staff."

The various members of the health-care team include the following.

- Veterinary assistant
- Veterinarian
- Veterinary technician
- Veterinary technologist
- Veterinary technician specialist
- Receptionist
- Office managers
- Groomers
- Kennel assistants

Veterinary assistants may be approved through the National Association of Veterinary Technicians in America (NAVTA)-approved veterinary assistant program or trained on the job (www.navta.net/assistants). The term *veterinary assistant* is used typically for a person who assists in the care of animals but is not a credentialed veterinary technician, laboratory animal technician, or veterinarian.

The roles and responsibilities of veterinary assistants will be covered in detail in the forthcoming chapters. The duties of the veterinary assistant may include restraining and exercising patients, cleaning hospital and boarding premises, setting up equipment and supplies, cleaning and maintaining practice and laboratory facilities, and feeding patients. They may also be responsible for other clinical support tasks assigned by the credentialed veterinary technician and/or veterinarian. Most veterinary assistants are trained on the job by a supervising veterinary technician or veterinarian, but some assistants complete 6–12 months of training in a formal course of study.

The veterinarian is a doctor of veterinary medicine. Veterinarians have graduated from a 4-year AVMA-accredited postgraduate doctoral program culminating in a doctor of veterinary medicine (DVM) or veterinary medical doctor (VMD)

Textbook for the Veterinary Assistant, Second Edition. Kara M. Burns and Lori Renda-Francis.
© 2022 John Wiley & Sons, Inc. Published 2022 by John Wiley & Sons, Inc.
Companion website: www.wiley.com/go/burns/textbookvetassistant2

degree. Veterinarians must also pass the licensing board in the state or province in which they wish to practice. Veterinarians have many responsibilities in the hospital, and they are licensed to perform surgery, diagnose diseases and conditions, give a prognosis relating to the diagnosis, and prescribe medication. These skills are the veterinarians' alone – no other health-care team member can do these tasks.

The veterinary technician is a graduate of a program in veterinary technology accredited by the AVMA Committee on Veterinary Technician Education and Activities (CVTEA). The technician typically has received an associate's degree and national credentialing through the Veterinary Technician National Examination (VTNE). Some states require a national as well as a state credential, verified by the state board of veterinary medicine. Only graduates of an AVMA-accredited program are allowed to take the national board exam. The duties of a veterinary technician are many and often include, but are not limited to, nursing care, anesthesia, surgery, dental, laboratory, radiography, etc.

A veterinary technologist is a graduate of a 4-year, AVMA CVTEA-accredited program who holds a bachelor's degree from a veterinary technician school. Alternatively, a veterinary technologist may be a credentialed veterinary technician who holds a bachelor of science degree in another program with studies in supervision, leadership, management, or a scientific area. The technologist's responsibilities are similar to but more in depth than those of veterinary technicians. Veterinary technologists may also pursue careers in hospital management, education, or research.

Veterinary technician specialists (VTS) are veterinary technicians who have pursued further education, experience, and training in one of 16 current areas of specialization recognized by the NAVTA. Credentialed technicians who choose to specialize must accumulate a specific number of hours within a particular specialty during a set number of years. VTS candidates are also expected to have a strong knowledge and skill set pertaining to their specific area of medicine and nursing as well as a minimum number of continuing education hours specific to their specialty. Their advanced education and training culminates in taking a board examination specific to their specialty showing their advanced knowledge and skills.

The following are the 16 veterinary technician specialty academies currently recognized by the NAVTA.

1. Academy of Veterinary Emergency & Critical Care Technicians and Nurses (AVECCTN)

2. Academy of Veterinary Technicians in Anesthesia and Analgesia (AVTAA)

3. Academy of Veterinary Dental Technicians (AVDT)

4. Academy of Internal Medicine for Veterinary Technicians (AIMVT)

5. Academy of Veterinary Behavior Technicians (AVBT)

6. Academy of Veterinary Zoological Medicine Technicians (AVZMT)

7. Academy Of Equine Veterinary Nursing Technicians (AEVNT)

8. Academy of Veterinary Surgical Technicians (AVST)

9. Academy of Veterinary Technicians in Clinical Practice (AVTCP)

10. Academy of Veterinary Nutrition Technicians (AVNT)

11. Academy of Veterinary Clinical Pathology Technicians (AVCPT)

12. Academy of Laboratory Animal Veterinary Technicians and Nurses (ALAVTN)

13. Academy of Dermatology Veterinary Technicians (ADVT)

14. Academy of Physical Rehabilitation Veterinary Technicians (APRVT)

15. Academy of Veterinary Ophthalmic Technicians (AVOT)

16. The Academy of Veterinary Technicians in Diagnostic Imaging (AVTDI)

For more information on veterinary technician specialties, please visit www.navta.net/page/specialties.

Like all other members of the health-care team, receptionists play a significant role in the success of a practice. Receptionists benefit the practice as the face and voice of the hospital. They greet clients, detail and clarify invoices, and receive money. They are professionals with great people skills. Receptionists answer the hospital phone and schedule appointments. They are responsible for acknowledging clients when they walk in and out of the practice. Because they typically make the first impression on clients, receptionists affect the clients' perception of the hospital and are thus critical to the success of the hospital.

Office managers are responsible for the management of the front office staff. Their duties include training receptionists on proper and excellent customer service and communication skills. Office managers often make important decisions on behalf of the practice and supervise the running of the practice. They are typically responsible for the banking needs of the practice and resolution of performance issues among the team members.

Groomers have experience and education in performing technical skills relating to the fur and dermis of the patient. Many breeds of animals require specific grooming techniques, and advanced training is necessary to acquire such skills. Training and good communication skills are important to meeting the needs of the patient and the client. Groomers must also take precautions to prevent injury to animals and to themselves. A number of courses and on-the-job training programs are available for groomers. Many groomers belong to the National Dog Groomers Association (NDGA). This association works in conjunction with groomers throughout the country to promote professionalism. In some states, licensing or certification is required. The NDGA educates all areas of the profession and the public with regard to the pet grooming profession.

The NDGA's goals are to:

- unite groomers through membership
- promote communication with colleagues
- set recognized grooming standards
- offer those seeking a higher level of professional recognition the opportunity to have their grooming skills certified.

Kennel assistants are responsible for the cleanliness of the patient and monitoring patient status and immediately alerting the team to any changes. The majority of kennel assistants receive on-the-job training where they learn the workings of a veterinary hospital as well as procedures and protocols crucial to the patients' health and safety. Kennel assistants are taught to interpret correct nutritional instructions, feed the diet prescribed in the right amount, and remove food from *preoperative* patients. They are responsible for reporting any and all behavior or condition changes to the immediate patient caregiver.

Ethics

Ethics is defined as the moral principles that govern an individual's behavior or the conducting of an activity. In the veterinary profession, the way we handle pet owners, patients, and their care is guided by ethics. Ethics provides a map which lays out the rules of best practices and standards in protocols, procedures, and practices. Ethics is the discipline of dealing with what is right and wrong or associated with moral duty and obligation. It is also the principles of conduct overseeing an individual or a profession. Ethics provides a map for people to do "the right thing" within our profession.

According to Dr Albert Schweitzer, "Ethics is the name that we give to our concern for good behavior. We feel an obligation to consider not only our own personal well-being, but also that of others and of human society as a whole."

Often the line between ethical violations and legal violations is thin. A breach of descriptive or official ethical values would not be enforced by a court of law but might be cause for dismissal from the professional association.

Laws set the boundaries to which individuals must adhere. They are a system of rules created and enforced through legislation to regulate behavior

Ethics is usually centered around principles even higher than legal requirements. Additionally, members of professions, especially medical professions, are expected to adhere to ethical standards above those considered appropriate for individuals not involved in a medical profession. Pet owners accept, without question, the decisions and judgments made by medical professionals because of their education and expertise.

The AVMA provides principles of veterinary medical ethics for licensed veterinarians and can be found at www.avma.org/resources-tools/avma-policies/principles-veterinary-medical-ethics-avma

Veterinary medicine has a code of ethics for health-care team members to follow. Both veterinarians and veterinary technicians have a code of ethics. Additionally, when entering the veterinary profession, after meeting all the requirements for becoming a licensed veterinary medical professional, veterinarians and veterinary technicians take an oath to use their skills and knowledge for the benefit of animal health, animal welfare, public health, and the advancement of medical knowledge. All members of the veterinary health-care team adhere to the medical profession's ethic of *Primum non nocere* – first do no harm.

The veterinary technician oath is as follows: "I solemnly dedicate myself to aiding animals and society by providing excellent care and services for animals, by alleviating animal suffering, and promoting public health.

I accept my obligations to practice my profession conscientiously and with sensitivity, adhering to the profession's Code of Ethics, and furthering my knowledge and competence through a commitment to lifelong learning."

The veterinary technician code of ethics and oath can be found on the NAVTA website: www.navta.net/page/TechnicianOath

Coinciding with the evolution of electronic communication are systemic changes in health-care delivery. An increasing amount of medical knowledge is necessary to deliver even the most basic care. Telemedicine, the use of technology in the delivery of medicine to advance clinical care at a distance, is increasing in use. However, since the SARS-CoV-2 pandemic, telemedicine has become more significantly utilized to provide care to pets while keeping the safety of owners and veterinary team members at the forefront. As has been seen to date, telemedicine has helped to continue medical care and has the potential to transform patient-centered care. Technology platforms allow veterinary team members to communicate with pet owners through a variety of means, including text, email, and mobile device applications. This technology is especially important when more members of the veterinary team are involved, as it can enable communications between members of the team, thus improving overall coordination of care.

However, in medicine as a whole – human and veterinary – there are concerns about the adoption of telemedicine and its potential impact on patient care. Ensuring that telemedicine is ethically acceptable will require anticipating and addressing possible drawbacks such as the impact on the veterinarian–client–patient relationship (VCPR), imposing one-size-fits-all applications, and the belief that new technology must be effective.

The veterinary team must consider the same ethical issues with telemedicine that have always been thought of when providing care for patients. Focusing on maintaining a strong VCPR, advocating equity in access and treatment, and seeking the best possible outcomes, telemedicine can enhance veterinary practice and patient care in ways that provide quality medicine and are ethical.

The veterinary health-care team comprises many positions, each with various roles and responsibilities. It is important that teamwork is emphasized, as good patient care is a result of great teamwork.

References

McCurnin, D.M. and Bassert, J.M. 2017. *McCurnin's Clinical Textbook for Veterinary Technicians*, 9th edition. W.B. Saunders Company, St Louis, MO.

Prendergast, H. 2011. *Front Office Management for the Veterinary Team*. Saunders Elsevier, St Louis, MO.

Sirois, M. 2017. *Principles and Practice of Veterinary Technology*, 4th edition. Mosby, St Louis, MO.

www.wiley.com/go/burns/textbookvetassistant2

Please go to the companion website for assignments and a PowerPoint relating to the material in this chapter.

Chapter **2** Medical Terminology

Medical terms are made up of many different elements. It is important for veterinary assistants to have a clear understanding of the various parts of a word. Understanding each part will aid in learning the meaning and spelling of that word. You will be expected to recognize, pronounce, spell, and utilize commonly used medical terms. It is helpful to note that there are four main parts to a word.

- Prefix
- Suffix
- Root
- Combining form of a root word

A *prefix* is placed at the beginning of a word and consists of one or more syllables. It will modify or alter a verb, adjective, or noun, thereby creating a new word. The prefix usually indicates number, time, location, or status.

A *suffix* is the ending of a word and consists of one or more syllables. Similar to the prefix, a suffix is added to a root word to modify or alter its meaning. The suffix usually indicates procedure, disease, disorder, or condition.

The *root* is the central part of the word and is the foundation or essential meaning of a word. It may be a complete word in itself or a part of a word.

A *combining form* of the root word is a root with a combining vowel. The purpose of combining forms of root words is to make the resulting word easier to pronounce. Examples of the combining form of a root word are shown in the following list. The word root is in italic letters, and the combining vowel is in parentheses.

- *orth*(o)pedic
- *bacteri*(o)static
- *quadr*(i)plegic

When we take a root word such as "derm-," which means "skin," and combine it with the suffix "-itis," it becomes "dermatitis." Dermatitis is an inflammation of the skin. If we take the same root word and include the prefix "pyo-," we create the word "pyoderma," which is defined as bacterial infection of the skin.

Medical terms

Words are made up of one or more of these parts. Medical terms deal with the diagnosis and treatment of disease and the maintenance of health. It is important for veterinary assistants to understand the meaning of the word parts in order to be able to dissect medical terms in a logical way.

Spelling

Correct spelling of medical terms is essential because a misspelled word may give an entirely different meaning! Changing just one or two letters can change the entire meaning of a word. For example, a macrocyte is an abnormally large red blood cell, but a microcyte is an abnormally small red blood cell. Two or more medical terms may also be pronounced in the same way but have different meanings. For example, ileum and ilium are pronounced in the same way. However, ileum is the distal part of the small intestine while ilium is part of the pelvis.

Tips for succeeding in learning medical terminology

Since students learn in various ways, it is important to utilize a variety of methods to learn medical terminology. For some students, writing words helps them to learn faster than simply reading them. Some students retain material better when they use

Textbook for the Veterinary Assistant, Second Edition. Kara M. Burns and Lori Renda-Francis.
© 2022 John Wiley & Sons, Inc. Published 2022 by John Wiley & Sons, Inc.
Companion website: www.wiley.com/go/burns/textbookvetassistant2

various learning methods. Speaking into a tape recorder and using it to practice pronunciation is helpful. Proper pronunciation of medical terms takes time and practice. Listening to how words are pronounced by medical professionals and using medical dictionaries and textbooks are the best ways to learn pronunciation. Making flash cards to quiz yourself may be another useful method. There are also online quizzes and flash cards available. The key is repetition. Learning and memorizing these terms will require time and concentration.

Now that you have a basic understanding of the different parts of a word, let's look at some commonly used prefixes, suffixes, and root words.

Prefixes

By learning the meanings of the commonly utilized prefixes, you will be able to break down unfamiliar words to find out their meaning. It may be helpful to divide them into categories according to their meaning. Below are the prefixes arranged into six categories.

1. Prefixes related to position regarding time and place
2. Prefixes describing position or location
3. Prefixes related to type
4. Prefixes related to direction
5. Prefixes describing number or quantity
6. Prefixes related to size, amount, and color

If we have the root word "operative" we can change the meaning by inserting different prefixes. For example:

- preoperative – before a surgery
- postoperative – after the surgery
- perioperative – around the time of the surgery

Prefixes related to position regarding time and place:

ana-	up, back again
ante-	before, in front of, forward
cata-	down, through
meta-	beyond, over, between, change, after
noct-	night
post-	after, behind
pre-	before, in front of
prim-	first
sym-, syn-	together, union, with

Prefixes describing position or location:

anti-	against, opposing
apo-	separation from or derivation from
circum-	around
contra-	opposite, against, opposed
dorso-	pertaining to the back
ecto-	outside, misplaced

endo-	within, inner
epi-	on, over, upon
extra-	outside of, in addition to
hyper-	above, excessive, beyond
hypo-	under, deficient, beneath
infra-	below
inter-	between parts
intra-	within parts
medi-	middle
para-	beside, beyond
peri-	around
pro-	for, in front of, before
pseudo-	false
sub-	beneath, under
super-, supra-	excessive, above, superior
trans-	across, through, over, beyond
ultra-	excessive, extreme, beyond

Prefixes related to type:

a-, an-	without, absent, lack of
auto-	self
bi-	two, double, twice
brady-	slow
co-, com-, con-	with, together
cry-	cold
crypto-	hidden
dys-	difficult, bad, painful, abnormal
eu-	good, normal
glyco-, gluco-	sugar, sweet
gyn-, gyneco-	female
hydra-, hydro-	water
mal-	bad

Prefixes related to direction:

ab-	away from
ad-	to, toward
de-	opposite, reverse, remove
dia-	apart, separate, between
e-, ex-	out of, away from
in-	in, inside, within, not
re-	back, again
retro-	behind, backward

Prefixes describing number or quantity:

ambi-, amphi-	both
bi-	two
di-	two, twice
hemi-	half

mono-	one
multi-	many
pan-	all, entire
poly-	many, excessive
quadri-	four
quint-	five
semi-	half, partial
tri-	three

Prefixes related to size, amount and color:

a-, an-	none
cyano-	blue
erythro-	red
leuko-	white
macro-	large
mega-	big
micro-	small
mio-	less, smaller
olig-	little, small
per-	excessive, through, by means of

Suffixes

By learning the meanings of commonly used suffixes, you will be able to break down parts of an unfamiliar word in order to find out its meaning. For example, if we take the root word "derm," which means skin, and add the suffix "-ology," we get dermatology which is defined as the study of skin. If we add the suffix "-itis" to "derm," we end up with dermatitis, which is an inflammation of the skin. So by changing the suffix we can create new words.

Below is a list of some of the suffixes commonly used in veterinary medicine.

-algia	pain
-centesis	surgical puncture
-cide	kills
-cyte	cell
-ectomy	cutting out, surgically removing
-emesis	vomit
-emia	blood condition
-itis	inflammation
-ology	science, study of
-oma	tumor
-otomy	creation of an opening
-penia	deficiency of, lack of
-phag	eating, devouring
-phobia	abnormal fear, intolerance
-pnea	breathing
-ptosis	prolapse, downward displacement
-rrhage	excessive flow

-rrhea	flow or discharge
-scopy	act of examining
-tomy	cut, incision

Root words

Below is list of commonly used root words. They are grouped according to their relationship to the anatomy – external or internal. External anatomy refers to any visible part of the body, and internal anatomy refers to organs, bones, and other tissues within the body.

External anatomy

blepha-	eyelid or eyelash
capit-	head
carp-	area corresponding to human wrist
cervic-	neck
dactyl-	digit, toe
dent-	tooth or teeth
derm-	skin
gingiv-	gums
gloss-	tongue
lapar-	flank or abdomen
later-	side
ling-	tongue
mamm-	mammary gland
nas-	nose
ocul-	eye
odont-	tooth or teeth
onych-	nail or claw
or-	mouth
stomat-	mouth
pil-	hair
pod-	foot
rhin-	nose
thorac-	chest or thorax
ventr-	belly or underside

Internal anatomy

arthr-	joint
balan-	penis
bronch-	bronchus
cardi-	heart
cost-	rib
cyst-	bladder

enter-	intestine
gastr-	stomach
hepat-	liver
hyster-	uterus
laryng-	larynx
metr-	uterus
myo-	muscle
nephr-	kidney
neur-	nerve, nervous system
oophor-	ovary
orchi-	testes
oss-	bone
ovari-	ovary
phleb-	veins
phren-	diaphragm
pneum-	lungs
proct-	rectum or anus
pulm-	lungs
ren-	kidney
splen-	spleen
stern-	sternum
thym-	thymus gland
thyr-	thyroid gland
trache-	trachea
urethr-	urethra
vas-	vessel or duct
ven-	veins

Common abbreviations used in veterinary medicine

Below is a list of abbreviations and acronyms commonly used in veterinary practice. Please note that this is not a complete list of all veterinary abbreviations. It is a list of the most common abbreviations that are of interest to the veterinary assistant. It is also important to mention that abbreviations and acronyms will vary among veterinary practices, and you should obtain a list of those commonly used at your workplace. You can also purchase a copy of the *Standard Abbreviations for Veterinary Medical Records*, 2nd edition, from the AAHA Press. It contains a complete list of standard abbreviations.

AD	auris dexter (right ear)
ad lib	freely, as wanted
AG	anal glands
AL	auris sinistra (left ear)
ASAP	as soon as possible
AU	auris unitas (both ears)
BAR	bright, alert, and responsive
BID	twice daily

BM	bowel movement
BUN	blood urea nitrogen
BW	body weight
C	with
CAP	capsule
CBC	complete blood count
CNS	central nervous system
CPR	cardiopulmonary resuscitation
CRT	capillary refill time
DOA	dead on arrival
DSH	domestic shorthair
DLH	domestic longhair
Dx	diagnosis
FeLV	feline leukemia virus
FIP	feline infectious peritonitis
FIV	feline immunodeficiency virus
FS	female spayed
HBC	hit by car
HCT	hematocrit
HW	heartworm
HWP	heartworm preventative
ICU	intensive care unit
ID	intradermal
IM	intramuscular
IO	intraosseous
IN	intranasal
IP	intraperitoneal
IV	intravenous
K-9	canine
LRS	lactated Ringer's solution
MN	male neutered
NPO	nil per os (nothing by mouth)
OD	oculus dexter (right eye)
OE	orchidectomy (neuter)
OFA	Orthopedic Foundation for Animals
OHE	ovariohysterectomy (spay)
OS	oculus sinister (left eye)
OU	oculus unitas (both eyes)
PCV	packed cell volume
per os	orally (by mouth)
PO	per os
PRN	as necessary
q	every
q2h	every 2 hours
q6h	every 6 hours
qd	every day
qh	every hour
qns	quantity not sufficient
QID	four times a day

QOD	every other day
RBC	red blood cell
R/O	rule out
SC	subcutaneous
SQ	subcutaneous
SR	suture removal
SID	once a day
SUSP	suspension
Tab	tablet
TID	three times a day
TNT	toenail trim
TPR	temperature, pulse, respiration
TX	treatment
UA	urinalysis
UNG	ointment
WBC	white blood cell

You may find some variations on specific abbreviations or terminology used. It is important to determine what specific abbreviations are used at your place of employment.

References

Birmingham, J. 1999. *Medical Terminology: A Self-Learning Text*. Mosby, St Louis, MO.

Chchron, P. 1991. *Student Guide to Veterinary Medical Terminology*. American Veterinary Publications, Goleta, CA.

LaFleur Brooks, M. 1998. *Exploring Medical Language*, 4th edition. Mosby, St Louis, MO.

Leonard, P. 2007. *Quick and Easy Medical Terminology*, 5th edition. Saunders, St Louis, MO.

McBride, D.F. 2002. *Learning Veterinary Terminology*, 2nd edition. Mosby, St Louis, MO.

Romish, J.A. 2000. *An Illustrated Guide to Veterinary Terminology*. Delmar Thomson Learning, Albany, NY.

Standard Abbreviations for Veterinary Medical Records. 2000. AAHA Press, Lakewood, CO.

www.wiley.com/go/burns/textbookvetassistant2

Please go to the companion website for assignments and a PowerPoint relating to the material in this chapter.

Chapter **3** Anatomy

It is very important for veterinary assistants to recognize and have a clear understanding of basic directional and *anatomical* terms and to understand and speak the language of anatomy. Like other veterinary professionals, veterinary assistants are expected to be able to communicate intelligently and precisely. When the veterinary technician or veterinarian asks you, the veterinary assistant, to restrain the animal so the distal portion of the radius can be bandaged, you will need to be able to understand and respond appropriately.

Anatomical directional terms

Directional terms should always be utilized because they accurately and concisely describe body locations as well as relationships of one body structure to another. Terms such as "up" and "down" or "forward" and "backward" should not be used as these terms can cause confusion among veterinary professionals. Consistent use of proper anatomical and directional terms ensures the clear and accurate communication of the intended message.

Directional terms and directional planes are references used to describe the position and direction of various body structures. Directions will generally refer to a relative location and not an absolute point. We must first understand the various anatomical planes utilized in veterinary medicine. The four basic planes are dorsal, median, sagittal, and transverse.

The *dorsal* plane is an imaginary line that divides the body into dorsal and ventral portions. The *median* plane is an imaginary line that extends directly down the middle of the body, dividing it into equal right and left portions (Figure 3.1). The *sagittal* plane is an imaginary line that divides the body into right and left unequal parts, and the *transverse* plane is an imaginary cross-section that divides the body into cranial and caudal parts.

The terms below are used to describe direction or the position of a body part. We will begin with the basic directional terms.

The term *cranial* refers to the head portion of the animal's body, while *caudal* refers to the tail portion of the body. For example, we might say that the tail is caudal to the head or the head is cranial to the tail.

The terms "anterior" and "posterior" are used to describe the front and rear ends of the body. *Anterior* refers to the front of the body and *posterior* refers to the rear end of the body (Figure 3.2). For example, if a *laceration* was near the tail of an animal, we might say that the laceration is located on the posterior portion of the body.

We stated that the median plane divides the body into equal right and left portions. The terms "medial" and "lateral" are used to describe the location as it relates to the midline. *Medial* is defined as nearer or toward the midline or median plane, and *lateral* is defined as farther from the midline or median plane or toward the side of the body (Figure 3.3).

The dorsal plane divides the body into dorsal and ventral portions. The terms "ventral" and "dorsal" are utilized to describe the location as it relates to the dorsal plane. *Ventral* is defined as pertaining to the belly or underside of the body, and *dorsal* is pertaining to the back of the animal or toward the spine. For example, the abdomen is ventral to the spinal column.

"Proximal" and "distal" are commonly used when referring to extremities, with the point of origin being the main body mass. *Proximal* is used to describe a structure nearer to the point of origin or closer to the body, and *distal* is used to describe a structure

Textbook for the Veterinary Assistant, Second Edition. Kara M. Burns and Lori Renda-Francis.
© 2022 John Wiley & Sons, Inc. Published 2022 by John Wiley & Sons, Inc.
Companion website: www.wiley.com/go/burns/textbookvetassistant2

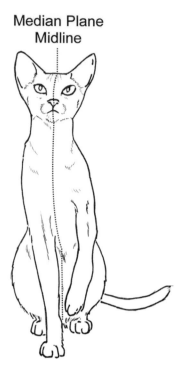

Figure 3.1 Median plane. Source: Courtesy of Dr Lori Renda-Francis, LVT.

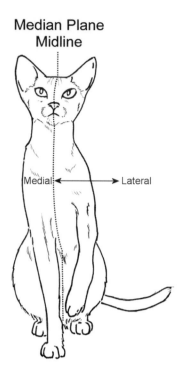

Figure 3.3 Medial/lateral. Source: Courtesy of Dr Lori Renda-Francis, LVT.

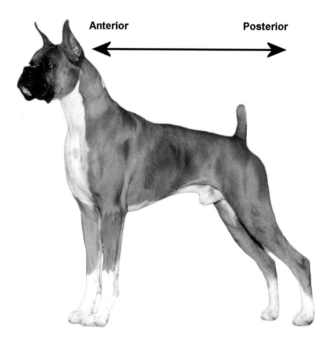

Figure 3.2 Anterior/posterior. Source: Courtesy of Dr Lori Renda-Francis, LVT.

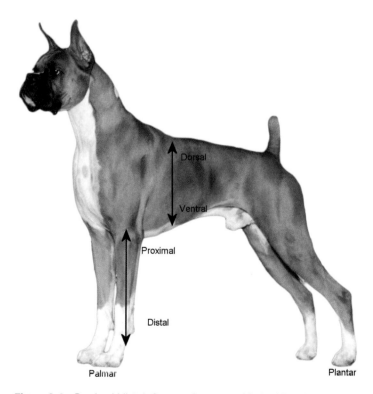

Figure 3.4 Proximal/distal. Source: Courtesy of Dr Lori Renda-Francis, LVT.

that is farther from the point of origin or away from the body (Figure 3.4). For example, the femur is proximal to the fibula.

The terms "palmar" and "plantar" are used when referring to the undersurface of the feet. **Palmar** is defined as the caudal surface of the forelimb below the **carpus,** and **plantar** is the caudal surface of the hindlimb below the **tarsus** (Figure 3.5).

"Internal" and "external" are used to describe a structure as it relates to the surface of the body. **Internal** refers to deep inside the body, and **external** refers to the outer surface of the body, which is more superficial.

Finally, the term **rostral** is defined as pertaining to the nose end of the head (Figure 3.6). For example, the nose is rostral to the eyes.

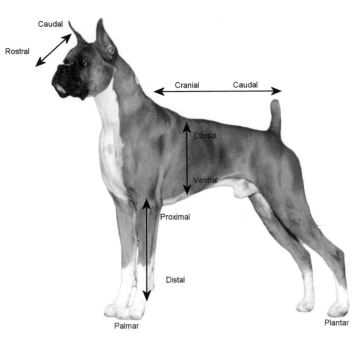

Figure 3.5 Anatomical terms. Source: Courtesy of Dr Lori Renda-Francis, LVT.

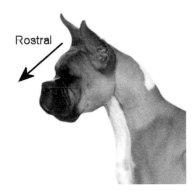

Figure 3.6 Rostral. Source: Courtesy of Dr Lori Renda-Francis, LVT.

Skeletal system

Skeleton is defined as the jointed framework of the bones. *Osteology* is the study of bones. Veterinary assistants will be expected to describe the bones of the body, which make up the skeleton, and have an understanding of the ways in which they connect and are moved.

The skeleton is divided into two main parts—the *axial* and the *appendicular*. The axial skeleton comprises the bones of the skull, the hyoid bones, the ribs, the sternum, and the vertebral column. The appendicular skeleton comprises the bones of the limbs: clavicle, scapula, humerus, radius, ulna, carpus, metacarpals, pelvis, femur, patella, tibia, fibula, tarsus, metatarsals, and phalanges.

Axial skeleton

The *cranium* is the portion of the skull that encases the brain. The mandible and maxilla are two significant facial bones. The *mandible*

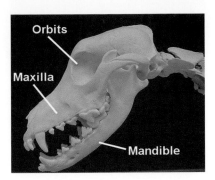

Figure 3.7 Cranium. Source: Courtesy of Jennifer Smith, LVT.

forms the lower jaw, and the *maxilla* forms the upper jaw. The eye sockets in the skull are known as the *orbits* (Figure 3.7).

The *hyoid bone* (also known as the hyoid apparatus) is made up of several parts that may be cartilage or bone. It is a U-shaped structure that is located above the larynx and below the mandible and is suspended by ligaments.

Ribs are pairs of flat, curved bones that attach dorsally to the thoracic vertebrae. The cartilage at the end where the rib attaches to the sternum is called the *costal cartilage*. The *sternum* is also known as the breastbone, and it forms the ventral midline of the rib cage. The ribs that are not attached to cartilage are known as *floating ribs.* Cats and dogs have 13 pairs of ribs.

The *vertebral column* is also known as the backbone and is made up of numerous vertebrae. There are five different types of vertebrae, and there are variations among species in the number of each different type. Here, we focus on the number of vertebrae in canine and feline patients.

The main functions of the vertebral column, also known as the spinal column, are to support the head and body and to protect the spinal cord. The vertebral column is made up of individual bones called vertebrae.

The *cervical vertebrae* are the vertebrae of the neck. There are a total of seven cervical vertebrae in all domestic mammals. The first one is called the atlas and the second one is called the axis. The *thoracic vertebrae* are the vertebrae of the chest. The ribs are attached to these vertebrae. There are 13 thoracic vertebrae in the cat or dog. The *lumbar vertebrae* are the vertebrae of the lower back. There are a total of seven in cats and dogs. The *sacral vertebrae* (also known as the sacrum) consist of three fused vertebrae to which the pelvis is attached. Finally, the *coccygeal vertebrae* are the vertebrae of the tail, and the number of coccygeal vertebrae can vary between six and 23 depending on the species and whether the tail has been docked.

Vertebral formulas are written in a specific format and vary from species to species (Figure 3.8). For example, the dog or cat vertebral formula would look like this:

C-7, T-13, L-7, S-3, Cy 0-23

Appendicular skeleton

As mentioned above, the appendicular skeleton is composed of the bones of the limbs, clavicle, scapula, humerus, radius, ulna, carpus, metacarpals, pelvis, femur, patella, tibia, fibula, tarsus, metatarsals, and phalanges.

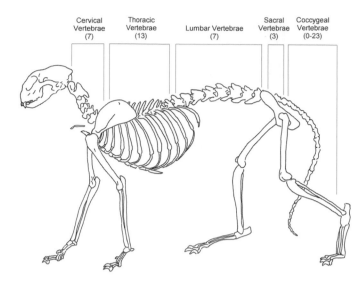

Figure 3.8   Vertebral formula. Source: Courtesy of Jennifer Smith, LVT.

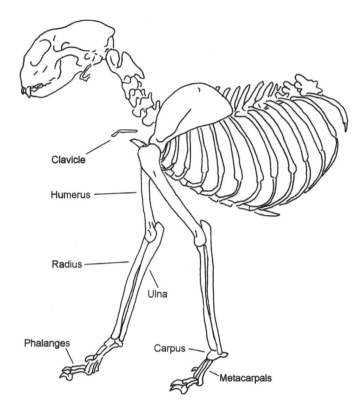

Figure 3.9   Bones of the forelimb. Source: Courtesy of Jennifer Smith, LVT.

Bones of the forelimb

Bones of the forelimb can vary depending on the species. The *clavicle* is also known as the collarbone and is a skinny bone that connects the sternum to the scapula. Not all species have a clavicle. The scapula is also known as the shoulder blade and is a triangular-shaped bone located on the side of the thorax. The *humerus* is the long bone of the forelimb that extends from the shoulder to the elbow. The ulna and radius are located distal to the humerus. The *radius* is the cranial long bone of the forelimb that runs from the elbow to the carpus, and the *ulna* is the caudal long bone of the forelimb that runs from the elbow to the carpus.

Just distal to the radius and ulna is the *carpus* which consists of the joint and several carpal bones. The carpal bones are two rows of irregularly shaped bones.

The *metcarpals* are long bones found just distal to the carpus. The number of metacarpals varies among species. Dogs have five metacarpal bones.

The most distal part of the forelimb are the phalanges. *Phalanges* are the bones of the digit. *Digits* relate to human fingers. The number varies in animals (Figure 3.9).

Bones of the hindlimb

The types and number of bones of the hindlimb can vary depending on the species. The information below refers to domestic animals such as dogs and cats.

The bones of the hindlimb consist of the pelvis, femur, patella, tibia, fibula, tarsus, metatarsals, and phalanges.

The *pelvis* and the coccygeal vertebrae articulate with the sacrum. The *acetabulum* is the hip socket in which the head of the femur sits. The *femur* is the longest bone in the body and is located just distal to the pelvis. The *stifle* is the joint located between the femur and the tibia. The *patella* is a large flat bone that is located over the stifle joint. In humans, this is referred to as the knee cap. Just distal to the patella are the tibia and fibula. The *tibia* is the larger of the two bones and is considered the more weight-bearing bone, and the *fibula* is a long, thinner bone.

The *tarsus* is located distal to the tibia and fibula and consists of numerous, irregularly shaped bones that are arranged in several rows. In humans, the tarsus is known as the ankle.

The *metatarsals* are the long bones found just distal to the tarsus. Similar to the metacarpals in the front leg, the metatarsals will vary among species. The most distal part of the rear limb are the phalanges. *Phalanges* are the bones of the digits (Figure 3.10).

Now that you are familiar with all the basic bones in the dog and cat and the basic directional terms, let's put them into use. For practice, use the information you learned above to complete the activity below.

1.   The skull is --------- to the pelvis. (cranial/caudal)
2.   The femur is --------- to the tarsus. (distal/proximal)
3.   The --------- is also known as the breastbone.
4.   The ---------vertebrae are the vertebrae of the neck.
5.   There are --------- lumbar vertebrae.
6.   The ------ is the long bone of the forelimb that extends from the shoulder to the elbow.
7.   The ------- is just distal to the radius and ulna.
8.   The ------- are the long bones found just distal to the tarsus.

Branches of science

Studying the animal body is a complex activity. There are six branches of science that deal with the study of the body: anatomy,

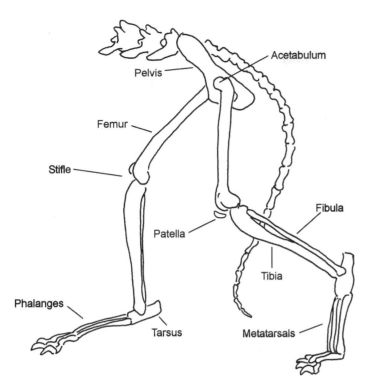

Figure 3.10   Bones of the hindlimb. Source: Courtesy of Jennifer Smith, LVT.

physiology, pathology, embryology, histology, and biology. We will define each of these branches even though this course focus mainly on anatomy and physiology.

- *Anatomy* – the study of the structure of the body and the relationship of its parts. Examination of the structures of various animal species is referred to as comparative anatomy.
- *Physiology* – the study of the normal functions and activities of organisms.
- *Pathology* – the study of the causes and effects of diseases or injury.
- *Embryology* – the study of the origin and development of an individual organism. It begins after conception, or fertilization of the egg, and continues through parturition, or birth.
- *Histology* – the microscopic study of the minute structure, composition, and function of cells and tissues.
- *Biology* – the study of all forms of life.

Body systems

The animal's body is composed of different systems. A system is a combination of organs that performs a particular function. The systems of the body and their functions are listed below.

- *Musculoskeletal system* – includes all the muscles, bones, and joints. It permits motion and movement of the body.
- *Integumentary system* – includes skin, hair, nails, sweat, and sebaceous glands. The skin is considered the largest organ in the body and has many functions. It covers and protects the

body, aids in temperature regulation, and has functions in sensation and excretion.

- *Cardiovascular system* – includes the heart and blood vessels. The main function is to transport the blood to the body.
- *Respiratory system* – includes the mouth, nose, trachea, and lungs. It is responsible for absorbing oxygen and discharging carbon dioxide. It also aids in regulating body temperature.
- *Digestive system* – includes the mouth, teeth, salivary glands, esophagus, stomach, intestines, pancreas, colon, liver, and gallbladder. Its function is to digest and absorb food and excrete wastes.
- *Urogenital system* – includes the kidneys, urinary bladder, genitals, ureters, and urethra. It provides for reproduction and urine excretion.
- *Endocrine system* – includes the thyroid glands, adrenal glands, and parathyroid glands. These glands are responsible for manufacturing hormones.
- *Nervous system* – includes the brain, spinal cord, and nerves. With the special senses, it processes stimuli and enables the body to act and respond.

External anatomy

The head consists of several different anatomical parts. The *forehead* area is just above the eyes and just before the stop. The indentation in a dog's forehead just above level of the eyes is the *stop*. The depth of the stop will vary depending on the breed of dog. The *muzzle* is the area between the stop and the nose. The length of the muzzle will vary depending on the breed of dog. The *nose* is located on the front of the face. It is black in most breeds. The mouth is located below the nose and, again, depending on the breed of dog, the shape and size will vary. Finally, the *flew* consists of the upper lips. The flew may be larger and longer in specific breeds such as the boxer or St Bernard. The *ears* are located on or near the top of the head and can vary in size, placement, and shape depending on the breed (Figure 3.11).

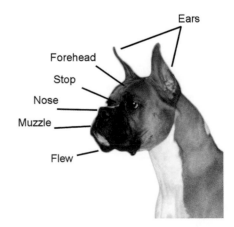

Figure 3.11   External anatomy of the head. Source: Courtesy of Dr Lori Renda-Francis, LVT.

Anterior portion

The **shoulder** is the muscular upper section of the upper arm, and the **point of the shoulder** consists of the front of the joint where the upper arm and shoulder blade come together. The **brisket** is the front portion of the body located between the forelegs and below the chest. The **forearm** is the top area of the upper front leg. The **wrist** is located lower on the front paw and is also known as the carpus. The **paws** include the toes, feet, and paw pads of all four of the dog's legs. The **elbow** is the joint that connects the upper arm and the forearm (Figure 3.12).

Posterior portion

The **stifle** is the joint that connects the lower thigh to the upper thigh. The **thigh** is the area of the hindquarters located between the hip and the stifle. The **tarsus** is the joint that connects the crus (the lower leg) to the metatarsals, which are the beginning of the foot. The back of the upper thigh is referred to as the **hamstrings**. The **tail** is just below the croup and comes in a variety of shapes and lengths depending on the breed. The **croup** is the area of the back from the root of the tail to the front of the pelvis. The **loin** is the area on both sides of the vertebrae between the last few ribs and the hindquarters (Figure 3.13).

Middle portion

The underside of the abdomen is the **belly**. The area from the withers to the root of the tail is the **back**. The **withers** are the top of the shoulder blade and the highest point of the body and are located just behind the neck. The **ruff** is the thick, dense hair located around the top of the neck. The **crest** is the upper arched area of the neck (Figure 3.14).

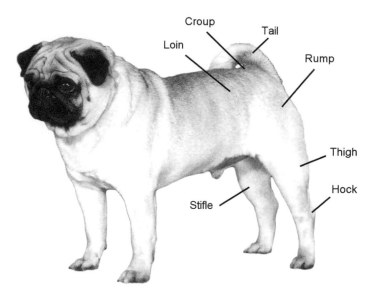

Figure 3.13 External anatomy, posterior portion. Source: Courtesy of Dr Lori Renda-Francis, LVT.

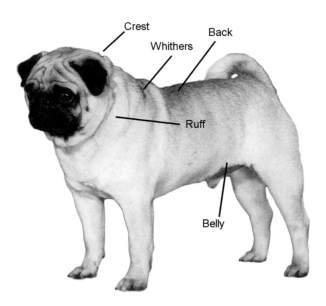

Figure 3.14 External anatomy, middle portion. source: Courtesy of Dr Lori Renda-Francis, LVT.

Common veins

While veterinary assistants do not perform venipuncture techniques, they do have a significant role in assisting the veterinarian or veterinary technician in successful collection. The main role of the veterinary assistant during venipuncture is to properly restrain the animal for the procedure. Therefore, it is important for the veterinary assistant to know which veins are commonly used and where they are located and to be able to describe them using correct anatomical terminology.

For dogs, the most frequently used sites for blood collection are the cephalic vein, the jugular vein, and the lateral saphenous vein. The most commonly used veins in cats are the cephalic vein,

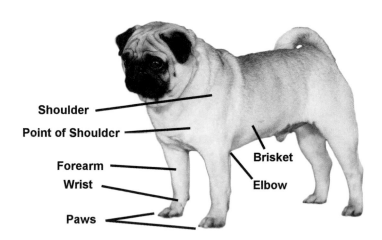

Figure 3.12 External anatomy, anterior portion. Source: Courtesy of Dr Lori Renda-Francis, LVT.

the jugular vein, the femoral vein, and the medial saphenous vein (Figure 3.15).

The **cephalic veins** are located on the anterior surface of the forearm. They run from the dorsomedial foreleg proximally along the foreleg. They are easy to locate and very accessible for venipuncture. The cephalic vein is used for collection of large volumes of blood in larger dogs.

The **lateral saphenous veins** are small, superficial veins that run diagonally across the lateral surface of the distal part of the tibia.

The **jugular veins** are large superficial veins located on either side of the trachea on the neck.

The **femoral vein** is used for blood collection in cats and extends from the groin on the medial aspect of the thigh.

The medial **saphenous vein** is also used in cats and extends from the hock to the stifle on the medial aspect of the calf. It becomes the femoral vein at the stifle (Figure 3.16).

Muscles

There are several muscles that can be utilized to administer intramuscular injections. Again, the veterinary assistant does not administer these injections but plays a large role in assisting the veterinarian or veterinary technician by properly restraining the animal. In order to properly restrain, it is important for the veterinary assistant to be familiar with the location of the various muscles (Figure 3.17).

- **Lumbodorsal** or **dorsal lumbar muscle** – located on either side of the midline.
- **Triceps** – located caudal to the humerus.
- **Quadriceps** – located anterior to the femur.
- **Biceps** – the posterior muscle of the hind leg.
- **Semimembranosus/semitendinosus muscle group** – located in the rear leg, also known as the hamstring muscles.

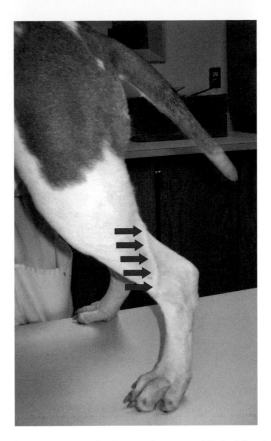

Figure 3.16 Saphenous vein. Source: Courtesy of Dr Lori Renda-Francis, LVT.

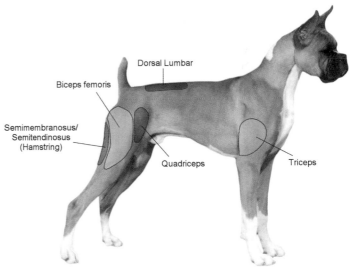

Figure 3.17 Muscles. Source: Courtesy of Dr Lori Renda-Francis, LVT.

Internal organs

Digestive system

The most cranial structure is the mouth. The **mouth**, or oral cavity, is a very important part of the digestive system in dogs. This is where digestion begins. The **tongue** and front **teeth** help a dog

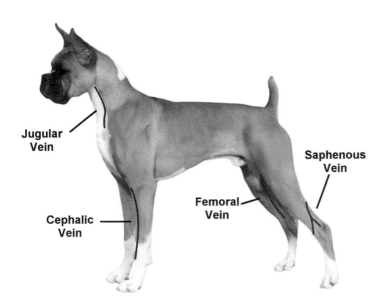

Figure 3.15 Veins. Source: Courtesy of Dr Lori Renda-Francis, LVT.

pick up pieces of food, and teeth in the back of the mouth grind the food into smaller particles. A dog has a total of 42 teeth, including incisors and canines, located in the front, and the pre-molars and molars, which are located in the back. As a dog chews, food is broken up into smaller particles for better digestion by enzymes in the stomach and small intestines. It passes through a small tube called the *esophagus* that connects the mouth to the stomach via the diaphragm.

The *stomach* is a sac-like structure that stores large volumes of food. From the stomach, the food enters the *small intestine.* There are three parts to the small intestine. The *duodenum* attaches to the stomach. The middle part is the longest part and is called the *jejunum*, and the last part is the smallest part and is known as the *ileum*. It connects to the large intestine. The *large intestine* connects the small intestine to the anus. Its primary function is to absorb water from feces as needed in order to keep the animal hydrated. Its other function is to store fecal matter that is awaiting passage from the body. The last structure of the intestine is the *rectum*, which leads to the most caudal structure – the *anus* (Figure 3.18).

The *liver* and *pancreas* are two essential organs that have multiple functions. Both have ducts that secrete special chemicals into the intestine to aid indigestion. They are next to each other anatomically, and a disease of one can sometimes affect the health of both. The *gallbladder* is a pear-shaped structure lying between the lobes of the liver (Figure 3.19).

Urogenital system

The canine urogenital system is a combination of the urinary and reproductive tracts. It includes the urinary and reproductive organs. The function is to provide reproduction and eliminate liquid wastes. The urogenital system is made up of the kidneys, bladder, ureters, and urethra along with the reproductive organs such as the testicles, penis, scrotum, uterus, ovaries, and vulva (Figure 3.20).

The *kidneys* are bean-shaped structures designed to excrete urea, uric acid, and other wastes. The *bladder* is a small, balloon-shaped structure that serves as a receptacle for fluid to be eliminated, and the *urethra* is the canal that carries the urine from the bladder. The urine enters the *ureters*, which are long tubes that funnel urine down into the bladder.

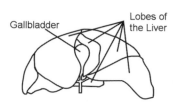

Figure 3.19 Gallbladder/liver. Source: Courtesy of Jennifer Smith, LVT.

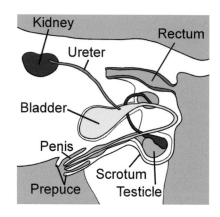

Figure 3.20 Urinary system. Source: Courtesy of Jennifer Smith, LVT.

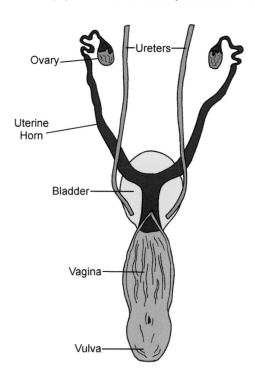

Figure 3.21 Female anatomy. Source: Courtesy of Jennifer Smith, LVT.

The male genital anatomy is mostly located on the outside of the animal. The *scrotum* is the sac that contains the *testicles*, which are responsible for producing sperm. The *penis* is the male sex organ and is covered by the *prepuce*. The female genital anatomy consists of the ovaries and the uterus. There are two *ovaries* that are located caudal to the kidneys. There are two horns of the *uterus*. The external opening of the female genital passage is the *vulva* (Figure 3.21).

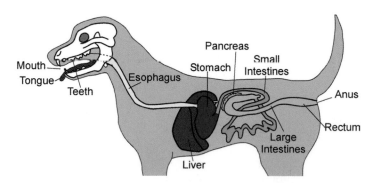

Figure 3.18 Internal organs. Source: Courtesy of Jennifer Smith, LVT.

Internal structures of the thorax

The **heart** is the main blood-pumping organ in the chest. The **trachea** is the tube that carries air to the lungs. The **lung** is the main respiratory organ and is composed of several lobes. The **diaphragm** is the muscle that divides the thoracic and abdominal cavities.

Conclusion

It is important for veterinary assistants to be familiar with basic anatomical directional terms and structures. This will allow them to properly communicate with other staff members.

References

Colville, T. and Bassert, J. 2002. *Clinical Anatomy and Physiology for Veterinary Technicians*. Mosby, St Louis, MO.

Sturtz, R. and Asprea, L. 2012. *Anatomy and Physiology for Veterinary Technicians and Nurses: A Clinical Approach*. Wiley-Blackwell, Hoboken, NJ.

www.wiley.com/go/burns/textbookvetassistant2

Please go to the companion website for assignments and a PowerPoint relating to the material in this chapter.

Chapter 4 Behavior, Handling, and Restraint

The entire veterinary health-care team is responsible for safety awareness in the veterinary hospital. In the hospital setting, this includes the safety of health-care team members, clients, and patients. Animals, not unlike people, may behave differently in unfamiliar surroundings. The goal of the veterinary health-care team is to insure that the veterinarian or technician examining the patient does not get bitten by a frightened and/or injured patient and that the patient does not suffer further injury. All animals have an innate fight or flight instinct that causes the animal to flee or stand ground and fight when faced with a stressful situation. It is important for veterinary assistants to remember that each patient will behave differently in different procedures and perhaps even from visit to visit. Remember, each patient has its own psyche and reacts to stress in its own individual way.

Social behavior

Canine

The social groups of today's domesticated dog are small and open to outsiders. They typically are not related individuals. There are also misperceptions regarding dominance in dogs and that dominance is a personality trait in dogs. In fact, we may see one dog take the dominant role in one relationship and a subordinate role in a different relationship. Additionally, the roles may change between individuals, depending on the context in which the interaction takes place. Oftentimes, dogs are incorrectly labeled by their owner as "dominant" when, in fact, they are fearful. The misconception that dog behavior problems are caused by dominance has led to the application of cruel and unwarranted forms of dog training. Dog owners do not need to and should not physically dominate their dogs and need to be educated regarding this mistaken belief. These types of behavior are likely to worsen the fearful dog's behavior problems.

Dogs use an assortment of visual and *olfactory* cues when initiating, forming, and maintaining social relationships. When unfamiliar dogs meet, they normally begin by sniffing each other. Commonly, sniffing begins at the head and moves toward the tail. Typically, the dog that approaches and begins sniffing first may resist being sniffed itself. Although the dog that is being sniffed is most likely to try to terminate the interaction, it is unlikely to attempt to sniff the other dog. A dog attempting to take the dominant role will usually approach the other dog in a "T position" in relation to the other dog's shoulder and begin sniffing. If accepting a subordinate role, the other dog turns its head away from the approaching dog. Dogs that do not want the subordinate role may resist being sniffed and may attempt to sniff the other dog. In addition, dogs may signal submission by rolling over on their back and exposing the inguinal region. This area is then sniffed by the dominant dog. Often, the dog will raise a paw loosely, wag its tail loosely, and exhibit a play face. Often this followed by the play bow indicating it is ready for play.

Feline

Domestic cats are often thought of as animals which do not socialize. However, this is not totally correct. Domestication of the cat has led to a highly adaptable animal that can modify its social organization according to available resources. Feral or free-ranging cats may live in large groups, especially when a food source may be near – a dump, a fishing village, or a farm. These groups are typically made up of related females which form a dominance pecking order. A dominant male cat's territory includes the territory of these females. The male is allowed when a female is in estrus. Other cats deemed to be "strangers" are chased away from the territory.

Domestic cats that live together may demonstrate cheek rubbing and tail rubbing. Even so, household cat aggression continues to be a problem for multicat households. Cat owners are unfamiliar with the visual signals used by cats, and their signals may be very subtle. Differentiating play from true aggression can be challenging for most pet owners.

Cats are not *asocial* animals; however, their tolerance of other cats is limited and is based on familiarity and individual temperament.

Introducing a new cat should be done in a gradual and systematic way rather than by simply releasing a new cat into the home. The veterinary team must educate clients about the challenges associated with adding cats to a household – behavioral and medical – before the owner gets a new cat. The tendency for a cat to be aggressive toward other cats appears to be an innate trait. Thus, cat owners must be educated that some cats simply do not like to live with other cats. Even if the addition of another cat has been done properly, there is no guarantee that the cats will eventually get along with one another. Tolerance of each other may be more likely in a larger home, where cats have plenty of litterboxes, food dishes, water bowls, etc., and are not forced to interact with each other because of close confinement. Those clients who want more than one cat find it easier to acquire two kittens and raise them together. Research demonstrates that aggression is less likely in pairs of cats, the longer they have lived together. Veterinary teams must educate clients that adding new cats to the home regularly and/or maintaining more than two or three cats at a time are more likely to lead to aggression and house soiling problems.

Animal body language

Canine

The *body language* of animals is a good indicator of their emotional state. It is imperative that veterinary health-care team members familiarize themselves with the body language of specific species and, when possible, a specific animal. Most dogs enjoy being with humans and exhibit behaviors that are associated with their happiness. This is indicated in dogs that initiate affection. Typically, these dogs wag their tail and approach people in a straightforward manner with a slightly lowered and/or cocked head. Although these dogs appear to be content, care must always be taken when the need to restrain arises. All dogs, even the happiest and most easy-going, have the potential to bite if treated too roughly or if they are cornered and feel threatened.

The veterinary health-care team must also become familiar with the body language of the fearful or anxious dog. The ears of a fearful dog are drawn down and back. These dogs make little to no eye contact and are typically cowering. There is a very high probability that they will bite if cornered or feeling threatened. Extreme caution must be exercised when trying to handle or restrain the dog exhibiting fearful or aggressive body language.

The dog will exhibit aggressive body language by lowering its head to the level of the shoulders, giving a level and intense stare, positioning its tail out straight (sometimes with a slight wag), and growling or baring the teeth. Dogs exhibit fear or aggression through body posture. Dogs might show that they feel threatened by a human looking directly at their eyes or approaching them from the front.

Dominance aggression can be defined as aggression toward other members of the animal's social group. This behavior is exhibited to prevent lower-ranking members of the social group from performing actions or engaging in activities for which the higher-ranking individual claims priority.

All dogs should be handled with the knowledge that they may bite at any time, and health-care team members must be prepared for this. In dogs exhibiting fearful and aggressive body language, this is especially true.

The fight or flight principle is quite evident when talking of the behavior of canines. A dog's typical defense mechanism will be to retreat (take flight) if it feels threatened. However, this is not true of all dogs, especially if the dog believes danger or threat is imminent. In this case, it may resort to the fight principle. We know that the canine dentition is designed for crushing and tearing and if a dog bites, that is the intent. Remember to observe the body language of the dog before restraining it. If the dog is baring its teeth, growling, curling its lips, and/or raising its hackles, the health-care team must take precautions and control the muzzle of the dog or risk being bitten.

The health-care team must also be prepared to control the dog's legs and/or paws. Although a dog's toenails are not generally thought of as dangerous, the dog may use them to attempt to ward off restraint. The dog's thrashing of the legs and paws may cause serious scratches on members of the health-care team, and these scratches have a high probability of becoming infected.

Appropriate steps must be taken by the health-care team to insure the safety of the patient and the health-care team. There are a variety of physical and *pharmaceutical* restraints that will aid in handling dogs to insure a safe hospital experience for the team and patient. It is important for the veterinary team to be familiar with physical restraint techniques. The veterinarian will diagnose and prescribe a pharmaceutical restraint when and if it is needed to insure the team's and the patient's safety.

The veterinary health-care team should always record the behavior of a patient in the medical record. Aggressive behavior should be clearly marked in the patient's record with a warning; this will help insure the safety of both the health-care team and the patient. It is important to abide by the following when approaching a dog in the hospital.

- Use the dog's name.
- Approach the dog quietly but confidently.
- Lower yourself to the dog's level but at a safe distance.
- Slowly offer the back of your hand for the dog to smell.
- Do not attempt to handle/restrain dogs in confined areas, as the dog may feel trapped.

Restraint

The health-care team should be aware of situations where a dog may not be handled safely and restraint equipment should be employed for the overall safety of the team and the patient. It is important to insure that all dogs have a collar and leash fitted during handling. The following list contains a variety of mechanical restraint devices that will be discussed in more detail.

- Leash
- Gauntlet
- Muzzle
- Catchpole
- Voice

One of the most readily available and simple tools for restraining dogs is the leash. Leashes in the hospital setting are typically a nylon rope with a handle at one end and a slip loop (for quick size adjustments) on the opposite end (Figure 4.1). The leash should be held open above the dog's head and readily available to place around the head or body when restraint is indicated. The slip loop allows for easy tightening or loosening when restraining or releasing the patient. It can be used cautiously on feline patients as well, although this use is not as common as with canine patients. All health-care team members should keep a rope or leash available at all times.

To protect health-care team members, heavy leather gloves known as gauntlets are often indicated. These are used to protect the hands and forearms when dealing with aggressive or fearful animals. Although gauntlets are made of thick leather, dogs, cats and birds have been known to bite or pinch through them. The thickness of the gloves typically allows the wearer to feel the bite or pinch before major injury occurs, thus enabling them to circumvent a potentially serious situation. Remember, the gauntlets may reduce the wearer's overall sense of touch and strength. Therefore, the wearer must take care not to exert excessive pressure on patients during restraint procedures. A decreased sense of touch and strength coupled with the restrainer's increased excitability and adrenaline can be a very dangerous mix.

Using a muzzle is another way to protect the health-care team, the owner, and the dog if the patient is nervous or aggressive.

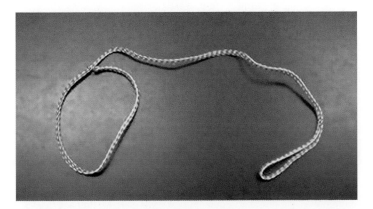

Figure 4.1   Rope leash. Source: Sheldon, C.C., Topel, J. and Sonsthagen, T. 2006. *Animal Restraint for Veterinary Professionals*. Elsevier, St Louis, MO.

There are a number of muzzles available and a recommendation of a type or brand should be given by the health-care team to the owner. The muzzles most often used are a wire/Baskerville muzzle, a nylon/Mikki muzzle, or a gauze muzzle. In place of a commercially manufactured muzzle, health-care team members can utilize a roll of gauze, a nylon sock, or even a piece of rope. However, the dog needs constant monitoring when it is muzzled to ensure there is no obstruction to the airway. Care must also be taken to ensure the muzzle can be removed efficiently and quickly. If the dog is thought to be likely to bite, its head should be safely restrained by a health-care team member while the muzzle is removed. Muzzles should be used only short term because they prevent dogs from panting and could thus lead to overheating if left on for extended periods. The health-care team should be especially prudent when using muzzles on **brachycephalic** breeds. Typically, a gauze muzzle is to be used for brachycephalic breeds. Scissors should be close at all times in case a muzzle needs to be cut off and quickly removed.

Care should be taken when applying muzzles. When applying muzzles to an animal on the floor, you should never kneel or sit, instead you should squat so that you can move away quickly if needed. Ideally, a second person should be restraining the animal when a muzzle is being placed. If you must place a muzzle alone, you should carefully approach the animal and apply the muzzle from the back or side of the animal.

Application of a gauze muzzle

When applying a gauze muzzle to a dog, you will want to utilize a nonstretch gauze. Cut a large piece of gauze to ensure that you have enough to wrap around the muzzle and behind the dog's head and still have enough to tie in a bow. It is better to have too much versus too little, since you may only have one good chance to muzzle the upset dog before someone gets injured. The dog should be in sitting or sternal or sitting recumbency.

Start by making a loop in the center of the gauze strip and cross one end under to create a half-knot. Once the loop is made you can carefully approach the dog from the back or the side. If the dog is being restrained you can approach him from the front. Bring the open loop down in front of the dog's muzzle and slide it on to the muzzle. Quickly tighten the gauze with the half-knot on top of the dog's muzzle (Figure 4.2). Keep your hands at a safe distance at all times, pulling the tie ends of the gauze down and around underneath the dog's muzzle and crossing them underneath the chin. Tighten the gauze again, and then bring the ends of the gauze back behind the dog's head, cross the ends behind the dog's ears, and tie in a bow (Figure 4.3).

Application of a leather, nylon or basket muzzle

It is important to select a muzzle that is the correct size. You will want to make sure that the dog is able to pant but not bite. You will also want to make sure it does not bunch the skin under the eyes and is not longer than the dog's nose length. The muzzle should end no closer than ½ inch from the eyes. Before trying to apply the muzzle, ensure that the fastener on the muzzle is

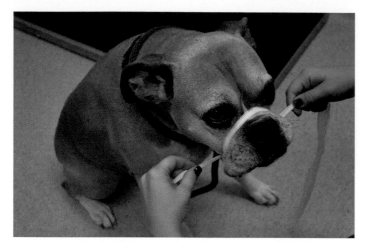

Figure 4.2   Application of gauze muzzle (1). Source: Courtesy of Dr Lori Renda-Francis, LVT.

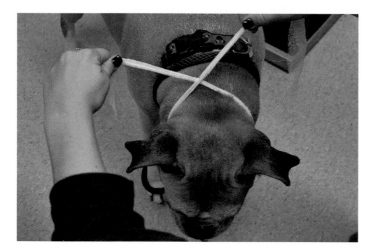

Figure 4.3   Application of gauze muzzle (2). Source: Courtesy of Dr Lori Renda-Francis, LVT.

adjusted to the approximate size of the dog's head. Approach the dog from the back or side. If the animal is being restrained, you may be able to approach him from the front. Hold the side straps out while slipping the material over the dog's nose. The longer part of the material should be under the jaw, so the straps fasten under the ears. The shorter part of the material should be on the top of the dog's nose. Clip the ends of the fastener together behind the dog's head and pull the straps tight against the head.

Using a catchpole

A catchpole is another commercially available device that may be used to restrain and move an aggressive or fearful dog. There are many names for this device – catchpole, dog catcher, rabies pole. This is a rigid pole that allows the health-care team member to remain at a distance from the dog while restraining it. The catchpole has a quick-release handle, which ensures that the dog does not become strangled. Care must be taken at all times to ensure

that the dog is not choking but that the loop is tight enough around the dog's head to prevent it from slipping out. The catchpole has a loop at one end that is placed around the animal's neck and tightened. Using this type of restraint allows for another team member to approach the animal from behind to administer medication or examine the animal.

Light restraint

Finally, the health-care team member can use his or her voice to help comfort and soothe a frightened or nervous animal. It is advised to use a soft tone. For some dogs, a higher pitched voice will be soothing, and for others, a voice tone that is deep and authoritative in nature should be used. The health-care team member should use the voice tone that makes the most sense with each dog. The use of a soft voice, regardless of the pitch, is calming to dogs. Many animals respond to a gentle serenade or shushing sound. Oftentimes, light restraint with a gentle voice is all that is needed to reassure a dog (Figure 4.4).

Kenneling

All health-care team members should be aware of the fight or flight principle when kenneling and restraining animals. If there is an opening to get out of the cage or out of a restraint hold, the animal will take it. Health-care team members must be aware of their surroundings at all times, insuring that no route is accessible for escape by an animal prior to opening a door to remove a pet and before releasing the restraint of a pet. When taking a pet from a cage or a kennel, the health-care team member must block the door opening with a knee or forearm to obstruct an obvious escape route.

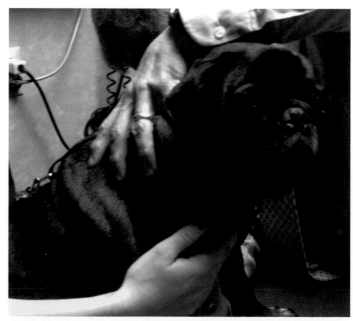

Figure 4.4   Light restraint. Source: Courtesy of Kara M. Burns, LVT, VTS (Nutrition).

A health-care team member can pick up a small-breed dog that is not fearful or aggressive by grasping the animal's scruff or by placing a hand under the dog's chin and placing the other hand under the thorax region. The dog's body should be kept close to the team member's, and a leash should be available to place around the dog's neck. At this point the dog is secure and can be placed on the floor. Large-breed dogs typically will be placed in a kennel or a larger cage closer to the ground. These dogs can be led out after the cage is opened, the escape route blocked, and a leash slipped around the dog's neck.

Fearful or aggressive dogs must be removed with caution from a cage or kennel. Common sense plays a huge role in the removal and restraint of aggressive dogs. The health-care team should muzzle or sedate an aggressive dog prior to placing it in the cage. The dog is protecting its territory, so cornering it will make it feel threatened. This is the perfect time to use voice as a restraint aid and offer approval and comfort. The use of a capture pole may be warranted, especially in instances where the dog is attacking the leash or the area of the kennel in which the team member is standing.

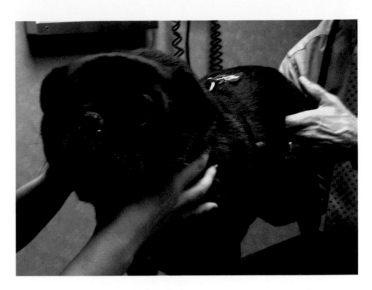

Figure 4.5   Tender hold during physical examination. Source: Courtesy of Kara M. Burns, LVT, VTS (Nutrition).

Lifting and positioning a dog

Always bend at the knees to pick up an animal. Do not bend over at the waist, as you put yourself at increased risk for back injury. Working with animals requires strength and proper posture. All health-care team members must adhere to proper lifting techniques for the good of the individual, team members, and patient. After bending at the knees and keeping your back straight, you can lift a small-breed dog by placing one hand under its mandible and your forearm under its abdomen. The dog should be carried close to your body for stability at all times. Medium-sized dogs should be held with one arm under the neck and the other arm under the abdomen or around the dog's hindquarters. For the safety of the pet and the safety and health and longevity of the team members, lifting large-breed dogs requires two team members who must communicate and work together to insure safety. One person should place his or her arm around the dog's thorax and the other arm under the dog's neck. The other person should place one arm under or around the dog's abdomen and the other arm around the hindquarters.

Placing a large dog on an exam table may produce anxiety for the animal, so the health-care team should attempt to examine the dog on the floor. Alternatively, hydraulic lift tables are becoming more popular. The dog may be placed on the table at ground level and secured, with health-care team members readily on hand. The table can then be raised to a level that allows the team to examine the dog.

Restraint while standing is necessary when the dog is undergoing a physical examination, anal sac expression, having its temperature taken rectally, or if a vaginal or rectal smear must be obtained. Restraint for these procedures involves placing one arm around the dog's neck or muzzle and the other arm around the dog's body. The dog must be pulled in close to the team member's body. Large and giant-breed dogs will require two team members to participate in the restraint. The restraint should not be a tight stranglehold on the dog but rather a tender hold with some softly spoken words. A tender hold with a well-behaved patient was all that was needed during the physical examination in Figure 4.5. The health-care team members must be ready at all times to tighten the grip if the patient starts to struggle or become aggressive.

Using recumbent restraint is necessary for many procedures. Procedures such as drawing blood from a cephalic or jugular vein, administering an IV injection, oral and **ophthalmic** examination, and administering medications are a few of the procedures that warrant restraint in sternal recumbency. In this kind of restraint, the health-care team member places one hand under the neck or muzzle region of the dog and the other around the hindquarters and pulls the dog in close to their body. If the dog is trying to scratch with its front paws, the team member can remove the arm from around the hindquarters and wrap it around the abdominal area with the hand coming from the underside of the dog to the front legs. The front legs should be grasped slightly above the carpal area.

Placing a dog on its side will allow for restraint in lateral recumbency. With the dog on its side, the front legs are held while the team member places one arm across its neck. The other hand is used to hold the back legs. This is a useful restraint for **urinary catheterization,** radiographs, suture removal, and for access to the **lateral saphenous vein**.

Restraint in dorsal recumbency calls for two team members. The dog is placed in lateral recumbency and is carefully rolled onto its back. The front paws are extended cranially with the back paws extended caudally. This exposes the thorax and abdomen of the dog. A V-trough or foam wedges may be necessary to prevent the dog from rolling. This technique is often used for radiographs or **cystocentesis**.

Feline

Prior to their domestication, cats were known to be solitary animals that follow an organized social structure. Cats are also known to be very territorial. In today's society, cats often live indoors and with other cats. Cats can and do get along with other cats, but they have a vast array of communication behaviors of which the health-care team should be well aware. Some of these behaviors are listed below.

Body posture of a feline

- **Relaxed** – the cat walks with its tail down, but its tail will rise when it greets other cats and humans it knows.
- **Fear aggression** – the tail will be held close to the body and oftentimes will be fluffed (to give the appearance of being bigger). The pupils are often dilated.
- **Aggression** – the ears are swiveled, displaying the inner pinnae sideways, and the pupils are oblong.
- **Frightened** – the dorsal area will be arched and the tail raised. Again, the fur along the back and covering the tail will be fluffed to give the appearance of being larger and more intimidating.

Facial expressions of a feline

- **Relaxed** – ears are upright, whiskers are on the side of the face, pupils of eyes are moderately dilated (Figure 4.6).
- **Aggressive** – ears are erect and facing back; pupils are constricted.
- **Frightened** – ears are flat against the head, whiskers are held stiffly out to the side, and the pupils are dilated.
- **Conflicted** – ears will alternate between the flattened and turned-back position.
- **Alert** – pupils are dilated, and whiskers are tensed.

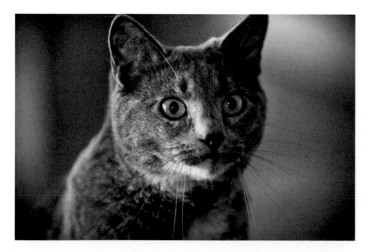

Figure 4.6 Relaxed cat facial expression. Source: Courtesy of Kara M. Burns, LVT, VTS (Nutrition).

For cats, scratching is a visual sign of territory ownership. The cat marks the area with the glands present around the paw pads. Scratching leaves a visual sign of territory ownership and maintains the claws.

Vocalization

- **Meows** – expression of needs to owners (often associated with feeding).
- **Loud yowls** – typically heard from queen in heat.
- **Growling** – range in volume; often in conjunction with aggression or fright.
- **Purring** – humans generally believe this is a sign of contentment, but it can also be a sign of low-grade pain.

Other feline body language

- **Glands on facial area** – the cat deposits secretions when it rubs itself on an object to be marked.
- **Urine** – sprayed by male cats at the height of the cat's nose, to mark territory for the next cat coming to the area.
- **Feces** – the cat may bury or leave feces to alert other cats to its territory.

When the veterinary health-care team is working with a feline patient, it is advisable to perform procedures quickly and efficiently. It is in the best interest of the patient and the team to avoid repeating procedures. If restraint is needed when working with felines, the team should start with the lowest amount of restraint necessary to finish the procedure quickly and efficiently. Should the cat begin to resist the restraint, the grip should be tightened only until control can be maintained. If the cat continues to resist, it should be released and other restraint options (i.e., chemical) should be discussed. Prior to releasing the cat, it is imperative that all team members know that the restraint is being slackened. One should attempt to relax the cat prior to restraining it through the use of touch (petting the cat) and voice (speaking to the cat). The cat is in an unfamiliar place surrounded by people it does not know. Kindness goes a long way! Rough handling and extreme restraint should never be used in the handling of cats, and cats should never feel as though they are fighting for life.

When cats become aggressive, the potential is high for them to use their claws and teeth. The teeth can leave deep puncture wounds that have a high risk of becoming infected. Also, cats are able to move in any direction. When the health-care team members think they have control, the cat may contort itself into an unexpected position. When cats are restrained, all doors and windows in the hospital should be closed to insure the cat will not escape from the building.

Restraint

When restraint of a cat is indicated, one of the best tools for the health-care team to have readily available is a large towel, which can be used to wrap the cat's body securely (Figure 4.7). It also allows for wrapping, and thus controlling, the cat's body, feet, and claws. For femoral or cephalic vein exposure, or if an **IM injection** is warranted, a front or back leg can be held outside the towel wrap. Also, the towel wrap restraint allows for oral or ophthalmic medications to be given without risk of the cat scratching a health-care team member. Some health-care teams have found that simply covering the head of the cat (paying careful attention to insure the cat can breathe) calms the cat down and enables them to perform procedures. Whichever method is used, insure that all team members involved are in agreement with the restraint plan.

Another tool that is very beneficial when cat restraint is needed is the cat bag or feline restraint bag (Figure 4.8). The cat bag should be make of a heavy canvas or nylon material and have a zipper or Velcro closure. The bag has openings for the cat's front and rear legs so one limb at a time can be removed for procedures. As cats come in all sizes, a variety of bag sizes are available. Health-care

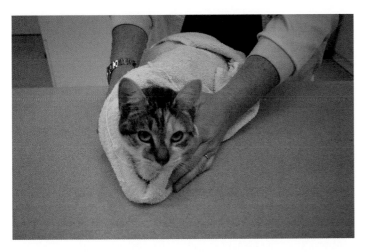

Figure 4.7   Feline towel restraint. Source: Courtesy of Dr Lori Renda-Francis, LVT.

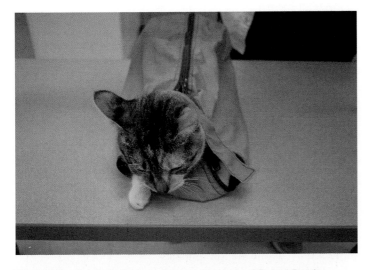

Figure 4.8   Cat restraint bag. Source: Courtesy of Dr Lori Renda-Francis, LVT.

team members should never leave a cat in a feline restraint bag unattended because the cat can easily roll off the table. When it is time to remove a cat from the feline restraint bag, the whole team must be alert and prepared. To remove the cat, the bag closure should be undone, and then the neck strap loosened. Cats typically walk out of the bag at this point, although they may be slightly put out by the procedure. If the cat is stressed and aggressive, health-care practitioners should draw their hands back quickly after loosening the neck strap.

As with dogs, muzzles are available commercially for felines. Feline muzzles typically cover the cat's eyes, leaving a small opening for the cat to breathe through. However, muzzles typically add to a cat's stress and anger, so thought and planning should be used prior to muzzling. Another restraint technique might be better.

Gauntlets can also be used when handling cats, as these heavy, thick gloves will help to protect from scratches or potential bite wounds from the cat.

Another method to use specifically with cats to help in their restraint is distraction. Heavy but gentle patting or rubbing of the cat's head can be used to draw its attention to the distraction and away from the procedure being performed. It is recommended to vary the stroke and the force (but never to the point of roughness). Another idea that is commonly used and typically successful is blowing air into the face of the cat. Light blowing onto the cat's face will help the health-care team to distract the animal from the medical procedure. The speed and direction of the air flow should vary, and as always, the utmost care should be taken when a health-care team member approaches the cat's face.

When physical examination of a cat is warranted, the health-care team member should hold the cat in a sitting or sternal recumbent position with one hand at the front of its chest and the other hand steadying the hind end. Team members should talk quietly to the cat and when possible gently pat it to try to ease its stress. As the examination of the cat moves to the head, one hand of the restraint should encircle the neck with the hand holding the mandible. The other hand can then move over the back to hold the front feet of the cat. This positioning allows the restrainer to hold the cat against his or her body. The less restraint, the better for everyone involved, especially the feline patient.

Another restraint technique often used for SQ or IM injections, temperature taking via the rectum, or for access to the saphenous vein is the lateral recumbency restraint. The team member should scruff the cat behind the neck/dorsal area, grasping as much fur as possible with one hand, while grasping the back feet of the animal with the other hand (Figure 4.9). The cat is held and slightly stretched at the same time. When in this position, most cats seem to believe they are unable to use their front feet to scratch.

Not all cats react to restraint in the same manner. All members of the health-care team must be familiar with the various restraint techniques. Most importantly, all team members must be prepared and have all equipment ready when performing any procedure on a feline patient. This helps to assure the success of the procedure and decreases the stress and impact on the feline patient.

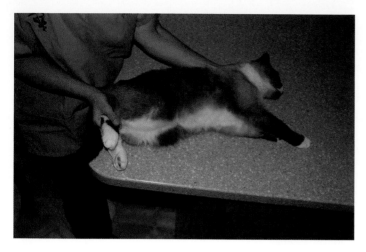

Figure 4.9 Lateral recumbency restraint. Source: Courtesy of Kara M. Burns, LVT, VTS (Nutrition).

Fear Free®

The mission of the Fear Free initiative is to ease fear, anxiety, and stress (FAS) in pets, in addition to educating and motivating the owners who care for them. Fear Free is about improving the health and welfare of animals.

Pets need members of the veterinary health-care team to look after their physical and their emotional well-being. Fear Free provides tools, protocols, procedures, and guidelines on how to decrease FAS in patients. Decreasing FAS in patients has a domino effect and we see a decrease in pet owners and veterinary team members as well.

The focus of Fear Free is on preventing FAS in every patient and the concepts should be used with all patients, whether they are relaxed and happy to be in your care or afraid and displaying avoidance or aggression.

Remember, animals and clients have specific preferences. The first step is noting these preferences in the pet's medical record. Also consider starting an emotional record for each individual patient, in addition to the medical portion.

Some of the key concepts of applying Fear Free while providing medical care include communication, considerate approach, gentle control, and touch gradient. Creating a plan of action for each patient can be a quick process that saves time and creates a more pleasant experience for the veterinary healthcare team, patient, and client.

Common behavior signs associated with fear, anxiety, and stress in cats and dogs (Figure 4.10)

Obvious signs

- Cowering/crouching
- Ear lowering
- Growling
- Hiding
- Hissing (feline)
- Lifting lip
- Tucking tail
- Trembling

Subtle signs

- Avoiding eye contact
- Blinking slowly or squinting
- Closing mouth tightly
- Dilated pupils
- Licking lips
- Lifting paws
- Pulling mouth back
- Pacing
- Panting
- Self-grooming
- Shifting eyes
- Staying close to the owner
- Tail flicking/thrashing (feline)
- Taking treats roughly, being pickier than usual about treats, or refusing treats
- Unable to settle down
- Yawning

Every member of the health-care team should be able to recognize signs of a relaxed or stressed patient, as this is critical to establishing a Fear Free environment. As noted above, some signs may be subtle, and the owner will not recognize these as being associated with FAS. It is imperative that the health-care team continually assesses the patient while at the veterinary hospital. The patient is actually communicating – we just need to be cognizant of the signs. Be aware of the patient's body language and what it is conveying. Being aware of the subtle signs will allow the team to adjust their behaviors accordingly to prevent the patient from escalating. Adjusting behavior may be simple – such as pausing briefly to let the patient acclimate to your touch before proceeding.

Remember to keep an emotional record alongside the medical record and detail what worked for the patient. This will help future visits to be less stressful for all involved. Examples of information to be captured include:

- types of rewards that were effective
- where the patient preferred to be examined
- the way a procedure was performed.

This way, when the patient returns for a hospital visit, the team will have an initial plan for care and the pet owner will be impressed with your thoughtfulness.

In addition, the veterinary team should use a considerate approach. This approach involves the interaction between the veterinary team,

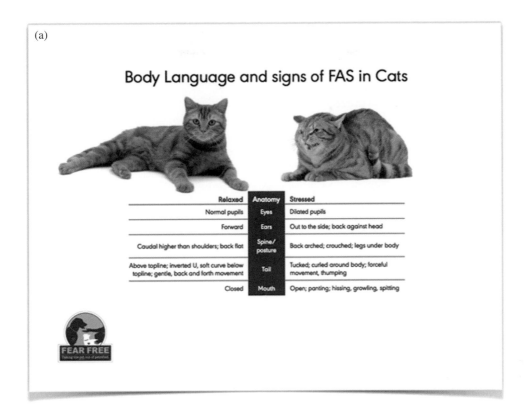

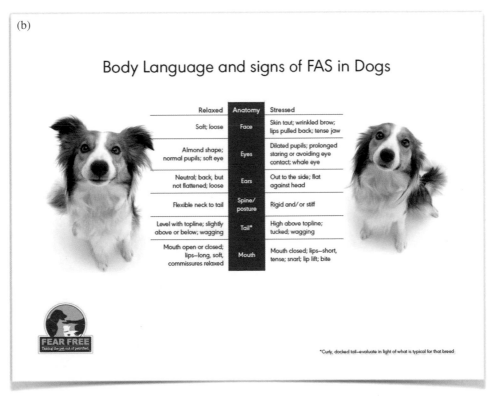

Figure 4.10 Fear and stress in (a) cats and (b) dogs.

the patient, and input from the environment while veterinary care is being administered. Creating this relaxing and satisfying experience involves establishing the environment keeping the patient and client in mind. The veterinary team should put themselves in the pet and owner's "shoes or paws." Minimize the stress – provide nonslip surfaces for pets to stand on, include calming scents and/or **pheromones**, use calming sounds, reducing odor, etc. These all help in providing a relaxing and calming environment for pets and owners alike.

Gentle control is another tool from the Fear Free toolbox. It incorporates how the veterinary team comfortably and safely positions the patient to allow the administration of veterinary care with minimal restraint. We discuss restraint above in this chapter, as we know it is frequently the restraint that frightens and stresses patients. As mentioned above, using distraction techniques while providing gentle guidance and support to a patient allows many procedures to be performed safely and with slight restraint and fewer team members.

For a greater understanding of Fear Free and the initiative which aims to make veterinary visits less stressful, visit https://fearfreepets.com/

Identification

If an animal is staying at the hospital and will be placed in a run, cage, or kennel, it must wear an identification collar around its neck, unless injury prevents it from doing so. The hospitalization collar must stay on for the duration of the hospital visit. The information on the hospitalization collar must include:

- patient's name
- owner's name
- hospital admission date
- attending veterinarian
- reason for admission
- allergies and/or warnings – large/bright for team to notice easily.

All patients admitted to the hospital must also have a cage or medical card. The information above should be on the patient's cage or medical card, along with observations/notes on the following:

- food fed
- type of food
- amount of food eaten
- water given and amount
- amount of water patient drank
- urination
- defecation
- body temperature and time taken
- medications administered, time administered.

Avian restraint

As with all animals, proper restraint techniques for birds are important for the safety of the handler and the person performing examinations or treatments, but most importantly for the safety and well-being of the patient. Restraint is a large stressor for avian patients, so knowing the avian patient and proper restraint and capture techniques will help to decrease pain and stress resulting from restraint.

All escape routes should be closed, and the room should be sealed. Hiding places to which the bird may flee should be identified and closed off. To capture and restrain an avian patient, it is recommended to use a towel. Towels of different sizes relative to the size of the bird are indicated. Using a towel to capture a bird helps to reduce fear of hands in the future. Gloves are *not* recommended, as a fear of hands may develop with gloves and the wearer loses much of their tactile sensation which is extremely important when handling birds. A slow approach with the towel in hand is best. Do not try to capture a bird that is sitting on the owner, as this may result in behavioral issues of the bird toward the owner and may result in the bird biting or attacking the owner. Remember to use a calm and soothing tone when approaching a bird. Confidence should be displayed, especially when trying to capture and restrain a large bird – they can detect fear and hesitation.

The hand (in the towel) should grasp the head of the bird toward the cervical (lower) end of the head but do not choke around the neck. Hold the sides of the head firmly, but insure the bird is able to breathe. Oftentimes, letting the bird bite the excess towel offers a distraction. For small birds, use the remainder of the hand to control the body and make sure the towel is wrapped around the bird to control the wings and feet (Figure 4.11). Larger birds should remain controlled with the opposite hand holding the towel that is wrapped around the body. The person restraining the bird should be monitoring the bird's respirations and stress level the entire time it is restrained. Observe the avian patient closely for signs of stress, **hypoxia**, and **hyperthermia**. Hands should be moved accordingly to allow the examiner to exam the bird at a faster pace.

Restraint is a very stressful experience for a bird. Allow the examiner to move as quickly as possible to insure the bird is restrained as little as possible. It is typical for a bird to show signs of stress when the restraint is released and the bird is placed back in its carrier. Open beak breathing, holding wings away from body, and fluffing of feathers may be exhibited so be aware if the bird exhibits these behaviors for a while after returning to its cage. However, normally the bird should recover rather quickly,

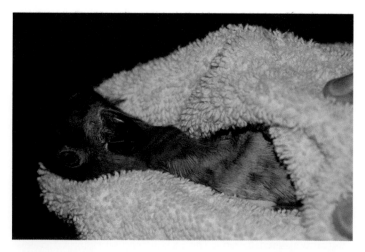

Figure 4.11 Restraining a bird with a towel. Courtesy of Kara M Burns, LVT, VTS (Nutrition).

Reptile restraint

Most snakes can be picked up in the transport carrier, especially when dealing with nonaggressive snakes. For aggressive snakes, a towel may be used by tossing the towel over the snake and finding the head of the snake. Once the head is located and restrained, it is safe to remove from the carrier. It is best to gently grasp the snake behind the head with one hand and support the body with the other hand.

Aquatic turtles, also known as chelonians, are considered easy to capture. However, restraining a chelonian involves controlling the head. To gain control of the head, the health-care team member should put their thumb on one side of the cranial neck portion and the index finger (or fingers if a larger animal) on the other side of the neck at the base of the skull.

Lizards typically can be held with two hands and removed from the transport carrier. However, some lizards are aggressive or the species' natural defenses will prevent one from simply picking up the lizard. In this instance, long-sleeved shirts, gloves, and a towel may be necessary. Frightened lizards may try to bite or scratch with their long claws. It is recommended to keep one hand on the neck, immediately behind the base of the skull, to prevent being bitten. Do not try to capture a lizard by the tail. Many species have a natural response to "drop" their tail to escape, and this may happen if they view the restrainer as a predator. Restraint of lizards can be obtained by placing one hand again around the neck and pectoral region and the other hand supporting the body near the pelvic region. Apply only enough pressure to keep the lizard restrained, as too much pressure may damage their spine.

Rabbit restraint

Physical restraint of rabbits needs to be carefully performed to avoid injury to the animal. Because rabbits have a well-developed muscular system and thin *cortical bone*, they are subject to vertebral and long bone fractures if restrained incorrectly. Because most skeletal injuries associated with incorrect restraint occur in the lumbar vertebrae, it is important to firmly restrain the hindlegs.

Rabbits should be handled in a manner similar to cats; place one hand under the forelimbs and use the other hand to hold the rear legs against the body. Always place the rabbit onto a nonslip surface to ensure that it has good footing. To restrain the animal, lightly scruff it and support its dorsum with the same arm. The opposite arm is used to support the body and rear legs.

Handling rodents

Guinea pigs

Most guinea pigs are docile and do not require aggressive restraint. Often a hand on the animal's dorsum is adequate to restrain a guinea pig patient on the examination table. When transporting a guinea pig, support the body with one hand under the thorax and abdomen while placing the other hand on the back to prevent the patient from falling or jumping.

Rats and mice

Rats and mice use their one means of defense – their teeth. Most rats and mice are easily handled and not very aggressive but they can bite if handled roughly or incorrectly. Mice have an increased tendency to bite if worried, stressed, or handled by an unfamiliar person. The best way of handling a mouse is to grasp it firmly by the base of the tail, lift it up carefully and then place it on to a nonslip table. Once it is placed on the table, grasp the scruff firmly between the thumb and forefinger. The mouse is now securely restrained for examination or for administration of any medication.

Rats tend not to bite unless roughly handled. The easiest way to pick up a tame rat is around the middle with one hand just behind the front legs, putting the other hand underneath to support the rat's weight. If you have an unfriendly or aggressive rat then the safest way to handle it is in much the same way as the mouse. Grasp it by the base of the tail, lift it on to a nonslip table, and then scruff it by the back of the neck with your thumb and forefinger. It is extremely important to remember that you should never grasp any mouse or rat by the end of the tail. This causes the skin to slough off, leading to severe damage and possible amputation of the tail.

Hamsters

Most hamsters are nocturnal and do not like to be woken up and handled during the day, especially by a stranger. For minor examinations or to move a friendly hamster, simply cup your hands around the animal and lift it up. For a more detailed examination or for an aggressive hamster, firmly scruff it at the back of the neck, ensuring that you grasp a lot of scruff between your thumb and forefinger. If you do not take enough scruff, the hamster may still be able to turn around and bite. Make sure the scruff is pulled cranially to avoid pulling it too tight around the eyes as hamsters are prone to prolapse if roughly handled. If you have an extremely aggressive hamster that you just cannot get a hold of then scoop it up into a clear plastic box, which will enable you to see if there is anything obviously wrong.

Gerbils

Gerbils are fairly docile animals and if socialized they are easy to handle. Typically, they only bite if frightened or stressed by rough handling. Gerbils move fast and are very good jumpers. To transport gerbils from one place to another, cup them in both hands underneath their bodies and gently lift them up. If a detailed examination is required or you have an aggressive animal, then firmly but gently grasp the scruff between your thumb and forefinger, lift the animal up, and support it underneath with your other hand and place it on a nonslip table for examination.

Never pick up a gerbil by the tail. The tail skin will slough the skin very easily, leaving only the vertebrae showing. This will never regrow and would have to be *amputated*.

References

Aspinall, V. (ed.) 2008. Handling and restraint. In: *Clinical Procedures of Veterinary Nursing*. Elsevier Butterworth Heinemann, Oxford, pp. 1–24.

Martin, D. 2017. The veterinary technician's role in implementing Fear Free. *Today's Veterinary Nurse*, July/August.

Sirois, M. (ed.) 2017. Physical restraint. In: *Principles and Practice of Veterinary Technology*, 4th edition. Elsevier Mosby, St Louis, MO, pp. 521–547.

Sonsthagen, T. 2020. *Tasks for the Veterinary Assistant*, 4th edition. Wiley Blackwell, Ames, IA.

Todd-Jenkins, K., Dugan, B., Remsburg, D.W., Montgomery, C. 2018. Restraint and handling of animals. In: *Clinical Textbook for Veterinary Technicians*, 9th edition. Bassert, J.M. Beal, A.D., Samples, O.M. (eds). Elsevier Saunders, St Louis, MO, pp. 166–206.

www.wiley.com/go/burns/textbookvetassistant2

Please go to the companion website for assignments and a PowerPoint relating to the material in this chapter.

Chapter 5 Office Procedures and Telephone Techniques

All veterinary health-care team members should have extensive knowledge of the workings of the hospital at which they are employed. Each employee should understand the process of making client appointments, the names of the employees at the hospital, the fee structure of the hospital, proper phone etiquette, products or brands that are recommended by the veterinarian(s), etc. This knowledge involves cross-training amongst positions within the hospital and is imperative for veterinary assistants and receptionists as the bulk of these procedures typically fall within their responsibilities.

Communication is the key to successful implementation and understanding of office procedures. Communication is also the key to a successful veterinary hospital.

Every client and pet should be greeted when they enter the veterinary hospital. Team members should have all the medical records prepared and available for the clients with appointments for that day. As clients and pets enter, greet them with a smile and a friendly greeting. Remembering the pet's name and greeting them upon entering the veterinary hospital makes the client feel important, remembered, and welcomed. They feel as though they are part of the health-care team – which, in actuality, they are. This one simple step forges the long-term relationship between client, pet, and health-care team (Figure 5.1).

Each veterinary hospital will have guidelines for professional appearance. This is based on the premise that "you never get a second chance to make a first impression." First impressions can be highly effective or may have devastating consequences. When meeting others for the first time, we want to establish comfort, trust, and rapport. A study from the University of Connecticut shows that first impressions turn out to be accurate 67% of the time. Clients will base their judgment of the practice and value of a veterinary hospital and its employees on the first appearance of the health-care team and the veterinary hospital. Personal grooming and professional appearance, appropriate language, and basic common courtesy are central to making a good impression and representing the veterinary hospital for which you work. When clients meet the health-care team for the first time, our clothing, manners, and etiquette are on display. Clients measure our self-confidence and our ability within 60 seconds of the first interaction. Health-care teams do not want to give the impression that team members are not self-confident and able to carry out their responsibilities.

When considering personal grooming and professional appearance, the health-care team must consider the safety of themselves, the patient, and their teammates and remember that each member of the veterinary hospital has the potential to have a very physically active position. Each individual must take into account everything from personal jewelry to professional clothing. Every veterinary hospital should have a ***standard operating procedures (SOP) manual***. This will review every procedure and requirement in the hospital and will include guidelines for personal grooming and professional appearance. Hospitals vary in regard to uniforms. Some may designate scrub tops and bottoms as the uniform of choice. Others may designate colors of scrubs to certain positions in the hospital. It is recommended to wear comfortable and durable clothing that is easily washable in hot water. To decrease the risk of disease transmission, clothing should be washed daily. Every member of the health-care team should wear a name tag which includes name, credentials, and job title (Figure 5.2). Remember patient and team member safety when choosing a name tag. Consider embroidery on the scrub top with a name or a name badge that is magnetic. Pin-style name badges have the potential to puncture the wearer and/or patient. Insure the required information is applied to whatever type of identification

Textbook for the Veterinary Assistant, Second Edition. Kara M. Burns and Lori Renda-Francis.
© 2022 John Wiley & Sons, Inc. Published 2022 by John Wiley & Sons, Inc.
Companion website: www.wiley.com/go/burns/textbookvetassistant2

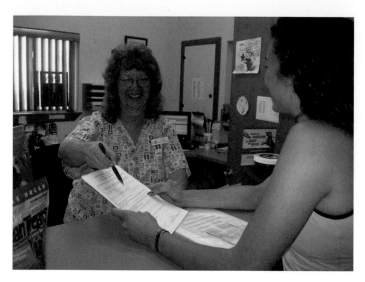

Figure 5.1 Health-care team member and client. Source: Sirois, M. (ed.) 2010. *Principles and Practice of Veterinary Technology*, 3rd edition. Elsevier Mosby, St Louis, MO.

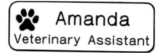

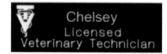

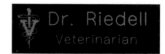

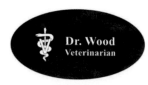

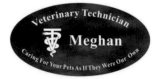

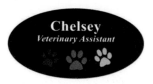

Figure 5.2 Name badge alternatives. Source: Courtesy of Kara M. Burns, LVT, VTS (Nutrition).

the hospital and the individual approve. Open-toed shoes should never be worn when working in a veterinary hospital. Many positions in the hospital require long days with short or nonexistent breaks, so it is important to wear comfortable and durable shoes. The SOP manual will also give guidance for wearing jewelry, including piercings. Remember, common sense plays a big part in choices of jewelry and piercings that are worn to work. The health-care team must think of patient and team member safety when considering jewelry. A watch that is waterproof with a seconds hand is needed when working in veterinary medicine. Other jewelry such as piercings, earrings, bracelets, and necklaces must be approved by the hospital owner or practice manager as directed in the SOP manual. There is high risk for a patient to catch their paw, claws, or teeth on jewelry, thus potentially injuring themselves or the individual. Rings pose a risk as described above in addition to potentially harboring bacteria. If rings are to be worn, the recommendation is a ring with a flat and smooth surface that may be taken off and washed frequently. Tattoo requirements will be detailed in the hospital SOP manual.

Part of working as a professional and portraying a professional appearance includes appropriate language and behavior. The language of every health-care team member should be professional at all times. Remember common courtesy. Swearing is NEVER appropriate. All health-care team members should be familiar with the appropriate language used when communicating about veterinary medicine.

Team etiquette should be established by the hospital and used by every member of the health-care team. Respect is the number one requirement in a professional working environment. Respect should be given to every member of the team with whom you work and to the client. All team members are important to the success of the hospital and the care of a patient. No one position is above another when patient care and successful hospital operation are involved.

Telephone techniques

The telephone is a very strong communication tool. It allows people at a distance and strangers to immediately access your hospital. Answering the telephone is the first impression that a client receives from your hospital. Improper phone etiquette may lead to the last interaction with your hospital as well.

The phone should be answered within the first three rings, otherwise the client may believe the hospital is too busy and impersonal to treat their pet. One should always be polite and courteous. Inaccessibility may drive existing and potential clients to another hospital. Always smile when answering the phone. Although the client cannot see you smile, they can hear it! This gives a warm and welcoming perception to the caller. Always introduce yourself when answering the call, identify the hospital name, and ask how you may help the caller. An example would be: "Hello, 123 Veterinary Hospital, Lori speaking. How may I help you?" Instantly a relationship is established because you have identified yourself and your hospital, and asked to assist the caller.

Always attempt to answer the call. Try not to put the caller on hold. There will occasionally be times when health-care team members may have to put a caller on hold. Again, common courtesy plays a big role. *Ask* the caller if you can put them on hold and *listen* for an answer. Do not ever simply ask and put the caller on hold without hearing their response. The caller may have an emergency that cannot wait. It is proper to not leave a caller on hold longer than one minute without returning to check on them. If you need them to continue to hold, take their name and phone number and give a time frame within which you will return their call. If a callback is necessary, it is imperative that the client is called within the agreed time frame. Not doing so gives the client the impression that they and their pet are not important to the hospital.

When answering a phone call, be sure to write down the owner's name and the patient's name. Repeatedly asking for this information suggests the hospital is not well organized and may imply that the owner and patient are not important. If this information is written down and the call is placed on hold, the caller feels as though the health-care team member remembers them personally when returning to the phone call.

There are certain phrases that team members should learn to use – and not use. To answer a question with "I don't know" gives the impression that the team member (and possibly the hospital as a whole) is not informed or educated. Even worse, it may give the impression that the veterinary team does not care enough to find or learn the needed information. Try using the phrase, "That is a great question, let me find out" rather than "I don't know." Also, the phrase "Just a second" signals abruptness and lacks compassion. Instead focus on a helpful response such as, "I will have that information for you in just a moment." Words, tone, and inflection all matter and we should choose to portray confidence, compassion, and understanding. Words and phrases such as "Absolutely!", "I know how much you care", and "I understand" are powerful assertions that help to create empathy with pet owners.

Every hospital should employ guidelines for health-care team members regarding what can and cannot be said. It is prudent to develop a list of frequently asked questions and appropriate responses. This insures consistency in answering questions and continuity from the practice manager and/or owner. Some of the more common situations include the following.

- Making appointments
- Emergency calls
- Updates for hospitalized pets
- Clients evaluating prices between hospitals – "price shopping"
- Angry callers
- Request for a refill of medication and nutrition

It is important to represent the hospital as compassionate and caring. Being a good listener is one way to do this. All health-care team members should be courteous and respectful when talking with clients on the phone. You will hear the same questions throughout your career, but remember the clients are asking because either they do not know or the situation is new to them. Health-care team members must be empathetic and calm and respond with common courtesy and proper etiquette.

Every telephone call has the potential to turn into an appointment. Remember your pleasant and confident communication can help a potential client to immediately feel comfortable and that they matter, and helps them to feel as though they can ask questions. Calls answered in a polite, educated, and unhurried manner are more likely to result in an appointment with the veterinary hospital. The team member should ask open-ended questions to generate conversation. Closed questions typically result in a one-word answer whereas open-ended questions allow for discussion. Providing value and education to a pet owner increases the likelihood that the veterinary hospital will gain a new patient and owner. *Always* ask if you can make an appointment at the end of a phone conversation. Additionally, end the call with compassion and ensure the caller's needs have been met.

Example: *"Mrs. Smith, thank you for calling AAA Veterinary Hospital. Have I answered all your questions today? My name is Lori; please call back with any other questions you may have."*

Scheduling appointments is a big and important task in the veterinary hospital. Appointments help to control the flow of the hospital – from the examination room, to boarding, to surgery, to urgent needs patients, to full emergencies. Scheduling also helps in scheduling the veterinary team, as well as improving the workflow of team members. By having the proper number of team members during heavily scheduled appointment times, hospital needs as well as client needs can be met.

Veterinary team members should understand and be trained on the hospital's appointment scheduling program. This includes understanding which appointments are scheduled for specific lengths of time, why those lengths of times are important, and how each appointment affects the entire team and the smooth functioning of the veterinary hospital.

Office procedures

Forward booking

If after a patient has received service at the veterinary hospital and another appointment is needed, best practice indicates that appointment should be made before the pet owner leaves the veterinary hospital. Booking appointments prior to the pet owner and patient leaving the hospital is known as **forward booking**. It is in the best interest of the patient for the hospital team to forward book medical progress examinations, booster vaccines, follow-up laboratory work, and annual examinations. These appointments should be made while the owner is still in the practice and prior to accepting payment for services.

It has been shown that the majority of clients return for follow-up appointments when they have been scheduled prior to checkout of the earlier appointment. This is similar to the practice in human dentistry. Most clients have an appointment for a 6-month cleaning while still with the hygienist. It is important that veterinary medicine follow suit, as this helps with the patient's overall health. The veterinary team should then provide pet owners with multiple reminders in multiple formats and allow for rescheduling when needed.

Whenever a client (or potential client) asks questions regarding the price of services, team members should be able to educate the client on service itself and "wow" the client with the value they will receive when coming to the practice.

Patient behavior upon arrival

Not all pets love to visit the veterinary hospital. The veterinary team must monitor patients as they arrive as they may be anxious and fearful. The team must monitor the patient's signs and implement stress-reducing approaches such as the following.

- Place patients expeditiously into the exam rooms to limit interactions with other patients.
- Place pheromones in examination rooms and allow time for the pet to acclimate prior to beginning the examination.
- Play soft, classical music in the examination room. This will aid with relaxation of both pet owners and patients.
- If appropriate for the patient, offer a few treats to help calm the pet.
- Thundershirts® provide pets with a sense of safety and have a calming effect. These can be applied to anxious pets in the exam room.
- Advise team members that a fearful or stressed patient is in the examination room.

Forms

There are a number of forms that are used in the veterinary hospital and all team members must be familiar with all forms. Clients may be asked to complete forms with their personal contact information, their pet's information, the pet's history, and potentially various release forms. The veterinary team is responsible for ensuring the forms are filled out completely and correctly. Owner contact information is essential for the veterinary team to connect with the owner regarding updates to the pet's health. Ensure the owner's address is correct at every visit to ensure reminders can be mailed for vaccines, tests, and medication refills. In addition, the client must sign the bottom of the form, which should state that they are responsible for any charges. Remember to ask clients if there is another caretaker who should be listed on the medical record. This helps to ensure that only the owner(s) with name(s) listed in the medical record can authorize treatment for the pet. Additionally, this allows for an overdue invoice to be discussed with those names listed in the medical record.

The patient's information is obviously an important section of the record. The form should include details regarding species, gender, neutered status, date of birth, breed, and color. It is important for team members to know the breeds within a species (see Chapter 7) as owners can be easily offended when team members are unfamiliar with the pet's breed or guess incorrectly. Be sure the documents are scanned into and become part of the patient's medical record, especially if a signature is included indicating the client agrees to payment terms.

Medical record

Every animal that is seen at the veterinary hospital should have its own medical record. The record should be dated each time an entry is made; the presenting problems should be listed, and the author must initial this entry. Veterinary hospitals vary – they may use paper medical records, be paperless, or paper light. Paper medical records must be kept on 8½ × 11 in. sheets of paper. It is important to note that index cards are no longer acceptable as the medical record. Every client interaction, every client conversation, consent form, laboratory report, consultation, physical examination, and medication administered and dispensed *must* be documented in the medical record. If it is not in the patient's medical record, then "it never happened." Many veterinary hospitals have moved to paperless medical records. Paperless hospitals have the benefit of being able to access client records, laboratory results, and radiographs at any computer station.

Consent forms

There are also a number of consent forms which pet owners may be asked to sign before various treatments and procedures can be performed on their pets. Every member of the veterinary team must be able to explain the meaning of every form that a client is asked to sign. It is important for team members to also read the consent forms aloud to the client, helping to ensure the client understands what he or she is signing. Consent forms are not required by law – their purpose is to protect the veterinary healthcare team. If the form is documented in the record, it can be submitted if a court case arises. If the form or conversation is not documented, the assumption is that the risks, benefits, or information were never discussed or provided. Again, "it never happened" if it is not in the medical record. Be sure all consent forms have the owner's and patient's name(s) along with the date and the initials of the team member helping the client sign the forms.

Rabies certificates

Rabies certificates today are often generated by the veterinary software system utilized by the hospital. The team member enters the rabies tag number, lot number, and manufacturer of the vaccine. Lot numbers or serial numbers of vaccines are crucial information and must be entered in the event of a recall. This information allows for hospitals to identify who received the recalled vaccine. The practice management software automatically populates client and patient information; veterinary signature and license numbers *must* be added to all printed certificates.

If a handwritten rabies vaccine book is used by the practice, the correct owner and patient information must be legible. The following information is required:

- date
- owner's name
- owner's address
- owner's phone numbers
- patient's name
- patient's age
- patient's breed
- patient's gender.

The rabies tag number and lot number are then entered, in addition to the veterinarian's signature and license number. It is imperative to ensure the information has been added correctly and legibly, as often the rabies tag and number help to identify lost pets.

Spay or neuter certificates

Once a patient has been neutered or spayed, a certificate is generated which provides the owner with proof that the pet has been neutered. There are times when city or county ordinances require that a pet is neutered and this certificate is proof.

Health certificates

When traveling with pets, airlines and various state and federal agencies require health certificates. Airlines want to ensure the pet is healthy and has seen a veterinarian prior to accepting the pet for transport. States want to ensure the pet is not importing any diseases if they are coming from a different state. Both federal and state agencies are responsible for the prevention of disease and have various regulations regarding the entry of animals. The majority of inter-state health certificates are good for ~10 days before shipment.

The pet must be fully examined by a veterinarian before the certificate is issued. The majority of the states in the nation require compliance with providing a copy of the health certificate. International health certificates are typically good for 30 days and require the signature of the state veterinarian. These certificates pertain to shipping pets out of the United States. Both forms of health certificates require the owner's name, address, and phone number along with the name, address, and phone number of the person who will be accepting and taking responsibility for the pet. All the animal's identifying information must be included, including age, breed, gender, and microchip or tattoo number. The animal's vaccines must be current, with the vaccination information stated visibly.

Small animal health certificates differ from large animal health certificates. A large animal certificate should disclose tests that are required (by state law) and have been completed – with the results on the certificate. It is important to verify regulations prior to shipping or transporting any animal to another state or country.

Invoices

A veterinary team member must review invoices with owners before collecting money. Services that have been provided should be detailed, and the team member should anticipate questions. The invoice should include every aspect of the services provided. Allow the client to review the invoice in detail after the team member explains the charges. Also, allow the client to ask questions. This detailed presentation allows the client to read and understand the services and charges. The value of client service can be increased when all procedures are explained thoroughly.

Payment

Most veterinary hospitals commonly accept payment in the form of cash (including debit card), check, or credit card. It is important to ensure that the signature on the credit card matches the signature on the receipt. The Federal Trade Commission created the Red Flags Rule which states that any credit card transaction should be verified with a picture identification. This rule was established to help decrease fraud and the use of stolen credit cards.

Another option for pet owners is pet health insurance. Many policies are set up so that the owners pay the hospital for the services their pet needs and are then reimbursed by the insurance company.

CareCredit is a health-care financing credit card that can be used for veterinary services. Clients can apply either online or while at the practice. A veterinary team member can enter the client's information online or through a telephone operator. Typically, the approval is received quickly – sometimes within 10 minutes. For more information, visit www.carecredit.com/vetmed.

In today's society, accepting cash has risks as cash can be counterfeit. Detecting counterfeit money is not easy. Best practices state having the local police department notify the hospital team if there has been passing of or suspicion of counterfeit money in the area.

Within the hospital, cash should be kept in a locked safe and out of sight from clients. Unfortunately, many businesses have realized the hard way that it only takes a second for a person to reach over the counter and grab money from the drawer. Cash drawers should have a lock and be locked immediately after they are closed. Never leave a cash drawer unattended, especially if it is unlocked. One moment of inattentiveness can result in the loss of a great deal of money.

References

Bixler, B. and Dugan, L.S. 2001. *5 Steps to Professional Presence*. Adams Media Corporation, Avon, MA.

Heller, R. 1998. *Communicate Clearly*. DK Publishing, New York, NY.

Prendergast, H. 2020. *Front Office Management for the Veterinary Team*, 3rd edition. Saunders Elsevier, St Louis, MO.

Sonsthagen, T. 2020. *Tasks for the Veterinary Assistant*, 4th edition. Wiley Blackwell. Ames, IA.

www.wiley.com/go/burns/textbookvetassistant2

Please go to the companion website for assignments and a PowerPoint relating to the material in this chapter.

Chapter 6 Nutrition

Members of the veterinary health-care team must have some understanding of nutrition and how it relates to the animals coming into the hospital each day. Nutrition is one area of veterinary medicine that affects every pet that comes into the hospital. Out of the three components that affect the life of an animal – genetics, environment, and nutrition – nutrition is the one factor that the veterinary health-care team can impact. Proper nutrition and feeding management are the foundation upon which healing and health maintenance rest.

Overview

A nutrient is any food constituent that helps support life. There are six major nutrient groups, three that supply energy and three that do not. The energy-producing nutrients are proteins, fats, and carbohydrates. The nonenergy-producing nutrients are vitamins, minerals, and water. In the wild, animals eat to satisfy their energy needs. Domestic dogs and cats rely on their owners to feed them. Consequently, pet foods must contain the nutrients and energy content balanced to the needs of the animal. When the pet consumes enough food to meet energy requirements, the proper amounts of proteins, fats, carbohydrates, vitamins, minerals, and water occur in the correct proportions. This is referred to as a "complete and balanced" diet.

Energy has no measurable size or dimensions but can be determined by completely burning a sample in a bomb calorimeter and measuring the heat produced, or "gross energy" content, of the food. We use the term "kilocalorie" in this measurement. A kilocalorie (kcal) is the amount of heat required to raise the temperature of 1kg of water by 1 °C. Typically, kilocalories are referred to simply as "calories" in discussions of food or exercise. The term "digestible energy" refers to the food's gross energy minus the energy that is nonabsorbable and lost in the feces.

"Metabolizable energy" is the food's gross energy minus the energy lost in the feces and urine; that is, the amount of energy that is actually available to the pet for metabolism following digestion and absorption.

Proteins

Proteins serve as the nitrogen source for animals that cannot utilize **atmospheric nitrogen**. Besides being the primary constituents of many body tissues, enzymes, hormones and necessary components of hemoglobin and antibodies, **plasma proteins** are needed to prevent **edema** and to transport substances in the blood. Proteins supply approximately 4 kcal of energy per gram and are composed of combinations of building blocks called amino acids. The essential amino acids cannot be synthesized and must be supplied in the diet at proper concentrations. Dogs require 10 different amino acids, while cats require 11. The additional amino acid cats require is taurine. The amount of protein required is dependent upon species, age of the animal, and quality of the protein.

The quality of a protein can be assessed by its digestibility and amino acid profile. Measuring the biological value of a protein is one way of determining quality. The more essential amino acids present in a protein, the higher its biological value and the better the quality of the protein source. The higher the quality of protein, the less protein is required. Protein supplied in excess of body needs is not stored as protein. The liver converts excess protein into energy, and the nitrogenous waste product (urea) has to be excreted by the kidney. Animal source proteins contain

Textbook for the Veterinary Assistant, Second Edition. Kara M. Burns and Lori Renda-Francis.
© 2022 John Wiley & Sons, Inc. Published 2022 by John Wiley & Sons, Inc.
Companion website: www.wiley.com/go/burns/textbookvetassistant2

more essential amino acids than some plant proteins, although combinations of the two are often complementary. When combined in proper proportions, they enhance the overall biological value of the protein in the diet. Cats, as true carnivores, require at least twice as much protein as dogs, and young animals require more protein than adults. Cats have a high protein requirement because they always use a given amount of protein for energy. Cats do not have metabolic flexibility where protein is concerned. This is one major reason why cat food is higher in protein than dog food. It is also the reason dogs should not be allowed to eat cat food and vice versa.

Carbohydrates

Cats and dogs have no minimum requirement for carbohydrates. However, carbohydrates are added to commercial pet foods as an energy source to supply calories and add variety, fiber, and palatability to the diet. Carbohydrates are typically less expensive ingredients in pet foods. Dietary carbohydrates provide approximately 4 kcal of energy per gram, and cereal grains are the most common source of carbohydrates in pet foods. Carbohydrates are classified into two segments based on their digestibility: soluble and insoluble. Raw carbohydrates are not digested well by carnivores (such as cats) or omnivores (such as humans, bears, and dogs), although simple things like grinding and cooking can increase digestibility. Soluble carbohydrates are also referred to as "nitrogen-free extract" (NFE).

Carbohydrates can consist of simple sugars (monosaccharides) and complex sugars (disaccharides and polysaccharides). Carbohydrates are digested with the help of enzymes such as maltase, sucrase, and lactase, which are found in the *intestinal epithelial brush border* and break down *disaccharides.* As a result, any disease process that impairs the intestinal epithelial brush border may affect the pet's ability to digest some forms of carbohydrates, disaccharides in particular. Soluble carbohydrates in excess of the amount needed to meet the animal's energy requirements are stored in the body as glycogen or fat and may lead to obesity. Cats inherently have a decreased ability to metabolize soluble carbohydrates due to low levels of glucokinase, the enzyme necessary in the first step of the breakdown of glucose and its entry into the energy-producing pathway.

Insoluble carbohydrates are sometimes referred to as "dietary fiber" and include cellulose, hemicellulose, and lignin, among others. Monogastric animals lack the intestinal enzymes to completely digest insoluble carbohydrate sources and rely on key bacterial flora to break down these fibers and permit partial assimilation. Various fiber sources have varying degrees of digestibility or solubility. Dietary fiber, especially cellulose, has been shown to normalize intestinal transit time. Components of dietary fiber have also been shown to alter fat and glucose metabolism and decrease the absorption of other nutrients. Diets high in insoluble carbohydrates are inappropriate for dogs and cats with high energy requirements such as animals undergoing growth, late gestation, lactation, stress, or work. Insoluble carbohydrates may be included in foods designed for weight control or reduction by promoting a sense of fullness without adding calories.

Fats

Fats serve as a more concentrated source of energy in a diet, providing 9 kcal of energy per gram. Fats are the primary energy source of most commercial pet foods. They also enhance palatability, are necessary for the absorption, storage, and transport of the fat-soluble vitamins A, D, E, and K, and are the source of linoleic, linolenic, and arachidonic acid, the essential fatty acids.

Essential fatty acids are constituents of cell membranes. They are responsible for the synthesis of *prostaglandins* and related compounds as well as the control of epidermal water loss. Cats require dietary sources of arachidonic acid found only in animal fats, which is another indication that cats are true carnivores, requiring meat tissue sources in their diet to survive. Dogs have the ability to synthesize arachidonic acid from linoleic acid. Essential fatty acid deficiencies occur in dogs eating low-fat dog food in which beef tallow is the sole source of fat, or when the food has been improperly stored for an extended period of time. Fat needs to be stabilized with an antioxidant or preservative to maintain the quality of the dry food to which it has been added. The same does not apply to canned foods, as canned foods are pasteurized and sealed. Fat deficiencies in cats and dogs may manifest as impaired wound healing, dry hair coat, scaly skin, and pyodermas or skin infections.

Vitamins

Vitamins are important in chemical reactions of metabolism, functioning as enzyme precursors or coenzymes. Vitamins are divided into two basic categories: fat soluble (vitamins A, D, E, and K) and water soluble (vitamins B complex and C). Fat-soluble vitamins can be stored within body fat and in the liver. Dietary excesses of fat-soluble vitamins may result in toxicosis. The water-soluble vitamins are not stored to any great extent in the body. The health-care team must be careful when excessive water loss occurs, such as when the patient is suffering from *polyuria* and/or diarrhea, as vitamin stores may be depleted and supplementation needed. Cats have additional vitamin requirements compared to dogs. Cats are unable to convert beta-carotene, present in plants, into vitamin A and thus require a dietary source of preformed vitamin A found only in animal tissues. In addition, niacin must be added to a cat's diet because cats cannot convert the amino acid tryptophan into the B vitamin niacin.

Minerals

Minerals can be divided into macrominerals, which are calcium, phosphorus, potassium, sodium and magnesium, and microminerals or trace minerals, which include iron, zinc, copper, manganese, iodine, cobalt, and selenium. The balance of all minerals in the diet is essential. Excessive intake of one mineral may be harmful, and any unabsorbed portion may bind with other minerals, adversely affecting their availability and resulting in a deficiency or imbalance. The best approach is to feed a diet known to contain the proper amount and balance of minerals for the animal's particular life stage or activity level.

Calcium is the mineral required in the largest amount in the diet, but it should be present in the proper proportion and amount in relation to phosphorus. Excess calcium intake in a pet's diet will result in a decrease in the absorption of phosphorus, iron, zinc, and copper and will delay bone growth and *maturation*. Dietary supplements such as calcium carbonate, dicalcium phosphate, bone meal or vitamin D given in conjunction with high-calcium diets or free-choice feeding are usually the sources of calcium excess. Calcium deficiency is primarily associated with phosphorus excess, such as in animals fed high levels of meat and organ tissue. The correct calcium-to-phosphorus ratio is approximately 1.1–1.4:1, and diets that are high in organ meats can have an inverse calcium-to-phosphorus ratio of 1:10 or higher.

Phosphorus plays an important role in cell metabolism and composition of bone and teeth. Excess dietary phosphorus increases glomerular filtration rate. Excess phosphorus in conjunction with calcium may result in soft tissue calcification, ultimately causing damage to the kidneys.

Sodium is the main cation of extracellular body fluids, while potassium is the main intracellular one. Sodium chloride or salt is a main taste factor in many pet and human foods. Excess dietary salt can contribute to hypertension and fluid retention and may potentiate cardiovascular and renal disease. While 4–8 mg/kg is adequate to maintain *homeostasis*, many commercial pet foods contain 10–40 times the amount needed, or 80–150 mg/kg of sodium.

The term "ash" has been used in the past in regard to pet foods, especially cat food and feline lower urinary tract disease (FLUTD). It is important to know that "ash" refers to all the minerals in a food; magnesium specifically seems to be the main contributing mineral in the manifestation of struvite-related lower urinary tract disease (LUTD), especially in cats. Low-ash foods could still contain excess levels of magnesium, making them inappropriate for urinary tract health. Veterinary assistants should recognize that the type and amount of minerals in the food and not the "ash" should be monitored when dealing with LUTD. Additionally, promoting production of urine with a mean pH (acidity) between 6.2 and 6.4 can inhibit the production of struvite crystals and urinary stones.

Water

Water is the most critical nutrient, and all pets should have access to fresh, clean water at all times. A 10% loss in total body water causes serious illness, while a 15% loss may result in death. The water requirement of a dog or cat, expressed in mL/day, is roughly equivalent to the animal's energy requirement in kcal/day. Veterinary assistants must ensure that patients have access to clean, fresh water at all times unless otherwise indicated by the veterinarian or credentialed veterinary technician.

Palatability

Palatability does not relate to the nutritional value of the food. Palatability is a measure of the degree to which an animal likes a food. Acceptability is an indication of whether the amount of food eaten will be enough to meet the animal's caloric requirements. A balanced food needs to be only palatable enough to ensure acceptability along with adequate nutrient intake, and a food's performance does not improve when an animal eats more of it. In fact, this type of behavior may predispose the animal to obesity. Pet owners, however, often judge a food by how quickly their pet consumes it. Some palatability factors include odor, temperature, texture, or feel of the food in the pet's mouth, fat content, water content, and salt content. When a client needs to improve the palatability of a diet without altering the nutritional profile of the food, simple things like moistening a dry food, warming a food to body temperature, hand feeding, or simply adding the canned version of the selected diet to the dry food in the bowl can be effective techniques.

Recommendations

Pet owners will look to the veterinary health-care team for recommendations as to what to feed their pet. The health-care team should be aligned with recommendations, and veterinary assistants should be familiar with diets available for managing both healthy and ill pets.

Therapeutic diets are formulated to aid in the management of certain disease conditions. These diets require a proper doctor/client/patient relationship, and recommendation of therapeutic diets can be made only by the veterinarian. It is important that veterinary assistants familiarize themselves with the therapeutic foods being recommended and the disease conditions that these diets manage. They should have a basic understanding of how the therapeutic diet aids in the management of the disease condition.

Nutritional management of pets is an iterative process. As recommended by the American College of Veterinary Nutrition (ACVN), nutritional management of pets includes assessment of the patient, the food, and the feeding method. Patient assessment is the first step and allows the determination of the patient's key nutritional factors and their levels. The key nutritional factors of the patient, as determined by the veterinarian and veterinary technician, become the basis for the second step, known as the feeding plan. The feeding plan consists of recommendations for food and feeding methods. The veterinarian will make the recommendation for the patient (in wellness nutrition, a nutrition technician may make the recommendation). The assessment of the current food and feeding method will help to indicate whether the current feeding plan is appropriate or not. The veterinary assistant plays an important role in this iterative process. Weighing patients when they enter the hospital and documenting all discussions with owners as they pertain to pets' nutritional status in the medical record are important responsibilities of the veterinary assistant.

The process is continually repeated in an attempt to determine the appropriateness or effectiveness of the feeding plan. If the feeding plan is found to be inappropriate, a new feeding plan is developed and implemented by the veterinarian and veterinary technician. This is the iterative or repetitive part of the process and depends on the needs of each patient. For example, a patient that is critically ill may need to be reassessed every few hours, whereas a normal adult dog or cat may be reassessed annually. The subsequent reassessment of the patient at each cycle is also referred to as "monitoring," and all members of the veterinary health-care team play a role in the continued monitoring of each and every patient admitted to or coming to the veterinary hospital.

Weight management

Obesity is the most prevalent form of malnutrition in North American pets. It is estimated that 58% of dogs and 60% of cats presenting to small animal hospitals in North America are overweight to obese. The health-care team, when evaluating overweight dogs and cats, divide the patients into two categories: pets that are 10–19% above optimal weight are considered overweight, and those that are 20% or more above optimal weight are considered obese.

Obesity is a disease that can complicate or exacerbate other disease conditions. Overweight pets are at increased risk for many other disease conditions, including heart disease, respiratory problems, diabetes, and osteoarthritis, to name just a few. The overweight pet is also at risk for a shorter life span. It has been found that pets that are lean or at optimal weight have the potential to live 1–2 years longer than overweight pets.

All members of the health-care team are responsible for assisting the veterinarian in the diagnosis of this dangerous disease and in addressing the detrimental effects of excess body fat with clients and pet owners.

Patient history

Obtaining the pet's history is the first step to evaluating overweight pets and determining the nutritional status of the patient. A complete history is typically taken by the veterinarian or veterinary technician and includes signalment (i.e., species, breed, age, gender, reproductive status, activity level, and environment).

A complete nutritional history should determine the quality and adequacy of the food being fed to the pet, the feeding protocol (e.g., meal fed, free choice, amount, family member responsible for feeding the pet), and a history of the types of food fed to the pet. A nutritional history should also include access to treats, number of treats a day, types of treat, supplements, or other foods. Again, the success of a weight management protocol depends upon all health-care team members familiarizing themselves with, understanding, and taking a nutritional history. When dealing with an overweight or obese pet, it is also imperative to include the following in the nutritional history.

- The brand of food the pet eats
- Types of snacks or treats offered
- Supplements
- Chewable medications
- Types of chew toys the pet plays with
- Whether human foods are given
- Access to other sources of food

Communication between the health-care team and client is crucial to successful management of obese pets. Clients often do not remember that a cup equals 8 ounces and will feed using a 16-ounce "cup." Overweight pets may have access to commercial foods fed to other species in the household. Pets also may be fed by more than one family member or receive numerous treats throughout the day.

All these findings from a nutritional history can indicate the cause of the pet's overweight or obese condition. Through the nutritional history, the health-care team can start to pinpoint breakdowns in compliance and begin to establish a feeding protocol to help reduce the pet's excessive calorie consumption.

Nutritional evaluation

Every animal that presents to the hospital, every time they present, should be assessed to establish nutritional needs and feeding goals, which depend on the pet's physiology and/or disease condition. Veterinary team members are involved in the patient's history, scoring of the patient's body condition, working with the veterinarian to determine the proper nutritional recommendation for the patient, and communicating this information to the pet owner.

The first step in evaluating a pet and determining its nutritional status is to take a thorough history, including signalment (i.e., species, breed, age, gender, reproductive status, activity level, and environment). Next, a nutritional history should be taken to determine the quality and adequacy of the food being fed to the pet, the feeding protocol (e.g., whether the pet is fed at designated meals or has free choice, the amount of food given, the family member responsible for feeding the pet), and the type or types of food given to the pet. Open-ended questions should be asked of the owner. This type of questioning helps to uncover more information, as it gets the owner talking; closed questions typically produce a one-word answer, thus potentially not uncovering everything the patient eats in a day. It also has the potential to put the pet owner on the defensive, thus sabotaging the relationship veterinary team members are trying to build with the pet owner – especially when it comes to nutrition.

Please see Box 6.1. Nutritional history questions to ask owners include the following.

- Tell me what your pet eats over the course of a day.
- Tell me what other pets and what other family members are in the household.
- Tell me about your pet's appetite.
- Tell me about any changes in elimination habits.
- Tell me about any supplements your pet receives.
- Tell me about any medications your pet receives.

The owner should also be asked about the pet's access to foods, supplements, and medications and how much of each the pet consumes each day. Pets also may be fed by more than one family member or receive numerous treats throughout the day. All these factors play a role in proper nutrition of pets.

All members of the health-care team should be familiar with taking a nutritional history. Through this mechanism, the team can pinpoint a breakdown in owner compliance (e.g., is more than one person in the household feeding the pet, is the pet getting more calories than is being recommended, etc.) and begin to establish a feeding protocol to insure the pet's proper calorie consumption.

Box 6.1 Nutritional history questionnaire

Date _____ Pet's name _____ Species _____ Breed _____

Date of Birth _____ Gender _____ Neutered/Spayed [ ] No [ ] Yes **Weight** [ ]

1. Tell me about your pet's living environment [ ] Indoors [ ] Outdoors [ ] Both
2. Tell me about your pet's activity level. Plays/walks [ ] 3 times/day [ ] 1-2 times/day [ ] Never
3. Do you have other pets? [ ] No [ ] Yes
   a. If yes, list here _____
4. Are pets fed separately? [ ] No [ ] Yes
5. Does your pet have access to other, unmonitored food sources? No Yes
   a. If yes, please describe _____
6. Tell me about your pet's appetite. _____
7. Who feeds your pet? _____
8. What changes have been made to your pet's diet in the past 30 days? _____
9. Please list the brands and product names (if applicable) and amounts of ALL foods, treats, snacks, dental hygiene products, rawhides, and any other foods that your pet is currently eating.

Food/Treat	Form	Amount	How Often	Date Started

10. Tell me what supplements your pet receives. _____
11. What medications is your pet taking and how is each administered? _____
12. Tell me about the toys your pet enjoys. _____
13. Tell me about food or treats not formulated for pets that your pet receives._____
    _____
    _____
14. Tell me what foods/treats are NOT tolerated by your pet. _____
15. If you are going on vacation and I am your pet sitter, tell me everything I need to do for your pet while you are gone. _____
    _____
    _____
    _____

© Kara M. Burns, LVT, VTS (Nutrition).

Body condition scoring

Body condition scoring (BCS) allows for health-care team members to evaluate a patient's fat stores, muscle mass, and weight changes (Figures 6.1 and 6.2). BCS also allows for consistent communication between health-care team members. The two most common BCS systems are a five-point scale and a nine-point scale. Both use a nine-point rating, with the five-point scale being scored to the nearest half-point and the nine-point scale being scored to the whole point. The entire health-care team should utilize the same scoring system from the outset so as not to confuse or miscalculate the patient's weight (Box 6.2).

To give a score, the team member begins at the head of the pet and works toward the tail. Fat cover is evaluated over the ribs, down the topline, around the tail base, and ventrally along the abdomen. The BCS scoring ranges from 1 to 5 with 1 being very thin and 5 being obese. A score of 3 is considered ideal. Body composition studies in cats and dogs have shown an optimal body condition of 15–25% body fat. Therefore, a BCS rating of "ideal" will estimate the pet to have 15–25% body fat.

A BCS rating of overweight will estimate the pet to have 26–35% body fat, and a BCS rating of obese will estimate the pet to have greater than 40% body fat.

Risk factors

Pets become overweight or obese when they are in positive energy balance for an extended period of time. In other words, they are taking in too many calories and not expending enough calories. Genetics, spaying and neutering, age, physical activity, and caloric composition of food are risk factors for positive energy balance, weight gain, and obesity. All health-care team members must help clients understand these risk factors to help treat or prevent obesity.

Assessing the food

Body weight and body composition in pets are determined by the nutrient composition of the food and the amount of food

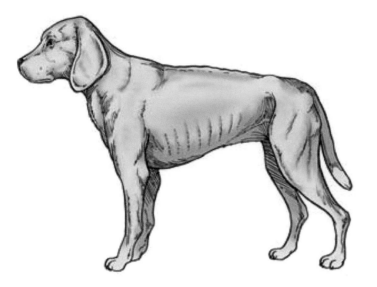

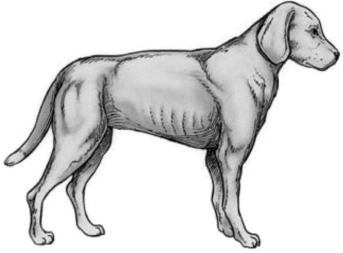

BCS 1. Very thin
The ribs are easily palpable with no fat cover. The tailbase has a prominent raised bony structure with no tissue between the skin and bone. The bony prominences are easily felt with no overlying fat. Dogs over six months of age have a severe abdominal tuck when viewed from the side and an accentuated hourglass shape when viewed from above.

BCS 2. Underweight
The ribs are easily palpable with minimal fat cover. The tailbase has a raised bony structure with little tissue between the skin and bone. The bony prominences are easily felt with minimal overlying fat. Dogs over six months of age have an abdominal tuck when viewed from the side and a marked hourglass shape when viewed from above.

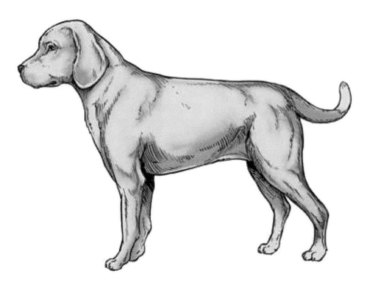

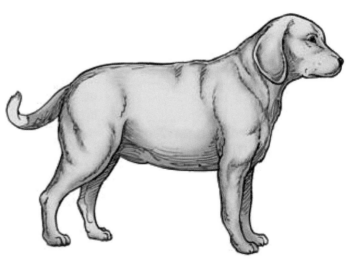

BCS 3. Ideal
The ribs are palpable with a slight fat cover. The tailbase has a smooth contour or some thickening. The bony structures are palpable under a thin layer of fat between the skin and bone. The bony prominences are easily felt under minimal amounts of overlying fat. Dogs over six months of age have a slight abdominal tuck when viewed from the side and a wellproportioned lumbar waist when viewed from above.

BCS 4. Overweight
The ribs are difficult to feel with moderate fat cover. The tailbase has some thickening with moderate amounts of tissue between the skin and bone. The bony structures can still be palpated. The bony prominences are covered by a moderate layer of fat. Dogs over six months of age have little or no abdominal tuck or waist when viewed from the side. The back is slightly broadened when viewed from above.

Figure 6.1   BCS descriptors for dogs in a five-point system. Source: Reprinted with permission from Hand, M.S., Thatcher, C.D., Remillard, R.L., Roudebush, P., Noventy, B. (eds). 2010. *Small Animal Clinical Nutrition*, 5th edition. Mark Morris Institute, Topeka, KS Public Domain.

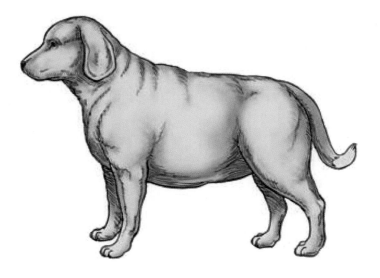

BCS 5. Obese
The ribs are very difficult to feel under a thick fat cover. The tailbase appears thickened and is difficult to feel under a prominent layer of fat. The bony prominences are covered by a moderate to thick layer of fat. Dogs over six months of age have a pendulous ventral bulge and no waist when viewed from the side due to extensive fat deposits. The back is markedly broadened when viewed from above. A trough may form when epaxial areas bulge dorsally.

Figure 6.1 (Continued)

Box 6.2 Body condition scoring anatomical descriptors.

BCS 1 – Very Thin
- Ribs prominent
- Tail base prominent
- Severe abdominal tuck
- Accentuated hourglass

BCS 2 – Underweight
- Ribs easily palpable
- No palpable fat
- Obvious waist
- Tops of lumbar vertebrae visible

BCS 3 – Ideal
- Ribs easily felt
- Tail base smooth
- Abdominal tuck
- Lumbar waist

BCS 4 – Overweight
- Ribs not easily palpable with moderate fat cover
- Noticeable fat deposits over lumbar spine and tail base

BCS 5 – Obese
- Fat over ribs
- Tail base layer of fat
- No abdominal tuck
- No waist

eaten in a day. A complete history, including the types and amounts of food eaten, must be taken before a treatment plan for weight loss can be developed. The nutrients making up the patient's diet should also be considered. The proportion and quantity of protein, fat, and soluble carbohydrate in the food will help determine its caloric density. Furthermore, the balance of these nutrients can help with the acceptability of the food which is imperative for reducing or maintaining the pet's body weight and body condition.

The pet owner should be educated on how to keep a food record or diary. This is very important when beginning a weight loss program for the pet. The food record should include the following.

- Amounts of food fed
- Types/forms of food fed
- Caloric content of food
- Who feeds the pet
- How the pet is fed – free choice versus meal fed
- What treats the pet receives and from whom
- Caloric content of consumable treats
- When the pet is fed
- Other animals in the home and patient's access to this food
- Access to other foods
- Type, amount, frequency of exercise
- Indoor versus outdoor pet

Clients should be instructed to keep all pets that are on a weight loss program away from the kitchen and dining areas during family meals. This will help reduce begging by the pet and reduce the urge from the owner to give in to the begging.

Exercise is extremely important and is one way to increase energy expenditure and widen the difference between energy consumed and energy expended. Exercise may also benefit obese patients by reducing the loss of lean muscle. Not unlike humans, exercise should begin gradually and increase slowly as tolerance improves. Owners are encouraged to take their pets for a walk and exercise with them. For overweight cats, there are a number of interactive toys such as laser pointers, feather toys, noisy balls, and so forth that will increase the activity level of the cat and increase the time the owner spends with the cat, thus strengthening the human–animal bond (https://indoorpet.osu.edu/).

Pet owners and health-care team members today have access to a lot of information regarding pet nutrition via the internet, news sources, blogs, etc. However, with this wealth of information comes sometimes confusing and incorrect nutritional information. As veterinary team members, we need to educate ourselves on proper companion animal nutrition and sort through the minutiae to educate well-intentioned owners on what constitutes proper nutrition for their beloved pet. There is a lot of misinformation regarding pet food; however, for the purpose of this discussion, we will focus on pet food regulation and interpretation of pet food labels.

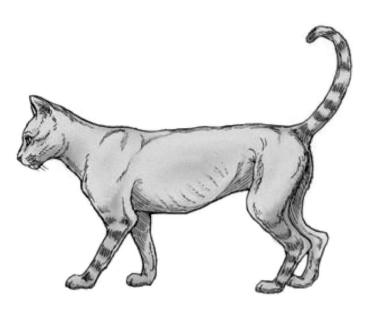

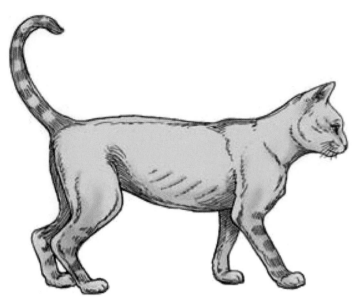

BCS 1. Very thin
The ribs are easily palpable with no fat cover. The bony prominences are easily felt with no overlying fat. Cats over six months of age have a severe abdominal tuck when viewed from the side and an accentuated hourglass shape when viewed from above.

BCS 2. Underweight
The ribs are easily palpable with minimal fat cover. The bony prominences are easily felt with minimal overlying fat. Cats over six months of age have an abdominal tuck when viewed from the side and a marked hourglass shape when viewed from above.

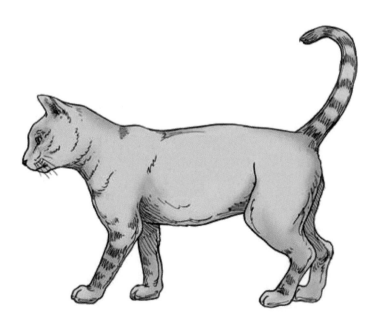

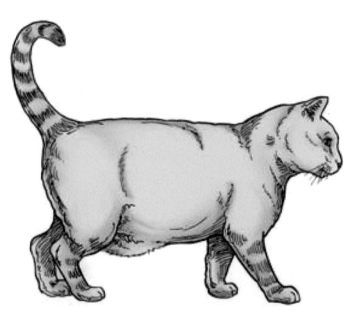

BCS 3. Ideal
The ribs are palpable with a slight fat cover. The bony prominences are easily felt under a slight amount of overlying fat. Cats over six months of age have an abdominal tuck when viewed from the side and a well-proportioned lumbar waist when viewed from above.

BCS 4. Overweight
The ribs are difficult to feel with moderate fat cover. The bony structures can still be palpated. The bony prominences are covered by a moderate layer of fat. Cats over six months of age have little or no abdominal tuck or waist when viewed from the side. The back is slightly broadened when viewed from above. A moderate abdominal fat pad is present.

Figure 6.2 BCS descriptors for cats in a five-point system. Source: Reprinted with permission from Hand, M.S., Thatcher, C.D., Remillard, R.L., Roudebush, P, Noventy, B. (eds). 2010. *Small Animal Clinical Nutrition*, 5th edition. Mark Morris Institute, Topeka, KS Public Domain.

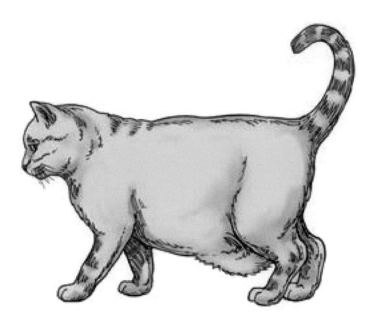

BCS 5. Obese
The ribs are very difficult to feel under a thick fat cover. The bony prominences are covered by a moderate to thick layer of fat. Cats over six months of age have a pendulous ventral bulge and no waist when viewed from the side due to extensive fat deposits. The back is markedly broadened when viewed from above. A marked abdominal fat pad is present. Fat deposits may be found on the limbs and face.

Figure 6.2   (Continued)

Pet food labels

The pet food label is the primary means by which product information is communicated from the manufacturer or distributor to pet owners, veterinarians, health-care team members, and regulatory officials. Reading and interpreting pet food labels is one method via which health-care team members and pet owners can obtain information about pet foods; however, labels do not necessarily provide information about food quality (e.g., digestibility and biological value). Owners and veterinary professionals should contact pet food manufacturers or nutrition experts for additional information that can be used to evaluate the quality of various pet foods.

Pet food labels not only communicate information about the product, they also serve as a legal document. A small number of agencies and organizations regulate production, marketing, and sales of pet foods in different countries. Each agency has different responsibilities with varying degrees of authority. Some of these agencies regulate information found on pet food labels whereas others influence the regulatory process. Pet foods are regulated at their point of sale (e.g., foods manufactured in the United States but sold outside the US must meet labeling requirements of the country in which the food is sold). Pet foods sold in the US must conform to Food and Drug Administration (FDA), Association of American Feed Control Officials (AAFCO), and state pet food labeling requirements.

Pet food labels include two main parts: the principal display panel and the information panel. Certain pieces of information are required on each part of the label, whereas others are optional.

Principal display panel

The principal display panel is defined by the FDA as "the part of a label that is most likely to be displayed, presented, shown or examined under customary conditions of display for retail sale." It is the primary means of attracting the customer's attention and should immediately communicate the product identity. The product identity must include a designator such as "dog food," "cat food," "for puppies," or "for dogs and puppies." The brand name is the name by which pet food products of a given company are identified. The product name is not essential and may be the same as the brand name; it is usually descriptive of the food and is subject to regulations dealing with composition of ingredients. The product vignette is a visual representation of the product and it must accurately depict the contents of the package (e.g., food pictured on the label cannot appear better than the actual product).

The amount of ingredients that must be present in order to use a certain product name are determined by percentage rules. For example, the term "chicken" requires that at least 70% of the product contain chicken; "chicken dinner/entrée," etc. must contain 10% chicken if moist and 25% chicken if dry; "with chicken" means that the product contains at least 3% chicken; "chicken flavor" means that chicken is recognizable by the pet (<3% chicken). A nutrition statement may be provided on the display panel; it is usually brief and may include such terms as "complete and nutritious," "100% nutritious," or "100% complete nutrition." The use of these terms implies that the product contains ingredients in quantities sufficient to provide the estimated nutrient requirements of a dog or cat or the product contains a combination of ingredients that when fed to a normal animal as the only source of nourishment will provide satisfactory results.

Information panel

The information panel is adjacent to the principal display panel and includes product information. The ingredient statement must be shown on the label and includes a list of ingredients (which must conform to AAFCO names), in descending order by weight. Ingredients are listed on an "as is" basis, which makes interpretation of ingredient lists difficult since many key ingredients are added with different moisture contents. Because meats contain more moisture, they may be listed first on the ingredient list, although the primary component of the food is a mixture of grains. This is often misleading to pet owners. In addition, the ingredient statement does not provide information about the quality of ingredients.

One limitation of the ingredient statement is that terms such as "meat by-products" are difficult to evaluate. Many owners are under the impression that "by-products" are not healthy and may even be harmful to their pets. However, the nutritive value of various meat by-products varies widely. It is often misinterpreted that foods containing meat by-products are inferior to foods containing whole meat. AAFCO defines meat on an ingredient label as any combination of skeletal, striated muscle or muscle found in the tongue, diaphragm, heart, and esophagus with or without the overlying fat and the portions of the skin, sinew, nerves, and blood vessels which normally accompany muscle. Meat must be suitable for use in animal foods and therefore excludes feathers, head, feet, and entrails. Meat by-products do not include hair, horns, teeth, or hooves. Nutritive values in meat by-products also vary greatly. For example, meat by-products such as liver, kidney, and lungs have excellent nutritive value, whereas udder, bone, and connective tissue have poor nutrient availability.

By-products are simply secondary products produced in addition to the principal product. Many human foods contain by-products, and most pet foods contain by-products. For example, by-products of human milk production would be ice cream, cheese, and butter. Many by-products are excellent sources of nutrients for pets as well as people.

The guaranteed analysis includes crude protein (minimum), crude fat (minimum), crude fiber (maximum), and moisture (maximum). Additional guarantees are optional and may be included by the manufacturer. The guaranteed analysis is a general idea of the nutrient content of a food but is of little value in comparing foods because specific nutrient contents are not given and values are listed on an "as is" basis. While crude protein is an accurate index of protein quantity, it does not indicate protein quality. Crude fat may be used to estimate the energy density of the food. Crude fiber is an estimate of the indigestible portion of the food; it usually underestimates the true level of fiber in the product. Foods that contain higher levels of fiber are generally lower in calories. The moisture content represents the water content in the food; it cannot exceed a maximum of 78% in the United States. Foods that are >78% moisture must use a different name such as "in gravy," "in sauce," or "in aspic." The dry matter contains all nutrients (except water) and subtle changes in moisture content may result in marked differences in dry matter, which subsequently affects amounts of nutrients in a food.

The nutritional adequacy statement on the information panel is often more detailed than the brief statements found on the principal display. Examples include "Complete and balanced nutrition for growth of kittens" and "meets . . . requirements for the entire life cycle of all dogs." The nutrition statement will help you determine if the manufacturer is making claims for a specific-purpose diet versus an all-purpose diet. Pet foods with no statement of adequacy include snacks, treats, and some therapeutic foods. Therapeutic foods have a statement that they are to be used by or under the direction of a veterinarian. No further nutrition statement is required since the complete nutritional profile is usually available to the veterinarian.

The basis of the nutrition claim is documented on the pet food label by one of two methods: the formulation method or the feeding trial method. The formulation method is simply a laboratory nutrient profile analysis and does not require any feeding or digestibility trials to prove availability of the nutrients in the profile analysis. This method is recognized on a label by a statement such as "Meets or exceeds the minimal nutritional levels established by AAFCO" or "Formulated to meet the AAFCO dog nutrient profile for. . ." AAFCO nutrient profiles are published for two categories: growth and reproduction, and adult maintenance. The feeding trial method is the preferred method for substantiating a claim. Feeding trials can result in adequacy claims for four categories: gestation and lactation, growth, maintenance, and complete for all life stages. A food that has successfully completed a sequential growth and gestation/lactation trial can make a claim for all life stages. The required wording for labels that have passed these tests is: "Animal feeding tests using AAFCO procedures substantiate that (brand) provides complete and balanced nutrition for (lifestage)." Pet foods that do not meet AAFCO requirements by either of the standard methods will have a nutritional statement as follows: "this product is intended for intermittent or supplemental feeding only."

Dog and cat foods labeled as complete and nutritious for any or all life stages must list feeding directions on the product label. At a minimum, feeding directions should include the instructions "feed (weight/unit) per (weight) of dog or cat" and frequency of feeding. These feeding directions are general guidelines and should serve as a starting point; adjustments may be needed to maintain optimal body condition.

Summary

Nutrients are important to the well-being of cats and dogs. Veterinary assistants must remember that nutrition plays a role in all pets, healthy or ill. This overview lays the foundation for the role of nutrition in pets and shows that proper nutrition and feeding management are the foundation upon which healing and the maintenance of health rest. The role of nutrition should be incorporated into each pet's life by all members of the health-care team.

References

Ackerman, A. 2008. *Companion Animal Nutrition: A Guide for Veterinary Nurses and Technicians*. Elsevier, Edinburgh.

Burns, K.M. 2013. Why is Rocky so stocky? obesity is a disease. *NAVTA Journal*, Convention Issue, 16–19.

Hand, M., Thatcher, C., Remillard, R., Roudebush, P., Novotny, B. (eds). 2010. *Small Animal Clinical Nutrition*, 5th edition. Mark Morris Institute, Topeka, KS.

Wortinger, A., Burns, K.M. 2015. *Nutrition and Disease Management for Veterinary Technicians and Nurses*, 2nd edition. Wiley-Blackwell, Ames, IA.

www.wiley.com/go/burns/textbookvetassistant2

Please go to the companion website for assignments and a PowerPoint relating to the material in this chapter.

Chapter **7** Breeds

Cat breeds

Cats are one of the most popular household pets in the United States, according to the American Veterinary Medical Association. In fact, there are nearly 10 million more cats living in US homes than there are dogs.

Many families are completely suitable for a cat. It is important to recognize and take into consideration the effects that a cat may have on the family. Overall, cats are affectionate and loving pets that tend to be independent and appear aloof. That does not mean that they will not require time, care, and attention. The responsibility and commitment of owning a cat can be long term as many cats live into their teens.

The job of veterinary professionals working within clinical settings may require a fair amount of client communication and the ability to educate potential cat owners about the numerous choices of cat breeds available.

During this discussion, the veterinary assistant is responsible for conveying important information to the future cat owners, encouraging them to research breeds of interest. It is important to find the perfect match for a client's lifestyle, household, and preference. Although cats are generally uniform in size and shape, each cat is uniquely different when it comes to personality, needs, characteristics, and temperament. Failure to properly educate clientele or providing misleading or false information regarding the responsibilities of cat ownership will often result in a less favorable outcome for both the cat and the family.

Coat color variations

Many people accidentally confuse cat breeds with coat colors. Each breed of cat has specific coat colors that are consistent within the breed. On the other hand, domestic shorthair cats of unknown breeds can have an array of different coat colors.

The term "tabby" is used to describe a coat pattern with different expression.

- Tabby color variations all have common variable striping over a base color of silver, red, or brown. The various patterns are as follows: classic or symmetrical curved markings – color pattern that occurs in many breeds; mackerel – an elongated striped fishbone pattern; ticked – overlay color at the tips of the fur resulting from ticking that is produced by the presence of an agouti wild-type gene; torbie – patched tabby.

- Tortoiseshell coloring is black, orange, and brown hairs admixed in a variable pattern. A range of dual colors is also possible. Most tortoiseshells, like most calico cats, are female. Tortoiseshell and calico males are rare and occur if the sex **chromosome** numbers are abnormal.

- Bicolor coat patterns are composed of a coat with a white background with solid patches interspersed.

- Parti-color is a pattern where more than one color is superimposed on a white background.

- Chocolate coat color results from a mutation of the tyrosine-related protein 1 and is expressed as a brown pigment that is the precursor of black.

- A dilute coat color is a pale version of a full-intensity coat; for instance, blue is dilute to black; cream is dilute to red.

- Harlequin patterning indicates a marking on the head and tail and three small patches of color on the body on a white coat.

- Marbled describes a coat pattern where spots have a dark outer edge and the inner part of the spots is lighter colored.

- Rex coats consist of wavy, curly, or crinkled hairs and are coded by genes found in the Cornish Rex and Devon Rex.

Textbook for the Veterinary Assistant, Second Edition. Kara M. Burns and Lori Renda-Francis.
© 2022 John Wiley & Sons, Inc. Published 2022 by John Wiley & Sons, Inc.
Companion website: www.wiley.com/go/burns/textbookvetassistant2

- Shaded patterns indicate color on the hair shaft with pigment distribution between chinchilla (light) and smoke (darker).
- Van patterning is a white coat color with a colored tail and colored markings on the head.

Cat Fanciers' Association

The Cat Fanciers' Association (CFA) is a great reference tool to share with future cat owners that will allow them to explore the world of cat breeds prior to their purchase. The CFA is the world's largest registry of pedigreed breeds. The registry currently recognizes 42 pedigreed cat breeds to be shown in the championship class and two breeds classified as miscellaneous that can be shown in the miscellaneous class. The CFA is a nonprofit organization that was established in 1906. It has registered over 1 million pedigreed cats and has over 600 member clubs.

New pedigree cats can be a result of spontaneous mutations, which occur when two domestic cats reproduce and create an offspring that looks different from both of the parents, or as a result of planned hybridization, when two preexisting cat breeds are bred to achieve a desired outcome.

Currently, the CFA has categorized purebred cats into natural, hybrid, established, and mutant breed groups. Pedigreed cats rely greatly on the interest of a particular person or group of people (club members) who are devoted to preserving or bettering a desired breed for many years to come. These people are also known as breeders or cat fanciers.

The CFA registry allows breeders to reference an ongoing history of different cats. In order for a breed to be considered purebred or pedigree, extensive breed criteria and standards established by the CFA must be met. The CFA uses preestablished registration rules that judge each individual breed precisely on its health, anatomical appearance, and physical beauty. The CFA's rules of registration may be used as a guide for future breeders interested in creating or registering a new breed.

The CFA's 42 cat breeds are listed below.

Abyssinian

The Abyssinian breed of cat is one of the oldest recognized breeds in history. Although the appearance of Abyssinians closely resembles ancient Egyptian artifacts, this sleek muscular cat's history is still up for debate. As stated by Carolyn Osier in *Kitten Buyers' Guide: A Handbook for the Potential Abby Owner*, "The Abyssinian breed is proclaimed to be one of the most intelligent animals ever created." The breed is also described as very people oriented. Abyssinians are described as "not a lap cat," which may make them more suitable pets for adult families that appreciate the company of an Abby without a lot of hands-on interaction.

American Bobtail

The American Bobtail is a very distinct, wild-looking breed of cat that has characteristics and features that resemble those of a wild animal. As portrayed in its name, this breed has a naturally short, "bobbed" tail that adds to its already wild appearance. The American Bobtail is a solid, athletic cat but is also a surprisingly calm, gentle creature that expresses love and affection and appreciates the same in return from human companions. Due to the American Bobtail's disposition, the CFA describes Bobtails as an "excellent household pet for a family of all ages." Bobtails, unlike most cat breeds, do not mind being picked up and carried around. They are very welcoming to new family additions whether they are two- or four-legged, making them a great fit for multiple household types.

American Curl

The American Curl is a truly magnificent-looking breed with a one-of-a-kind appearance and remarkable characteristics. American Curls have an incredible fluffy tail and bizarre ears that literally curl back, making this breed truly unique. But don't let the sophisticated "designer" appearance fool you! American Curls are actually perceived as very people oriented, faithful and affectionate soulmates that adjust quickly to other pets, children, and new situations, according to the CFA.

American Shorthair

The American Shorthair, which closely resembles domestic shorthaired cats, was established as a breed of its own in the late 1960s. This "all-American" breed is a well-rounded cat that is known for its long life span, strong health, impressive looks, and great compatibility with dogs and children. American Shorthairs have gained huge recognition at a national level, as they have been declared "Kitten of the Year" and, of course, "Best in Show," which surely make this fuzzy companion animal great for most any household setting.

American Wirehair

The American Wirehair breed is the result of two American domestic cats mating. The American Wirehair, as its name implies, has a rare short and wiry coat, differentiating it from all other breeds. Wirehairs are "easy going, disease resistant and good producers," according to the CFA.

Balinese – Javanese

The Balinese breed is a spitting image of its ancestor breed, the Siamese. The only difference between these two cats is the luxurious ermine-like coat and gorgeous fluffy tail plume of the Balinese. Like the Siamese, the Balinese are very long, slender cats. Balinese have similar personalities to the Siamese. Their affectionate, curious, and intelligent personality has earned them a reputation of inspiring breed enthusiasts to spout "glowing monologue[s]," as reported by the CFA.

The Javanese is a spectacular breed of cat characterized by a gorgeous silky coat, much like the coat of the Balinese, that comes in a wide array of colors as seen in the Colorpoint Shorthair breeds. The Javanese also carry the most desirable personality traits of the Siamese breed. The Javanese have been around for as long as the Balinese and received their name from the island located next to Bali. However, there is one significant difference between these two breeds, and that is the Javanese's multiple coat colors accepted by the CFA. By appearance, the Javanese may look like a delicate cat, but once you lay your hands on one, you will appreciate its impressive muscular physique. Javanese cats are people oriented and love to follow their owners around and cause mischief by using their paws to explore closed cabinets and drawers. They are real talkers and are never shy or hesitant to inform you when it is time to eat or play with their soft, adorable voices. As if that weren't enough, they are also very playful as they enjoy games that involve throw and retrieval. In addition to their spectacular breed appearance and personality, the Javanese require minimal upkeep.

Birman

The Birman cat breed originally came from Burma, where it was once considered a sacred companion animal. Aside from the Birman's remarkable legacy as the "cat of the Kittah Priest," Birmans have a bold royal appearance characterized by blue, almost round eyes, a full chin, and, of course, a "Roman nose." In the personality department, Birmans surely make their way to the top of the list as they are gentle, playful, and active – traits that make them a great option as a companion animal.

Bombay

The Bombay breed was created by careful selective inbreeding and outcrossing of different cat breeds to ultimately produce a distinct shorthaired black cat with captivating copper eyes. The primary goal behind the creation of the Bombay was to form a cat that closely resembles a "mini panther." The developmental process of the Bombay started in the 1950s and resulted in huge success thanks to the efforts of renowned cat breeder Nikki Horner. The Bombay achieved champion status in 1976. Bombays share many similarities with their cousin breed, the Burmese. These two breeds are sturdy and well structured with compact bodies.

Bombays also share many character traits with the Burmese. Bombays are described as lap-loving social and inquisitive cats. They are also known to be compatible with other four-legged family members as they have an easygoing personality.

British Shorthair

The British Shorthair may be one of the oldest English cat breeds with ancestry that relates all the way back to when the British Shorthair were known as the domesticated cats of Rome. British Shorthairs are known as calm and loyal cats with recognized endurance. Although "Brits" are rarely found in the United States, they are often imported in an attempt to expand the gene pool for American breeders.

Burmese

The Burmese, like many other cat breeds, stemmed from the creative process of selective cat breeding. The story behind the Burmese revolves around a San Francisco man by the name of Dr Joseph Thompson who acquired and bred a unique walnut-brown female cat from Burma with a Siamese in the early 1930s. The process resulted in the establishment of the Burmese cat breed.

Although the Burmese comes in many color varieties, the CFA recognizes sable, champagne, blue, and platinum when it comes to breed standards. This surprisingly hefty breed has adorable characteristics, from its persuasive eyes encompassed by a cutely rounded head down to its rounded yet well-muscled silky smooth-coated body.

Aside from appearance, the Burmese also come equipped with smashing personalities. Burmese are an extremely people-oriented breed. In fact, many Burmese will try to communicate with their owners upon encouragement. As the personality of Burmese cats almost mimics that of dogs, they may not appreciate a new canine friend in the family unless introduced to the Burmese during the early life stage. Unbelievably, most Burmese enjoy car rides, which makes them a perfect pet for frequent travelers.

Cats of this affectionate breed should not be allowed outdoors as they have poor survival instincts, if any at all, predisposing them to the great dangers of the outside environment. The females tend to be more opinionated when compared with the males. Male Burmese cats are perfectly content cuddling on their owners' laps whereas the females enjoy trying to take control over the household. The versatile personality of the Burmese makes them a great companion for feline-orientated households.

Burmilla (Miscellaneous Breed)

The Burmilla is one of the many cat breeds created by the efforts of humans. According to the CFA, this breed is said to have originated in the United Kingdom nearly 25 years ago as the result of a chance mating between a beautiful male Persian and a female Burmese.

Burmillas are nothing short of spectacular when it comes to personality. This breed is known to display the desirable qualities of a Persian cat by being quiet, affectionate, and calm-mannered. However, the Burmese side of the Burmilla is also displayed in its tendency to seek attention and get into mischief.

According to the CFA, the female Burmilla can weigh up to 7.5 lb with the male weighing up to 11 lb. These cats have a captivating quality in their eyes alone. Their eyes can range in color from gold-yellow to a beautiful green as they age. Their facial structure is short and is accompanied by small ears. Furthermore, the Burmilla's soft, silky long or short coat accentuates its muscled, cute body. This accident of a breed would surely dazzle in most any family setting with its striking appearance and playful and affectionate behavior.

Chartreux

The Chartreux may be one of the oldest cat breeds recently recognized by the CFA. As legend has it, the Chartreux once lived among and were named for the Carthusian monks of France many moons ago. However, recent research provides reason to believe that the name "Chartreux" was derived from the name of a popular wooly Spanish rug from the 18th century which closely resembles the wooly fur coat of the Chartreux. The Chartreux is known for its one-of-a-kind smiling facial appearance. In addition to this, it is the only cat breed that boasts a medium-length blue wooly fur coat. Chartreux are known to exhibit dog-like behaviors and can be taught how to play fetch. Because the Chartreux are very people oriented, it won't take long before they become quickly attached to their owners.

Unlike most cat breeds, the Chartreux usually enjoy being handled and chirp rather than meow. They also may take as long as 3 years to reach physical maturity which is a considerably longer time compared to most other cats. The behavior of an adult Chartreux is completely reliant on the degree of attention it receives. It also requires suitable environmental conditions during maturation. Although tempting, the double wooly coat of a Chartreux should never be brushed, but rather worked through with fingers on a daily basis. This process will not only keep it looking good but also helps with socialization. Unfortunately, in the interest of breed preservation, Chartreux are being returned to French breeders, which has minimized their availability in the Unites States.

Chinese Li Hua (Miscellaneous Breed)

The Chinese Li Hua breed is relatively new to the CFA as it was accepted in 2010. Although the Chinese Li Hua were just recently welcomed into the CFA, they are known to be one of the oldest domesticated cats in their native country, China.

Chinese Li Hua cats come in one color only, a beautiful brown mackerel that goes perfectly with their green, yellow, or brown almond-shaped eyes. These interesting cats may take up to 3 years to fully mature, much like the Chartreux. The females are typically smaller than the males which can weigh over 11 lb. In addition to appearance, the Chinese Li Hua also have a striking personality. They are described as gentle, quiet cats that get along with other household pets. Altogether, there is no doubt the Chinese Li Hua would make a great pet for many different family types.

Colorpoint Shorthair

Colorpoint Shorthairs are truly a bundle of astonishing personality, features, and breed characteristics. Colorpoints are affectionate and display loyalty and devotion to their owners. They possess many interesting qualities, for instance, their ability to adapt to the owner's mood and provide comfort when needed. In addition to their known intelligence, Colorpoints quickly pick up fetch-like games with mice and are very in tune to what their owners are doing around the house. They may even insist on talking in their cute raspy voices very frequently as they usually have a lot to say.

Like many other breeds, Colorpoints fall into the category of man-made breeds. As a result of breeding, mixing, and matching a sealpoint Siamese with a red tabby American Shorthair, the Colorpoint Shorthair was created. Currently, the CFA recognizes 16 colors for the Colorpoint Shorthair breed. In close resemblance to their cousin, the Siamese, Colorpoints have long solid bodies, big ears, and, of course, gorgeous blue eyes. Colorpoints also require a small amount of grooming along with a commonly recommended diet that is high in protein to keep up their muscular body physique.

Cornish Rex

The Cornish Rex cat breed originated in Cornwall, England, arising from a litter of barn cats back in the 1950s. Although they may look like odd creatures with their huge ears, "egg-shaped heads," and high cheekbones, they have a lot to offer when it comes to personality. Cornish Rex cats are very affectionate and people oriented. Just from the look of their amazing body with long and skinny yet strong legs and muscular torso, you can tell the Cornish Rex is meant to be an extremely agile cat with quick jumps, turns, and stops. As stated by the CFA, the Cornish Rex "is a perfect pet for the owner who wants an active cat to participate in the family."

Devon Rex

The Devon Rex was discovered by an English woman who found a rather strange-looking kitten birthed from a cat she was taking care of. It was thought that the father of the litter was a tomcat with distinct curly hair. This resulted in a kitten that had a truly rare curly hair coat. The Devon Rex has multiple characteristics, which include big ears, a "pixie-like face," bright, large eyes, and the one-of-a-kind wavy or curly fur coat. Let's just say it's easy to spot them in a crowd.

The personality of the Devon Rex is just as unique as the breed's physical characteristics. Devon Rex cats are intelligent, very friendly and playful, and get involved with everything and anything as they like to explore.

Another interesting fact about Devon Rexes is that they are known as "heat seekers." They are warm to the touch because their coat provides poor insulation. For this reason, warm surfaces such as televisions and heater vents are favorite hang-out spots of the Devon Rex. Devons truly are a versatile, amusing, and low-maintenance cat breed, which makes them a great consideration for families looking for a fun, loving cat.

Egyptian Mau

The Egyptian Mau is an over-the-top cat breed when it comes to both appearance and personality. The Egyptian Mau nearly perfectly resembles artwork created by ancient Egyptians which indicates that it is a domesticated subspecies of the African wildcat. The Egyptian Mau is truly special in that it is the only naturally spotted domesticated feline. The characteristics of the Egyptian Mau – wild spontaneous spots, strides of a cheetah, and dazzling green eyes – can easily grab the attention of the whole room. The Egyptian Mau is a great pet for an extremely cat-oriented family willing to devote a great amount of time, affection, and attention to this spectacular breed. Maus are characterized as "fiercely" loyal and devoted to not only their feline family but their human family as well.

European Burmese

The European Burmese and the Burmese cat breed found in North America originated from the same place but the offspring of the European Burmese is characterized by solid and color points. Although the Burmese and European Burmese were created from the same source, they differ in appearance. According to the CFA, the European Burmese is an "elegant cat with gently rounded contours" whereas the Burmese has a "well-rounded, compact body appearance" with subtle differences in their eyes. Although they may look different, the European Burmese and Burmese share similar personality traits. The European Burmese enjoys living with other pets, but they manage in a single-pet household as well. They are known to be just as affectionate and loyal as the Burmese, making them overall a great family pet.

Exotic

The Exotic cat breed is pretty much the spitting image of the well-known and loved Persian breed. This is exactly what breeders intended to achieve by mixing the two breeds but with one major difference, which revolved around changing their coat type. There is no doubt that Persians are adorable and have held the title of one of the most popular cat breeds for many years now, but they have one major drawback which is their requirement for daily grooming. Maintaining the coat of a Persian requires time and commitment that most families struggle to provide. Exotics have a short, thick, fluffy coat that significantly lessens their grooming requirements. Although the Exotic and Persian are classified as two different breeds, they are identical when it comes to personality. Exotics are sweet cats that very rarely voice their opinion. Other admirable characteristics of the Exotic include their playfulness, love for people, affectionate behavior, and last but not least, their overall peaceful presence.

Despite popular belief, male Exotics are actually more affectionate than the females. Females are known to be more aloof and noticeably less affectionate than the males. Because Exotic cats mature more slowly than most other purebreds, spaying and neutering is typically done at a young age, making these cats less likely to display behavioral issues arising from adult instincts. Needless to say, Exotics have earned an outstanding reputation for being the "perfect pet," and they would make a great addition to most any household and family type.

Havana Brown

The Havana Brown is known as a hybrid or man-made breed. History suggests that these brown Siamese look-alikes were documented in Europe and England back in the late 1800s. On the other hand, the self-chocolate Havana Browns were created by a careful selective breeding process. These dreamy chocolate-coated breeds are known for their color coat. There is not much else to be said about their personality.

Japanese Bobtail

The Japanese Bobtail is a naturally occurring breed that is very special to Japanese culture. In fact, the Japanese view these cats as a symbol of good luck. Documentation provides almost certain evidence that these cats found their way into Japan from Korea or China at least 1000 years ago.

Japanese Bobtails were imported into the United States in 1968 and accepted into the CFA in 1993. Their flawless coats come in long and short lengths and display almost any form, with Me-Ki being the most popular. Japanese Bobtails are strong, resilient cats with health attributes that reflect low mortality rates in their offspring. The tails are very different from other bobbed-tail breeds, such as the Manx. The Japanese Bobtail's tail is covered by a large, fluffy array of tail plume and is expected to contain kinks, angles, curls, or possibly a combination. Along with their unusual tail, Japanese Bobtails also have appealing personality traits. They are described as intelligent, active, and extremely vocal cats that can nearly hit every tone on the scale.

Japanese Bobtails are sure to dazzle in most any home as they enjoy human interaction and get along well with children and other pets.

The coats of a Japanese Bobtail tend to never mat or shed. It is easy to see why the Japanese Bobtails are an all-round awesome companion animal for any family.

Korat

The Korat is truly an over-the-top breed with exceptional hearing, scent, and sight capabilities. Korats are known for their extraordinary, glistening, large green eyes. Korat kittens' eyes start out blue, as is true of most kittens, then over time turn a vivid green color when they reach 2–4 years of age. Their hair is nicely bound to their skin, which dramatically reduces the amount of shedding, which makes them a very appealing breed for cat lovers who suffer from allergies. These native-to-Thailand silver cats are considered to be symbolic of good fortune to the

Thais. Korats tend to be easily spooked, so it is important to incorporate loud noises, handling, and other fearful experiences into their life when they are kittens in order to avoid complications in the future. Korats have a pleasing personality as they are very affectionate and devoted to their owners. They also get along well with other cats but are known to take charge. The Korat's gentle personality also makes this cat highly compatible with children. With a glowing background, they are sure to please most any kind of family.

La Perm

The La Perm cat breed started out in 1982 as a bizarre mutation on a farm in Oregon, where one of a litter of six domesticated barn kittens was born hairless, unlike its furry siblings, according to the CFA. This mutant kitten was born with uniquely bald "blue print" skin which surprisingly developed into a soft curly coat within the cat's first 8 weeks. The owner of the bald kitten initially thought nothing much of the baldness but came to realize the "mutant" kitten was actually a hidden gem in the world of cat breeds as bald kittens started appearing more frequently in litters and attracted a lot of attention. Furthermore, the owner investigated the breed and discovered that the baldness gene was found in both the male and female. It didn't take long before the owner took advantage of the situation and decided to selectively breed the cat. The outcome was a great success as these cats were accepted into the CFA and declared a breed of their own. La Perm means wavy or rippled and these cats are sure to dazzle in any coat variation from tight ringlets to corkscrew curls. From their generalized good personality and unmistakable cool coats, the La Perm really has it going on.

Maine Coon

The Maine Coon is a mysterious breed surrounded by numerous myths, legends, and fantasies. Maine Coon cats are larger in stature than most other breeds. They are intelligent, trainable, and often referred to as "dog-like." They offer hours of enjoyment with their antics but can at times be intrusive. Without question, they want to be part of everything, and maintaining your privacy may require a closed door between you and your cat. Most Maine Coon cats have a fondness for water – to be in it, watch it, wash their food in it, or just plain play in it – so don't be surprised if you have an uninvited guest in your shower or help washing the dishes one day.

The Maine Coon has a silky and somewhat oily coat but it is not dense and its upkeep is much easier than that of other long-haired breeds. The coat will require occasional grooming. Because they love attention of any kind, grooming is easily accomplished.

Manx

The Manx is yet another gorgeous long- or shorthaired tabby that is said to have come from the Isle of Man well over 100 years ago.

Records suggest that the Manx was recognized by the CFA back in the 1920s. The Manx is known for its unusual tail variations. Since the tailless gene in the Manx is dominant, the offspring could be born with short tails, a rise, no tail, or the litter may be mixed with all of the above.

Although all the tail types are extremely cute, only the "rumpy" (no tail) and rumpy rise (raised tail) meet the CFA breed standards. Aside from the Manx's tail features, the breed is known for its adorable rounded face and body appearance.

Manx cats greatly enjoy playing, whether it involves a game of fetch or burying their toys like a dog. Manx cats' powerful rear legs allow them to be extreme jumpers with quickly executed agile movements, making them very amusing to watch.

They are divided into two different personality types – the one-person cat or the whole-family cat. Once a Manx has attached itself to a family or owner, it is less likely to find happiness with anyone else when placed in a new home. Overall, the Manx is a delightful cat breed that would sparkle in a loving family that can provide a permanent home.

Norwegian Forest Cat

The Norwegian Forest Cat is a magnificent cat breed for multiple reasons. Norwegians have vivid "emerald" green eyes accentuated by a band of gold with a heavenly silky soft fur coat. Interestingly, Norwegian Forest Cats also change their appearance in the winter and summer seasons by adjusting the thickness of their fur coat in relation to the climate. Another astonishing feature of Norwegians is their unbelievably long tail, which can measure up to a whopping 12 inches when fully extended. Surprisingly, Norwegians require minimal grooming, if any at all. They were created by the marvelous wonders of Mother Nature, making them truly wild.

Owning a Norwegian Forest Cat may require a little more work than most other cat breeds. Since Norwegians actually came from the forest, instinctively they do not appreciate the company of people right off the bat. This does not mean they are feral but they are not considered to be the cat breed that is most interested in people. Owning a Norwegian Forest kitten will take some time and dedication in order to mold it into a favorable loving family pet further down the road. It is critical to properly expose Norwegian Forest kittens to different experiences around children, other pets, and human interaction in general. The Norwegian Forest Cat would fit perfectly in a family setting that is dedicated to and understanding of this special cat breed.

Ocicat

The Ocicat is an eye-catching breed with fierce spots that imitate the appearance of cats found in the wild. Judging by the Ocicat's looks, it's hard to believe these cats were created by the process of selectively breeding Abyssinians, American Shorthairs, and Siamese cats. Ocicats are typically large with a muscular body covered in a short, "satin sheen" coat that complements their musculature.

Although the Ocicat may have a fierce, wild appearance, its personality is empowered by "dog-like" behaviors. In fact, many Ocies can be taught how to play fetch, walk on a leash, and are even responsive to their name being called. Ocies are also known as a social and active cat breed and completely devoted to their family. However, they like to check out strangers as well. The Ocicat's great personality and appearance surely make it an awesome family pet for most households. These cats adapt well to change. However, because they have an intense social behavior and devotion to their family, single-pet households or families pressed for time may want to consider a different breed.

Oriental

The Oriental breed was created to explore the many possibilities of color variations. Orientals are not only neat looking but also have a splendid personality. They will surely amaze with their undying devotion and affectionate behavior. They love to observe and sometimes help their family with day-to-day activities. As a result of Orientals being intelligent and curious in general, it is almost expected to see some menace-like behaviors. Long after kittenhood, Orientals remain entertaining and playful as adults.

The appearance of the Oriental is just as interesting as its personality. These cats are slender, short- or longhaired, with skinny yet muscular "tubular" bodies that come in almost any color. Overall, Orientals are bound to please most any family with their fun-loving personalities.

Persian

It is easy to see why the Persian, with its adorable squished facial features, luxurious long coat, and loving personality, is one of the most popular breeds out there.

Persians are quiet cats which grab attention with their large eyes rather than by using their pleasant voices, like most other cats do. They have a small body with short, heavy-boned legs and of course a long, fluffy coat to top them off. Unlike most cats, Persians enjoy relaxing on furniture and peering out of the windows rather than rambunctious play involving jumping and climbing.

Unfortunately, Persians have a few potentially undesirable traits associated with the breed. Due to their long, flowing coat, it is wise to keep them strictly indoors. This coat will also require daily grooming in order to avoid inevitable matting and hairball complications. Routine bathing is a must and should be started when they are kittens to ensure that the cat is accustomed to the process by adulthood. Last but certainly not least, as a result of Persians having large captivating eyes, it is common to see tears run down their face. For this reason, periodic facial cleansing is highly recommended. Persians are a very sweet, inactive, and loving cat breed that will steal the hearts of any family willing to take on the challenge of keeping them pristine, healthy, and looking good.

Ragamuffin

The Ragamuffin is one breed that will have you saying "Aw"! Ragamuffins have a massive body with a beautiful, long coat that comes in all types of patterns and colors. These amazing cats also have large, endearing eyes. Based on their appearance, one might never guess that the Ragamuffin actually requires minimal maintenance.

According to the CFA, these striking, large cats typically reach weights of 10–15 lb for females and 15–20 lb for males! In addition to their impressive body weight, these heavily boned cats fully mature at roughly 4 years of age. Although Ragamuffins are slow to mature, they are known to have a long life span with strong overall health.

Ragamuffins have pleasing and calm personalities. They love to be on their owner's lap whenever possible. There is no doubt that Ragamuffins would make a spectacular family pet with their loving and affectionate personalities and great ability to get along with other pets and children.

Ragdoll

The Ragdoll is a large, pointed breed with amazing blue eyes. The Ragdoll is a man-made breed that is a nicely balanced cat. Ragdolls are rather big, weighing in at 15–20 lb for males and 10–15 lb for females as stated by the CFA.

Like several other cat breeds, Ragdolls are slow to mature, with their coat reaching full color at 2 years of age and their full body size and weight at 4 years. In addition to their stunning appearance, Ragdolls have wonderful personalities. They are very people oriented and enjoy partaking in "dog-like" activities such as a game of fetch. Also like dogs, they are receptive to voice commands. Ragdolls might be one of the few cat companions considered to be perfect, with their laid-back and well-behaved personality.

Russian Blue

The Russian Blue is truly a color-defying breed said to have come from the isles of Archangel in northern Russia. Unlike many other breeds, the Russian Blue is a cat of natural beauty. As the legend goes, Russian Blues were once captured for their rare "double plush" coats which are said to closely resemble the coat of a beaver or seal. Once known as the "foreign blue" or "Archangel" cat, the breed is said to have made its way from Archangel to northern Europe and England in the late 1800s. Russian Blues have a dense bright blue coat garnished with silver tipping. And don't forget their gorgeous green eyes and clean-cut, fine-boned, and well-muscled body to go along with it.

Aside from their appearance, Russian Blues also have a glowing reputation when it comes to personality. They are gentle, affectionate, and smart creatures that may enjoy exploring closed cabinets in their free time or an occasional game of fetch, not to mention that they are also mood-sensitive and self-motivated entertainers; what more could you possibly ask for?

Their outstanding compatibility with children and other pets and their undemanding personalities make them a perfect match for pretty much any family type.

Scottish Fold

The Scottish Fold was first spotted on a farm by a shepherd in Scotland, according to the CFA. These unique cats are known for their attention-grabbing ears that fold down and forward, unlike the ears of any other breed. Despite their name, Scottish Folds can also have straight ears as the folded-ear gene is incomplete, making its presence unpredictable.

Scottish Fold kittens are born with straight ears, then at approximately 3 weeks of age, some of the kittens' ears will fold while the other kittens' ears remain straight. Judging by their appearance, it is easy to understand why Scottish Folds are described as "hardy cats," but they are sweet-natured cats with soft elegant voices that are rarely heard. They are comfortable in homes filled with children, dogs, and other animal friends.

Scottish Folds are a unique option for a spectacular and unmatchable looking family pet. However, these guys are in high demand due to their folded ears.

Selkirk Rex

The Selkirk Rex breed was derived from a dominant gene found in a shelter cat in Montana, according to the CFA. Soon after, the naturally curly cat was bred to a black Persian and thus the Selkirk Rex was established.

Selkirk cats come in long and short coat types and naturally look adorably scruffy and untamed, giving them a special look only a mother could love. They are a heavy-boned large breed with a profoundly fluffy tail.

Although their appearance may be a little rough, these cats definitely make up for it in the personality department. Selkirks are very tolerant and loving cats that enjoy giving and receiving affection. The Selkirk Rex would make a wonderful family pet, as long as their owners can handle their permanent crazy hairdo.

Siamese

The Siamese is an ancient cat breed that was exported from Thailand in the late 1800s, possibly making it one of the oldest breeds in the CFA. Siamese cats wow people with their striking appearance characterized by vivid, closely set blue eyes, "tubular" well-muscled body, long neck, and cutely wedge-shaped head.

Furthermore, Siamese cats are also astonishing creatures when it comes to personality. They are known for their impressive intelligence, communication skills, and unconditional love for their family. This radiant loyal bred is sure to bring joy and love to any family looking for a beautiful, smart companion cat.

Siberian

The Siberian cat breed is said to have been around for at least 100 years, according to the CFA. Although the Siberian is a naturally occurring breed and was declared Russia's national cat, supporting documentation on the breed is hard to come by in Russia. Therefore, there is not a whole lot to be said about the Siberian's personality.

However, Siberians are described as having a thick plush coat that changes between winter and summer and can come in multiple colors. The Siberian is extremely hard to locate in the US, which may be a major setback for people interested in acquiring one of these rare beauties for an exotic family pet.

Singapura

Singapura is Malay for Singapore, and this breed is native to the streets of Singapore. It is part of the minority of naturally occurring cat breeds, according to the CFA. The appearance of the Singapura is characterized by a brown coat accentuated by a ticked pattern that coincides with its southeast Asian origin. In the early 1970s, Singapura breed experts worked quickly to perfect this breed in order to make it pedigree worthy. The process was successful as the Singapura was accepted by the CFA in 1982. These cats are comparably smaller in body size than an average cat, with large prominent eyes, large ears, and a uniquely colored beige coat that covers their petite, muscular body.

Interestingly, Singapura cats will not reach full size until approximately 15–24 months of age, meaning they are slow to mature. Their adult body weight is 5–6 lb for males with females weighing in at 6–8 lb, according to the CFA.

The personality of Singapuras is described as very people oriented, almost to the point where they may even become a little obnoxious. In addition to their nuisance-like behavior, they are also known as playful and intelligent cats. It is important to note that inexperienced cat breeders should never attempt to breed Singapuras due to their overall difficult-to-match breed standards as stated by the CFA. Singapuras are an all-around cool cat with distinct attributes, such as their tiny body size. They would make a great family cat for those who do not mind a very playful, personable cat.

Somali

Everything about the Somali is breathtaking, from its eye-catching vividly colored ticked coat to its voluptuous tail plume. From appearance to personality, the Samoli has got it going on! These alert cats are masters at balancing their life with love and devotion to their family and finding time to carry out their playful antics such as cupboard exploring and games of fetch.

The Samoli is a man-made breed that has a medium-sized body, impressive musculature, and large captivating eyes that range in color from green to copper. Their medium-length, silky-smooth coat requires minimal upkeep. Somalis are pretty much "it" when it comes to the most desirable companion cats.

Sphynx

The Sphynx is an unmistakable, radical-looking naturally hairless breed that showed up in a litter of domestic kittens in Canada in 1966. Though Sphynxes are known for their nakedness, some can come covered in fine hairs, much like "peach fuzz."

Not much is known about the personality of the Sphynx, but it is said that in cold weather conditions, these uniquely bald cats have no problem borrowing heat from alternative sources such as humans, dogs, or even other cats.

Tonkinese

The Tonkinese is a gorgeous cat breed composed of all its ancestors' most desirable features. Tonkinese are medium-sized with nice muscular bodies that can have the coat pattern and captivating gold to green eyes of a Burmese. They can also come in color-point patterns with glistening blue eyes like the Siamese. Either way, they are bound to end up beautiful creatures. Tonkinese cats are not only smart and goofy, but they also show a tremendous amount of love for their owners and are not afraid to let it be known. They are known for their "dog-like" behaviors – a keen sense of smell, impressive memory, and affectionate personality.

Caring for these marvelous cats is considered to be relatively easy. It is best to keep Tonkinese cats indoors with tons of toys and scratching posts to keep them busy as they are known to get into mischief when bored. Having two Tonkinese to keep each other occupied may be a great idea to avoid undesirable behavior issues, especially for busy homes. Overall, these versatile, enthusiastic, and loving cats make delightful companion animals.

Turkish Angora

The Turkish Angora is said to be one of the most outgoing and affectionate cat breeds of all. In fact, the Turkish Angora is a national treasure in its native land. Owners in the United States perceive these outstanding cats as treasures also.

Turks are graceful cats with nearly perfect personalities. They are not only smart, playful, and affectionate, but they have the great ability to adapt to change, unlike many other cats. They also get along great with children and other household animals, although they have been known to take the role as "alpha" pet.

These cats have a silky-soft medium to long coat that should be combed through a couple of times per week to prevent matting. This natural breed is said to have originated in the mountains of Turkey, and their history can be traced as far back as the 16th century in France, according to the CFA. Their sparkling appearance and personality make them a delightful family pet.

Turkish Van

The Turkish Van is an ancient breed that originated in southwest and Central Asia, a region that incorporates the present-day countries of Iraq, Iran, southern Russia, and eastern Turkey. New to the United States, the ancient Turkish Van is said to be the first breed to carry the special "piebald" gene that creates white cats with a medium to long coat accentuated by terrific colored markings present only on the head and tail.

Unlike the majority of other cat breeds, Turkish Vans love water! They even come fully prepared with a water-resistant coat. These interesting cats take 3–5 years to fully mature into a large, impressive, agile animal. These intelligent cats will bring excitement, love, and amazement to a respectful home environment.

Most popular breeds

According to the CFA, the 10 most popular cat breeds in 2012 were:

1. Persian
2. Exotic
3. Maine Coon
4. Ragdoll
5. Abyssinian
6. Sphynx
7. American Shorthair
8. British Shorthair
9. Siamese
10. Devon Rex.

Needless to say, both domesticated mixed breeds and purebred cats have an equal ability to make exceptional companion animals.

Health

Like dogs, cats are prone to various health problems. Some health problems are more commonly seen in purebred cats compared with nonpurebreds. As a veterinary professional, it is important for you to have a thorough understanding of common health problems seen in cats in order to properly educate owners on how to recognize when their cat is experiencing illness and disease.

According to the Veterinary Pet Insurance Co. (VPI), the top 10 reasons cats were brought to the veterinary clinic in 2011 were as follows.

Bladder infections (feline lower urinary tract disease)

Feline urinary tract disease is a catch-all name for many issues that occur within the urinary tract system. Feline lower urinary tract disease (FLUTD) can be characterized by small amounts of urine being produced, frequent urination in small amounts, blood in the urine, or straining to urinate. There may be several causes related to feline lower urinary tract disease such as urinary tract infections or the presence of stones or crystals, which is especially dangerous in male cats as it can lead to blockage and possible death.

Chronic kidney disease (chronic renal failure)

Chronic renal failure (CRF) is a type of kidney failure commonly seen in older cats although it may occur in cats of any age and, on rare occasions, dogs. Causes of chronic kidney failure can be related to infections, urinary stones, toxins, and thyroid disease. Cats experiencing chronic kidney failure often present with symptoms of increased water consumption, decreased food intake, loss of weight, lethargic behavior, constipation, diarrhea, and vomiting. CRF is frequently seen Maine Coons, Abyssinians, Siamese, Russian Blues, and Burmese breeds.

Overactive thyroid (hyperthyroidism)

Hyperthyroidism in middle-aged to older cats is usually caused by a thyroid nodule that is overactive. In some cases, cancer may also be a cause of hyperthyroidism. Cats that have hyperthyroidism typically present with clinical signs of weight loss, increased appetite, and vomiting.

Upset stomach (vomiting)

Vomiting in cats can be related to inflammation of the stomach (gastritis). Common causes of gastritis and vomiting in cats can be related to hairballs, eating foreign material and the consumption of nonfeline foods. Bacteria, parasites, and viral infections have also been known to cause vomiting.

Dental disease

Dental disease is a general name for multiple conditions of the oral cavity. Periodontal disease starts with inflammation of the gum tissue (gingivitis) leading to loss of the tooth attachment and eventual tooth loss if left untreated. Gingivitis is caused by an accumulation of tartar build-up on the surface of the teeth. When the tartar remains on the teeth for a period of time, the harmful bacteria found within the tartar start to produce enzymes that break down the tooth's attachment, eventually leading to tooth loss unless intervention takes place.

Diabetes

Diabetes is a disease that can affect both cats and dogs. Overweight cats are especially at risk for developing diabetes, much like humans. Cats will usually acquire non-insulin dependent (Type II) diabetes. This form of diabetes does not require the use of insulin therapy to manage the disease. Cats with diabetes often show signs of increased water consumption, increased urination, weight loss, and dehydration.

Intestinal upset (diarrhea)

Acute diarrhea (sudden onset) is one of the most common health issues seen in small animal practices. Acute diarrhea can be related to several causes such as diet change, foreign bodies, drug therapy, stress or a bacterial imbalance within the small intestines. Other causes of diarrhea may be related to the presence of parasites, bacteria, or a virus. Clinical signs associated with diarrhea may include **lethargic** behavior, lack of appetite, dehydration, bloody or nonbloody stools, and abdominal discomfort or pain.

Ear infections

Ear infections are commonly caused by the presence of yeast, bacteria, or ear mites. Cats that develop ear infections can have clinical signs that include itchy, red or inflamed ears, wax accumulation within the ear canals, head tilt, painful ears, or the ears may give off a bad odor.

Skin allergies

Cats can develop allergies just as humans do. Allergies come from substances typically found in the environment that may be harmless to most cats, but some will develop severe reactions when they encounter these substances. Cats with severe reactions to allergens have an immune system that is overly sensitive which in turn identifies the substances (allergens) as dangerous. Once the substance is recognized as an allergen, the cat's body will try to fight off the invasion. During this time, cats will display signs of itchy skin, ears, and eyes, runny eyes, ear infections, vomiting and diarrhea, swollen paws, and coughing, sneezing, or wheezing. Some causes of allergies include food, grass, weeds, mold, mildew, dust pollens, prescription drugs, perfumes, cleaning products, cigarette smoke, fabrics, rubber and plastic materials, and fleas.

Lymph node cancer (lymphosarcoma)

Lymphosarcoma is one of the most commonly seen malignant cancers affecting cats. It is described as cancer of the lymphocytes (a type of white blood cell) and lymphoid tissues found throughout the body. Lymphoid cancer or "lymphoma" can be classified by its location. This type of cancer usually has a poor prognosis. Cancer treatment is available and may slow down the cancer's progression.

Dog breeds

Dogs are one of the most popular household pets. Dogs provide unconditional love, laughter, and happiness to their family which makes them a wonderful companion animal.

As a veterinary assistant, you will come in contact with many different breeds of dogs. It is important to be able to recognize each breed and to be aware of their specific behavioral characteristics. It is also important to be familiar with any unique characteristics of each breed and with any specific conditions or diseases.

All domestic dogs are members of the same species, *Canis familiaris*. When we see different breeds, it appears we may be looking at very different animals. Canine registries, such as the American Kennel Club (AKC), bring order to the diversity of dog breeds. They keep studbooks and pedigree records in addition to categorizing the breeds into groups.

American Kennel Club (AKC)

The AKC is a nonprofit organization that was established in 1884. Its main functions are to maintain a purebred dog registry, sanction dog events, and promote responsible dog ownership. It also advocates for the purebred dog as a family companion, advances canine health and wellbeing, and works to protect the rights of all dog owners. The mission of the AKC is to uphold the integrity of its registry, promote purebred dogs, and breed them for type and function.

As a veterinary professional, you may be asked to help potential pet owners decide on the type of pet that would be best for them and/or a specific breed of dog. Deciding what breed of dog to obtain is extremely important. The AKC recognizes over 160 different breeds of dogs, and each breed has its own appearance, activity level, unique characteristics, and specific needs. Potential pet owners need to dedicate serious consideration and research to determine which breed of dog is right for their family and lifestyle.

According to the AKC, there are several areas to consider when deciding on a specific breed. They include temperament, size, grooming needs, sex, age, and health considerations.

- *Temperament* – specific breeds have different personalities. It is important to match the personality of the dog with the personality of the family. Some dogs are more active while others are very laid back. Some will need a great deal of attention from their family while others may be content to be left alone.
- *Size* – all puppies are small, but they will grow. It is important to know how large each breed is expected to grow to make sure the family has enough space in their home and yard to meet the needs of the dog.
- **Grooming needs** – some breeds need very little coat care while others with long luxurious coats will need daily care to keep them looking good and healthy. Even shorthaired dogs will shed, so it is important for pet owners to decide how much hair they are willing to put up with.
- *Sex* – according to the AKC, in general, there is no significant difference in temperament between male and female dogs. In general, unless the pet is to be shown or bred, they should be spayed or neutered which helps eliminate most minor temperament differences.
- *Age* – there are advantages to obtaining either a puppy or an adult dog. One disadvantage of a puppy is the amount of training required for it to be properly socialized. Puppies require a large amount of time and patience, and should not be left alone for more than a few hours at a time. They will also require plenty of trips outside and a great deal of interaction with people. Adult dogs tend to be calmer, and many have already had basic obedience training in addition to being potty trained.
- *Health* – both pedigree and nonpedigree dogs may be predisposed to certain health diseases or conditions, some of which may be more commonly seen in purebred dogs. There are many factors that can contribute to health issues in dogs such as inherited background, environmental factors, living conditions, diet/nutrition, and weight.

Breed groups

The AKC has placed specific dog breeds into one of seven different breed groups. These groups were designed based on what the breed was originally bred to do and what its overall purpose was. The seven breed groups are the sporting group, hound group, working group, terrier group, toy group, nonsporting group, and herding group. There is also a miscellaneous group composed of specific breeds that have been placed there while they wait for final recognition by the AKC.

The AKC registers only purebred dogs that have come from a registered litter. Puppies born to AKC-registered parents but which have yet to be registered by their owner should come with an individual Dog Registration Application from their breeder. The application is to be filled out by the seller and the new owners and asks several questions such as the puppy's sex, color and markings, and registration type. It should be understood that the AKC does not recognize the quality of the dog and will not be held accountable for any health issues that may arise. The AKC describes itself as a body of different dog registries that provide certification to offspring with a known birth date, mother and father.

The sporting group

Members of the sporting group tend to be naturally active, alert, and enjoy outdoor activities. Breeds included in the sporting group consist of pointers, retrievers, setters, and spaniels. They are sometimes referred to as gun dogs or bird dogs because they were bred primarily to assist their owner by finding and retrieving various types of game in fields and in the water.

The pointing and setting breeds are naturally encouraged to locate game. They achieve this by stopping and "pointing" midstride. The spaniel breed is known to move the game closer to the hunter for a more accurate and accessible kill. The retriever breed is utilized by hunters to locate and retrieve killed game. They are proficient at traveling through both water and dry terrain.

Although working breeds live to work, they are great companion dogs for nonhunting family homes, but they will require a fair amount of exercise to keep them satisfied.

The hound group

The members of this group were bred to help capture game by tracking prey using their acute senses of sight or smell. Most hounds share the common ancestral trait of being used for hunting. Scent hounds have a strong appearance with a solid body build whereas sight hounds have a more lean body which makes them quicker. All dogs of the hound group share an interest in mammalian prey. Unlike the sporting group, the hound group are self-motivated hunters that are known to lead the way during hunting expeditions instead of waiting patiently for their owner's cue.

The working group

The dogs in the working group were bred to help humans with a variety of jobs. These include things like pulling carts or sleds, guiding the blind, serving as watch dogs and police dogs, aiding in water rescues, guarding, and tracking. Most are powerfully built and display unusual intelligence.

The terrier group

The terrier group is composed of feisty and energetic breeds that were bred to seek out and kill vermin such as badgers, woodchuck, foxes, weasels, and rats. They do this both above and below ground. In fact, the word "terrier" refers to *Terra* or earth. Unfortunately, some terriers have also been used to fight against each other. Based on the description, terriers may be placed into a category of long or short legs. They are strong-headed powerful breeds that also require a lot of attention and obedience training. Terriers also appreciate being put to work mentally and physically.

The toy group

Members of the toy group were bred for the very important role of making loving companions for their owners. Toy breeds are very interesting as they are an exact replication of their larger breed in both appearance and breed mentality. In general, the toy breeds are a fun group of dogs that is very easy to get along with.

The nonsporting group

The nonsporting group comprises a diverse group of dogs with an array of different sizes, shapes, personalities, coat types, and overall appearance. At one time, members of this group consisted of all dogs who did not hunt.

The herding group

The herding group consists of dogs bred to assist people in the control and movement of livestock. They commonly herd sheep and cattle. They accomplish this task by using barking, nipping, or body language to communicate with the animals being herded. In addition to their natural herding instinct, these dogs are highly intelligent and work precisely to their owner's command when properly trained.

Health

Nearly all dogs will encounter some sort of health issue at some point in their life. Some dog breeds are predisposed to certain diseases or conditions. Nonpedigree dogs may also be predisposed or affected by common health conditions and diseases.

According to the Nationwide Pet Insurance Co. the top 10 health conditions that brought dogs and cats into the veterinary hospital in 2018 were as follows.

Skin allergies

Dogs are notorious for developing skin allergies. Allergies are caused by a specific substance (allergen) coming in contact with the dog's body that recognizes the substance as dangerous. Some of the more common allergies affecting dogs are caused by foods, atopy (predisposed hypersensitivity to inhalant allergies), bacteria, contact, and fleas. Dogs with allergies will often develop skin infections, hair loss from scratching, itchy skin, redness, and inflammation.

Ear infections

Ear infections may be caused by the presence of yeast, bacteria, and ear mites. Dogs with ear infections often show signs of itching at the ears, head shaking, head tilt, pain associated with the ears, redness, inflammation, brown debris within the ear canals, and foul odor.

Noncancerous skin mass

Noncancerous (benign) skin growths can develop anywhere on the body of younger and older dogs. Young dogs will often develop benign skin growths called histiocytomas. Clinical signs of histiocytomas are rapidly growing, "button-like" pink nodules, found on the face, lips, abdomen, and legs. Older dogs, especially those that are overweight (obese), will tend to develop multiple benign growths called lipomas. Lipomas (fatty tumors) are more frequently seen in females than males and are characterized by being round or oval in shape, slowly growing, freely movable, and soft in texture.

Intestinal upset/diarrhea

Diarrhea is one of the most common conditions seen in dogs that present to the veterinary clinic. Diarrhea can be caused by diet change, eating foreign bodies, stress, oral medications, parasites, viruses, or bacterial imbalances within the intestines. Clinical signs of diarrhea may include vomiting, bloody loose stools, dehydration, weight loss, and appetite loss.

Skin infections

Skin infections are commonly caused by the presence of bacteria. Some skin infections can have a rapid onset and are characterized by moist dermatitis (hotspots). Other forms of skin infections can develop in a dog's skinfolds. This is where excess skin traps moisture and bacteria that will eventually lead to infection. Also, it is common for some skin infections to lead to acne and lesions in the affected areas. Typically, the infected skin is the only affected area on the dog's body whereas the rest of the body is usually not affected and remains looking normal. Irritated or itchy skin infections may develop ulcers due to self-trauma from itching or licking at the infected skin. Clinical signs related to skin infections often include hair loss, irritation and inflammation to the skin, lesions, acne, and odor.

Vomiting/upset stomach

A common cause of upset stomach in dogs is acute gastritis (inflammation of the stomach). Dogs can develop upset stomach (gastritis) for several reasons such as change in diet, eating foreign materials, eating spoiled food, consuming toxins, or the presence of a bacterial, parasitic or viral infection. Clinical signs seen with upset stomachs in dogs include vomiting, loss of appetite, painful abdomen, lethargic behavior, and the presence of dehydration.

Arthritis

Inflammation of the joint (arthritis) in dogs causes stiffness in the joints and surrounding muscles. Arthritis can affect both young and old dogs. However, arthritis is typically seen in older dogs that have experienced wear and tear to their joints over time. Obese dogs may be predisposed to early arthritis issues due to excess weight on their joints. Clinical signs of arthritis are painful joints, exercise intolerance, decreased activity, loss of joint mobility, and difficulty standing up and lying down.

Dental disease

Dental disease is one of the most common medical conditions. Over 80% of dogs over the age of 3 years have active dental disease. Periodontal disease is an infection and inflammation of the periodontium (the tissues surrounding the tooth). There are four tissues that make up the periodontium: the **gingiva**, cementum, periodontal ligament, and **alveolar bone**. Periodontal diseases starts with gingivitis and if not treated, the infection will spread deeper into the tooth socket, destroying the bone.

Anal gland inflammation

Anal gland disease is common in dogs. The anal sacs may become **impacted** due to inflammation of the ducts. The secretion within the impacted sacs can thicken and the sacs become swollen and distended, thus making it painful for the dog to pass feces.

Bladder infection

Bladder infections in dogs are commonly caused by the presence of bacteria entering the urethra and then advancing into the bladder. Once the bacteria enter the bladder, they colonize and attach themselves to the mucosal lining of the bladder where they cause great discomfort. Clinical signs of bladder infections include increased water intake and urination, blood present in the urine, decreased urination, foul-smelling urine, cloudy urine, and frequent licking of the urethral area.

References

Bell, J.S., Cavanagh, K.E., Tilley, L.P., Smith, F.W.K. 2012. *Veterinary Medical Guide to Dog and Cat Breeds*. Teton New Media, Jackson, WY.

Nationwide Pet Insurance. 2019. Common medical conditions for dogs and cats can lead to costly veterinary visits. https://news.nationwide.com/common-medical-conditions-for-dogs-and-cats-can-lead-t-costly-veterinary-visits/ Accessed July 2021.

www.wiley.com/go/burns/textbookvetassistant2

Please go to the companion website for assignments and a PowerPoint relating to the material in this chapter.

Chapter **8** Breeding and Genetics

Introduction

As a veterinary professional, you will be expected to know and understand the common terms pertaining to theriogenology (animal reproduction) that may be used on a daily basis in a clinical setting. It is recommended that you familiarize yourself with the following terms prior to reading this chapter as doing so will help you to better understand the material.

- *Bitch* – a female canine that is intact
- *Brachycephalic* – a description of canine breeds that are characterized by a wide, short head
- *Colostrum* – the first milk produced by the mother after parturition
- *Copulation* – the sexual behavior of animals in which the sperm from the male is deposited in close range of the eggs of the female
- *Dam* – a female animal that has produced an offspring
- *Dystocia* – a slow or difficult birthing process
- *Estrous cycle (heat)* – the phases of reproduction that start at the beginning phase of puberty and reoccur at various intervals depending on the animal species, which prepare the female's uterus to accept a fertilized ovum (egg)
- *Estrus* – the period of the female's heat cycle during which she is receptive to the male
- *Parturition* – the birthing process
- *Proestrus* – the phase within the canine estrous cycle that occurs right before estrus

- *Queen* – a female cat that is intact
- *Stud* – a male animal that is used for breeding purposes
- *Tie* – the time period in which the male and female dogs become "tied" together as a result of enlargement of erectile tissue that occurs during copulation
- *Tom* – a male cat that is intact
- *Whelping* – the act of giving birth to canines

Dogs

Breeding dogs is a very involved, complicated, and costly venture. There are numerous risks that involve the health of the dam and the puppies. Before a female is bred, she will need to be tested for temperament, conformation, and overall genetic health. Special care should be taken to avoid or decrease the chance of genetic or hereditary problems in the offspring. Most breeds have specific diseases, conditions, or predispositions, and dedicated breeders will test for and not breed any animal that may produce such conditions. This can be expensive but is a necessary step to quality breeding. There should be only one reason to breed, and that is to improve the breed.

Occasionally pet owners will want to breed their dog so that their children can experience the birthing process or because they like their dog and want another one just like it. These are not realistic expectations, and it is the veterinary professional's responsibility to educate the owner on the advantages and disadvantages of breeding as well as the time commitment involved so that the owner can make an educated decision. Breeding a dog

Textbook for the Veterinary Assistant, Second Edition. Kara M. Burns and Lori Renda-Francis.
© 2022 John Wiley & Sons, Inc. Published 2022 by John Wiley & Sons, Inc.
Companion website: www.wiley.com/go/burns/textbookvetassistant2

requires a great deal of time, space, money, and knowledge and needs to be considered seriously. Once owners are informed or conduct some research, they sometimes realize that breeding their dog may not be a good decision.

Owners of female dogs who decide not to breed their dog should consider having it spayed. There are many health benefits associated with spaying, such as decreased chance of mammary tumors. Additionally, spaying eliminates the possibility of unwanted litters as well as diseases such as *pyometra* and *metritis*. The spay (an ovariohysterectomy, OHE) may be done while the animal is in heat, but it may be best to wait until the heat cycle is over to decrease the chance of complications.

If it has been decided that the dog is worthy of breeding and serious research has been completed on the male, it is time to get started. Finding a compatible male is crucial to successful dog breeding and requires a great deal of time and knowledge. One must first understand the heat cycle of a female dog so let's start there.

The heat cycle

The heat cycle can also be referred to as the estrous cycle or coming "into season."

Prior to the start of the estrous cycle, there may be some changes in the temperament of the bitch. Some bitches become more affectionate and clingy while others become grumpier. It is common during this time for her to mount other females and allow them to mount her. This happens quite often and will stop once the canine heat cycle is completed. Her appetite may begin to increase, she may urinate more frequently, and she may frequently lick her vulva. A few days to a week prior to the start of a heat cycle, the vulva will begin to swell and will remain swollen until the end of the cycle. The first day of the heat cycle is characterized by a bloody discharge from the vulva.

A female dog will usually come into heat about every 6 months. Most dogs begin their first heat cycle between the ages of 6 and 12 months, and the cycle lasts for 3 weeks. The bloody discharge continues through the first week but tends to get lighter as the week goes on. This period is referred to as "proestrus."

The next part of the heat cycle (estrus) is the time in which the bitch will allow a male to breed with her. The vulva will still be swollen, but the discharge should be clear to straw colored. This stage can last from 4 to 14 days but averages about 7 days. Owners who do not want their dog to be bred must make sure to keep her away from all male dogs for the full heat cycle (3 weeks after the first bloody discharge appears).

Breeding

When breeding should take place

Once the decision to breed has been made, and both male and female prospects have been checked as healthy and worthy of breeding by a veterinarian, the breeding process is ready to begin. The correct timing of this introduction is critical for optimal

fertility to take place. The bitch will generally ovulate around 48 hours following a surge of the reproductive hormone secreted by the anterior pituitary gland. This surge will usually take place during the second day of the estrous cycle. *Ovulation* typically occurs on the fourth day. After ovulation has taken place, the immature eggs (oocytes) will need 1–3 days to further develop. After 1–2 days, the eggs are fully mature and fertile, so the bitch is and will remain fertile from the fifth to the ninth days of the estrous cycle. This period is referred to as "standing heat." The sperm from the male will also require a maturation (capacitation) time of 7 hours inside the uterus of the bitch. Once the sperm has entered the uterus, it can remain viable for 4–6 days.

In order to achieve proper timing, the following concepts should be taken into consideration and followed in the order suggested.

Determine the start day of proestrus

Breeders traditionally mate or *inseminate* the bitch 10–14 days following the proestrus onset. This is not followed by all breeders, and alternative days are also used. Determining the mating time solely based on the start day of proestrus is associated with poor conception rates due to the increased variability of proestrus length and/or owners failing to recognize the early signs of proestrus.

Pay close attention to behavior changes

This method is considered to be successful in producing high and reliable conception rates in dogs. This technique is performed by using a male dog to "tease" the bitch, starting on the fifth day of proestrus. After the bitch shows signs of standing for the male (the "acceptance period"), the breeding process should begin and continue for 2–4 days. This method works with most dogs, but if the bitch is unwilling to stand for the male, artificial insemination may be a better choice to achieve conception.

Check for vaginal discharge or perform vaginal cytology

Checking for vaginal discharge is actually an unreliable indication of when to breed the bitch as some bitches never expel bloody discharge whereas others bleed throughout the estrus stage. Vaginal cytology is beneficial in providing information on where the bitch is within the heat cycle. In this method, vaginal cells are examined with a microscope, and the guidance and assistance of professionals such as the veterinarian or veterinary technician are required for useful and reliable results.

Measure hormonal levels in the bitch

The measurement of hormonal levels in the bitch is also considered a reliable way to help the breeder determine when the bitch has reached the optimal time for breeding. This procedure is usually performed by in-house veterinary test kits that analyze the hormonal levels present in the bitch by testing a small sample of blood. This is done on a daily basis from the start of proestrus.

How the natural breeding process works

When breeding the canine, the bitch is usually taken to the male as females tend to be less stressed out by new environments. According to the American Kennel Club, breeding young male dogs with experienced bitches typically yields a smooth process. On occasion, the assistance of human attendants is needed during the breeding process, especially if the male and female dog are anatomically challenged or incompatible. For example, English bulldogs have a very heavy front end and can actually be too heavy for the female's back end.

During the actual breeding process, the male dog mounts the bitch from the rear and holds her in position by clasping his two front logs over her midsection. The male then displays rapid thrusting movements that allow penetration and ejaculation to occur. After the thrusting pelvic motions come to a stop, the male and bitch will remain together for an additional 10–30 minutes, a period referred to as "the tie." The tie is formed by the swelling of the bulbus glandis (swollen portion of the penis), which occurs while the penis is still located inside the female. It is critical to allow the bitch and stud to separate on their own. Manually separating them can seriously injure both animals. It is normal for the stud to move around during the time of the tie, which may result in the bitch and stud ending up rear to rear, which is also considered normal. Eventually, the bitch and stud will part on their own, concluding the breeding process.

Whelping

Whelping puppies is not always easy and stress free. Whelping requires experience and should include collaboration between the pet owner and veterinarian. Some breeds whelp easily, and others are known to have difficulties. For example, some brachycephalic breeds such as the bulldog or pug (Figure 8.1) may need

to be delivered by *cesarean section*. Their large shoulders and heads make it difficult for the bitch to pass them through the birth canal, thus predisposing the bitch to *dystocia* (a difficult birthing process). This situation causes a delay in the birthing process, which becomes increasingly dangerous for the neonate's chance of survival as time passes.

Labor can be divided into three stages. The first stage of labor occurs about 24 hours following a decrease in the bitch's temperature. This stage often goes unnoticed. The bitch's temperature (normally between 100 and 101 °F) will usually drop to 98 °F 8–10 hours prior to the onset of contractions. At this time, the bitch may begin to show some signs of labor. She may become more restless and seem to find it difficult to get comfortable. She may begin to spend more time in her whelping box. Frequent urination is common, and the bitch may vomit or have frequent bowel movements due to the pressure on her organs. She may refuse to eat, and there may be mucous discharge from her vulva.

During the second stage of labor, the bitch may begin digging or "nesting" in her whelping box. She will also pant and shiver, and it is not uncommon for her to vomit, urinate, or defecate during this stage.

The third stage of labor is when the water sac is present (Figure 8.2) and breaks. The shivering, panting, and digging will continue and may get stronger during this phase. As time goes on, the contractions will become stronger and will come closer together. The bitch will be visibly pushing to try to expel the puppy (Figures 8.3 and 8.4).

Necessary human interaction with newborn puppies

On occasion, veterinary assistants will need to share advice with owners on what materials are needed and what to expect during the birthing process if it takes place in a home setting. This discussion usually occurs when the bitch is brought in to the veterinary hospital for her pregnancy check-up or during a spontaneous call from home if the owner was unaware the dog was pregnant and/or going into labor. Either way, clients will

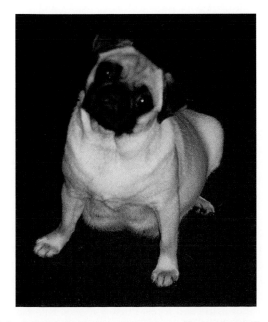

Figure 8.1 Pregnant bitch. Source: Courtesy of Dr Lori Renda-Francis, LVT.

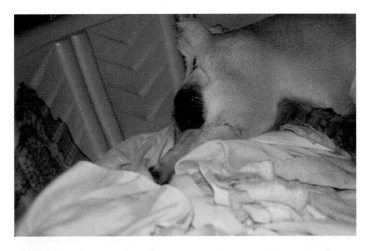

Figure 8.2 Water sac presented. Source: Courtesy of Dr Lori Renda-Francis, LVT.

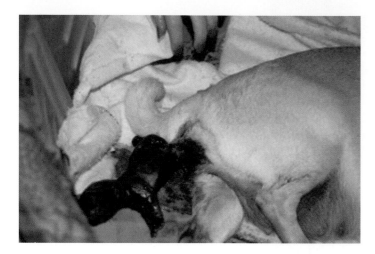

Figure 8.3 Puppy being born. Source: Courtesy of Dr Lori Renda-Francis, LVT.

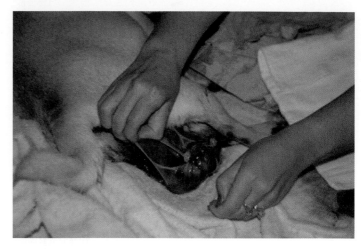

Figure 8.5 Breaking sac. Source: Courtesy of Dr Lori Renda-Francis, LVT.

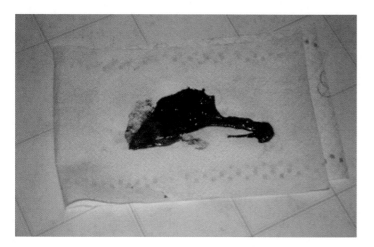

Figure 8.4 Placenta. Source: Courtesy of Dr Lori Renda-Francis, LVT.

should be helping with this process at home as newborn puppies are delicate and vulnerable to injury.

The help from human personnel begins once the first pup has been expelled from the bitch.

- If the mother has failed to break open the sac upon delivery, human intervention may be required (Figure 8.5).

- After they are birthed, puppies will need to have the mucus removed from their mouths with the bulb syringe.

- If the mother has failed to chew through the umbilical cord, the owner or helping individual will need to tie off the cord in two locations, leaving a space of at least 1 inch between the tie and the body of the puppy. Once the ties are placed, the umbilical cord should be severed or crushed using a hemostat, by the attendant. The blood expulsion from the cord will be greatly reduced if the umbilical cord is ligated in advance.

- The puppy should then be vigorously rubbed in order to stimulate a breathing and crying response.

- The puppy should be kept adequately warm throughout this process.

- The puppies should be encouraged to nurse (Figure 8.6). They may be placed on the mother's nipples to encourage them to receive their mother's first milk (colostrum), which is packed with antibodies and vitamins vital to the puppies' survival. At this time, the noses of the puppies may need to be rubbed across the mother's nipples to increase their interest in sucking or their mouths gently pried open so that they can attach to a nipple.

- After nursing, the newborn puppies will need to be stimulated to urinate and defecate. A responsible mother also helps with this process, but to make sure every puppy is taken care of, human interaction is necessary. In order to stimulate urination and defecation in a puppy, a warm, moist cloth is used to gently rub on the penis or vulva and anus to stimulate release of urine and feces. Pups will need this assistance for the first 3 weeks of their life.

need to be properly educated on how to manage the delivery process in their home.

Clients should be encouraged to obtain the following materials needed during the delivery process: a bulb syringe (used to remove mucous build-up present in the pups' mouths); dental floss or suture material that can be used to tie off the cord; sterile scissors; warm blankets (to hold the newborn pups in during the rubbing process); and a warm cloth (to stimulate the puppies' first urination and defecation).

The birthing process of puppies is truly a fascinating event, but it does require a small amount of human intervention at home to help it go smoothly. Veterinary professionals must possess a thorough understanding of the birthing process in order to relay crucial information to clients at home seeking advice over the phone.

During stage 2 (the delivery stage) of labor, the bitch will start to expel pups. This stage is characterized by contractions that can occur every 30–60 minutes between pups, or the pups may be delivered in quick succession. For this reason, it is important to recognize the signs of labor and be fully prepared to tend to the newborn pups. Only experienced and knowledgeable personnel

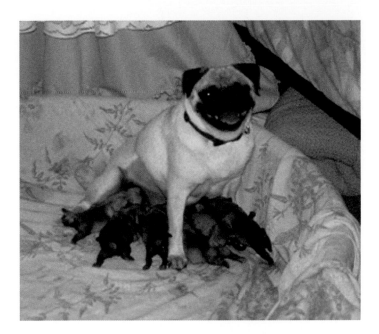

Figure 8.6   Bitch nursing pups. Source:Courtesy of Dr Lori Renda-Francis, LVT.

Warning signs (when to call the vet)

There are several complications that could occur during the birthing process that may cause the bitch to experience dystocia. It is critical for veterinary professionals to recognize signs and symptoms of dystocia. Professionals may need to interpret the information owners are providing over the phone and advise the owner to bring the pregnant bitch into the clinic. Dystocia requires the help and support of the veterinarian and veterinary professionals for healthy delivery of pups. Miscommunication between the veterinary assistant and the owner over the phone could pose serious health risks to the puppies and the bitch during the birthing process.

There are numerous reasons why dystocia may occur. Some of the more common causes are related to uterine inertia, psychological problems, pelvic abnormalities, abnormally large fetal size, abnormally positioned puppies, and the presence of dead fetuses.

Uterine inertia is characterized by the inability of uterine muscles to contract. Contraction of these muscles is essential for the bitch to successfully push the fetal puppies out of the uterus. This is often experienced by bitches that are obese, have poor exercise stamina, are of older age, or have infection present in the uterus.

Psychological problems that can occur during the birthing process are often caused by the overzealous involvement of the owner. Lingering around the bitch or the nesting box during labor is a common mistake many owners make which can cause the bitch to become overly nervous and ultimately result in delaying the birthing process, which can decrease the chances of the puppies' survival.

In some cases, dystocia may be caused by pelvic abnormalities present in the bitch. These may be due to previous pelvic fracture, obstruction in the vaginal canal caused by the presence of tumor, or an abnormally small pelvis.

Another cause of dystocia could be related to the size of the fetus. The presence of oversized fetuses is usually related to a small litter size. A small litter size allows the fetuses to grow larger than normal due to the excess space within the uterine horns. If the fetus is too large, the bitch will have a difficult time passing it through the birth canal, resulting in dystocia.

In rare cases, the bitch will experience mild dystocia due to the abnormal positioning of the puppies inside the uterus. This problem occurs when the puppies are faced in a transverse (sideways) position in the uterus. Both breech and anterior (head first) presentations are considered to be normal positioning in the bitch. Other malpositioning issues are associated with the abnormal posture of the puppies and the positioning of their limbs. Puppies are normally positioned inside the uterus with their backbone adjacent to the upper surface of the uterus with their limbs fully extended outward.

Last but certainly not least, dystocia can be caused by the presence of dead fetuses. Dead fetuses can bloat and cause a blockage in the birth canal.

The clinical signs associated with the previously mentioned conditions related to dystocia include:

- obvious decrease in blood pressure
- fetal delivery has not occurred within 24 hours of active labor
- vaginal discharge with a foul odor is expelled from the bitch
- fetal delivery exceeds 2–4 hours between pups.

If any of these conditions appear, the owner should seek veterinary care immediately as the bitch may require an emergency cesarean section to safely deliver the pups. There is no time to waste in such circumstances as the lives of the puppies and the bitch may be in jeopardy.

Cats

Heat cycle

The reproductive anatomy of a queen is similar to that of the bitch. Shorthaired queens will generally reach sexual maturity around 6–9 months of age or when they reach a body weight of 5–6 lb. However, the Manx and some longhaired breeds develop at a later age, between 11 and 21 months.

Queens are known as "spontaneous ovulators," which means their ovulation is induced by *copulation*. The estrous cycle of queens is uniquely influenced by the condition of the queen, the time of year (photoperiod), living quarters, and whether or not they are stimulated by the male. In the northern hemisphere, queens typically begin their heat cycle in January or February and go through a cycle every 4–30 days unless conception has occurred. During the summer season, the heat cycle intervals will increase in queens that are not bred. During the months of September and October, the heat cycle of the queen will begin to slow down.

The estrous cycle of all mammals is composed of five stages: anestrus, procstrus, estrus, postestrus, and diestrus.

During the first stage of the estrous cycle (anestrus), the cycling activity of the queen is temporarily absent. This coincides with decreased daylight.

The second stage of the estrous cycle (proestrus) in the queen is characterized by the increase of estrogen in the bloodstream and lasts for 1–2 days. At this time, the queen may become more affectionate and exhibit head and neck rubbing behavior.

The third stage of the estrous cycle (estrus) is when the queen is sexually receptive. During stage three, the queen will frequently vocalize in attempt to attract males to mate. The queen will display several different mating gestures in the presence of a male such as crouching and holding the tail off to one side to expose and elevate the vulva. This position is also known as "lordosis." If the male cat is absent at this time, the queen will display other behaviors such as tail deviation, treading with the rear legs, rolling and rubbing in addition to lordosis. If the queen is not bred, stage two estrous can last from 2 to 19 days. In queens that have not been bred, this stage will be slightly shorter.

The fourth stage (postestrus) is the stage between estrous cycles in queens that have not ovulated during the second stage. At this time, the queen's blood estrogen levels are low and sexual behavior is absent. On average, the fourth stage can last from 8 to 10 days.

The fifth stage of the estrous cycle (diestrus) takes place in queens that have been induced to ovulate. The fifth stage, also referred to as pregnancy, is characterized by a series of events that take place within the reproductive organs or the queen. In a pregnant queen, this stage may take up to 60 days. In a nonpregnant queen, this will last 40 days.

Feline breeding process

Under the appropriate circumstance, it is necessary to provide certain clients with helpful information with regard to the breeding process of cats. In order to properly breed cats, the estrous queen should be taken to the male (tomcat). In colony breeding, one male is placed in a group of 15–20 queens. If one female is subjected to multiple males during the mating process, she will produce a litter sired by multiple males. It is normal for the male cat to show behaviors of biting the female during the mating ritual. Within a few minutes of introduction, the male will mount and straddle the queen, followed by a quick intromission, ejaculation, and dismount. During this time, the queen may vocalize in a loud cry. After mating has taken place and the male has dismounted, the queen will jump away from the male and emit another loud cry, after which she will proceed to rolling or stretching on the floor and licking her vulva. Optimal conception can be achieved by multiple breeding sessions over 2–3 days. The queen may object to another male mounting her for up to 5 hours after successful intromission.

Queening

Unlike dogs, queens (female cats) will rarely encounter problems while giving birth (queening). Pregnant queens often prefer to give birth in an isolated area. Owners should provide the queen with adequate nesting materials such as blankets or towels along with a cozy box or cage for the queen to give birth. Within 12–48 hours of parturition taking place, the queen will start to show signs of nesting behavior. Around 12 hours before parturition occurs, the body temperature of the queen will typically decrease to below 99 °F, although many variables can affect the queen's temperature, rendering this an unreliable method of evaluation. There are several behaviors displayed by queens that are almost always in active labor, such as pacing, restlessness, nesting, and hostile behaviors directed toward other cats and strangers. Once contractions have started, the queen will typically place her body in a half-squatting position.

The next step of parturition in the queen is characterized by the breaking of the water bag (allantochorion membrane), indicating that a kitten has entered the birth canal. Normal positioning for kittens entering the birth canal is head first or feet first. Once the head or feet of the kitten have appeared at the vulva, it may take up to 5 minutes for the queen to complete the delivery. Once the kittens are expelled from the birth canal, the queen will begin to vigorously clean them by licking off any remaining placenta. The following may sound disturbing, but it is important to allow the queen to tend to the kittens without interruption. Once the kitten has been sufficiently licked clean, the queen will chew through the umbilical cord and then eat the placenta. On average, queens have a litter of four offspring, but the litter size can range from one to 10 kittens. The average time of queening will usually last around 14 hours from start to finish, but some queens may take as few as 4 or as many as 42 hours to complete the birthing process.

Determining gender in puppies and kittens

Determining the sex of a newborn puppy is much easier than determining the sex of a kitten. You can lay the puppy on its back to look at the ventral abdomen. Males and females have obvious differences. The scrotum of the male puppy is located just below the anus. The scrotum contains the testicles but they may not be palpable until the puppy reaches about 8 weeks of age. The penis is enclosed in the prepuce and is located anterior to the scrotum. The female puppy will have a vulva which looks like a slit-like structure located above the anus.

Determining the sex of a newborn kitten is a little more difficult. First, you should lift the kitten's tail and then locate the anus. The opening just under the tail is the anus. You will see the genital opening below the anus. In a male kitten, it will look like a small round hole. In female kittens you will see a vertical slit (Figure 8.7). Another difference is that the distance between the anus and the genital opening is greater in the male than in the female.

In young male kittens, the testicles will be hard to see. As the kitten grows, the testicles will become more apparent. To see the penis more easily, you can apply pressure to both sides of the genital area.

The color of kittens may also suggest their gender. A large majority of kittens that are calico colored (black, white, and

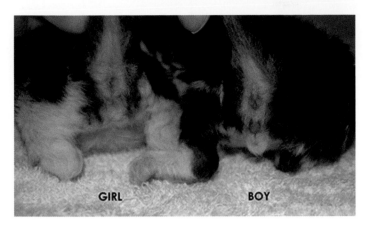

Figure 8.7 Gender identification. Source: Courtesy of Dr Lori Renda-Francis, LVT.

orange), dilute calico (gray, white, and tan), tortoiseshell (black and orange), or dilute tortoiseshell (gray and tan) are female. However, this method should never be relied upon for determining sex because it is not true for all cats.

Breeding management

As previously mentioned throughout this book, veterinary assistants are required to learn the importance of certain topics related to the veterinary field in order to convey accurate information to clients who seek advice or answers to the numerous questions they have in regard to owning a pet.

One subject in particular which veterinary assistants should pay close attention to is breeding. Breeding is a huge commitment that is often underestimated by many pet owners who fail to recognize the time, money, effort, and consequences associated with the process. Breeding of cats and dogs should be done by professional breeders who have an established name, not only for themselves but their purebred pet as well. This process does not happen overnight. It requires years of experience, knowledge, and passion from an individual to become a respectable breeder. Breeders often reproduce their purebred pets in an attempt to preserve the quality and standard of the overall breed type. Individuals who inquire about breeding their pets with the sole intention of making a profit or recreating offspring with the same disposition and personality as their current pet should be strongly discouraged and advised to reconsider.

References

American Kennel Club. 2013. *Guide to Responsible Dog Breeding*. www.akc.org/breeder-programs/breeder-education/akcs-guide-responsible-dog-breeding/

Bauer, M. 2010. *The Veterinary Technician's Pocket Partner: A Quick Access Reference*. Delmar, New York.

Campbell, K.L. and Campbell, J.R. 2009. *Companion Animals: Their Biology, Care, Health, and Management*, 2nd edition. Pearson, Hoboken, NJ.

Renda-Francis, L. 2004. Canine whelping management. *Working Dog Digest*, March, 25–28.

Romich, J.A. and Herren, R.V. 2000. *Delmar's Veterinary Technician Dictionary*. Delmar, New York.

www.wiley.com/go/burns/textbookvetassistant2

Please go to the companion website for assignments and a PowerPoint relating to the material in this chapter.

Chapter 9 General Nursing Care and Physical Exams

The nursing care of patients is typically performed by credentialed veterinary technicians in the hospital setting with help from veterinary assistants. It is important to know what nursing care entails and the role of the various health-care team members.

As an assistant, one of your duties may be bringing the owner and patient into an exam room and obtaining a thorough history. Prior to entering the exam room, you should review the record and learn the pet's name and sex. Nothing irritates pet owners more than when others refer to their female pet as "he" or "him" or vice versa. Each veterinary hospital may have a different form for taking history and performing a physical exam.

Taking a history

The history will involve asking questions of the pet owner to obtain information regarding their pet. The first question should be "What is the reason for the pet's visit?" If it is not already noted on the chart or check-in form, you should always record the signalment – the age, breed, and sex – of the patient.

Next you will determine what the owner's chief complaint is about the pet's health. You should ask questions that do not lead the owner to a certain answer. You may ask questions pertaining to certain body systems or past medical history. The questions can be tailored to each individual complaint. Some sample questions are listed in Box 9.1.

Remember that your job as an assistant is to merely record observations, not to interpret what may be wrong with the pet.

Box 9.1 Sample questions to ask pet owners.

- Tell me what you have observed with your pet.
- How long has the pet been sick?
- Has there been any vomiting or diarrhea?
- How is the pet's appetite and water consumption? Has there been an increase or decrease?
- What other animals reside in the house? Are they showing signs of illness?
- What could the pet have eaten or ingested?
- Has there been any coughing or sneezing?
- Are they up to date on vaccines?
- Has the pet shown these signs in the past?
- What diet is the pet currently on?
- Has the pet traveled recently?
- Has the pet had surgery in the past x months?
- Is the pet currently on any medications?

Physical exam

In many hospitals your duties may include the initial physical exam. Many hospitals will utilize a physical exam form. Initial observations include the pet's weight, general appearance, body condition score, mentation, posture, and gait. The body condition score is used to determine if a patient is over- or underweight.

Mentation determines the patient's overall mental status. There are numerous ways to describe mentation, several with corresponding abbreviations to record the status. They include: bright,

Textbook for the Veterinary Assistant, Second Edition. Kara M. Burns and Lori Renda-Francis.
© 2022 John Wiley & Sons, Inc. Published 2022 by John Wiley & Sons, Inc.
Companion website: www.wiley.com/go/burns/textbookvetassistant2

Table 9.1 Body system abnormalities.

Body system	Abnormalities
Eyes	Inflammation, discharge, uneven pupils, cloudiness of corneas
Ears	Discharge, debris, odor
Nose	Discharge (one or both nares)
Mouth	Gum color, growths, tartar, gingivitis, broken or missing teeth
Skin	Growths or masses, wounds, hair loss, pustules, parasites, discharge from mammary glands
Legs	Swelling at joints, wounds, deformities, pain
Thorax	Labored breathing, wheezing, coughing
Abdomen	Distension, painful when palpated
Urogenital	Discharge, swelling, masses or growths, verify gender

Box 9.2 Converting Celsius and Fahrenheit.

Celsius to Fahrenheit: (°C × 1.8) + 32

Fahrenheit to Celsius: (°F − 32) ÷ 1.8

alert, responsive (BAR); quiet, alert, responsive (QAR); aggressive; lethargic; depressed; comatose; moribund (near death).

Posture and gait refer to the animal's ability to stand and walk. Watch the animal as it is led to the exam room by the owner. Look for limping, incoordination, unsteadiness, and abnormal limb placement. Posture and gait abnormalities are more difficult to notice in cats. Most are brought in to the hospital in carriers, and cats tend to be more subtle in their posture and gait abnormalities. Therefore, posture and gait abnormalities in feline patients are usually left to the technician or veterinarian to determine.

Once initial observations are made, you will proceed to the full physical exam. Always perform a physical exam in an orderly fashion to avoid overlooking a body system. Many people use the "head to toe" approach. Start at the patient's head and work your way back to the extremities. Make sure all the body systems are addressed. The physical exam you perform as an assistant will not be a detailed one. That is the job of the veterinarian. Your job is to note obvious abnormalities as laid out in Table 9.1.

Any abnormalities noted on initial physical exam should be brought to the attention of the technician or veterinarian.

Determining and recording vitals

The five vital assessments taken on every patient are temperature, pulse, respiration, pain, and nutrition. The first three vitals listed are commonly referred to as TPR.

Upon initial examination, the veterinary health-care team should always assess the vital functions of a patient. These assessments are typically performed by the credentialed veterinary technician with the veterinary assistant helping the technician.

Temperature

Core body temperature is vital information when assessing the health status of a patient. Alterations in body temperature may be an early sign of metabolic instability and should be monitored on each hospital visit; while the patient is hospitalized; and during surgery or while the pet is anesthetized. Body temperature should be taken rectally with a mercury thermometer, a battery-operated digital thermometer, or in cases of longer-term continuous monitoring, an electronic probe. Care should be taken to utilize disposable thermometer covers as these help to reduce the potential of a *nosocomial infection* developing. When taking a rectal temperature, the thermometer should be left in the rectum for approximately 2–3 minutes.

Temperature is usually measured in degrees Fahrenheit in the United States. Most other countries use the metric system and thus record temperature in degrees Celsius. Degrees Fahrenheit is abbreviated °F (e.g., 101 °F). Most digital thermometers used in veterinary hospitals will record temperatures in both units. Care must be taken to ensure that the temperature is consistently taken in the same unit with each reading. If the temperature is taken in the wrong units, the number obtained can be converted into the other unit of measure (Box 9.2).

The resulting temperature should then be written in the medical record. Below are normal ranges for rectal temperatures:

- dogs: 101–102.5 °F or 38.33–39.2 °C
- cats: 100.5–102.5 °F or 38.1–39.2 °C
- horses: 99–101.5 °F or 37.2–38.6 °C.

Pulse

The pulse is the beat of the heart as felt through the walls of an artery. What is felt is not the blood pulsing through the artery but rather a shock wave that travels through the arteries and is generated by the contraction of the heart. The pulse and heart rate are often interchanged when describing vital signs. These two measurements differ in the sense that the heart rate is the number of contractions of the heart per unit of time while the pulse is the resulting shockwave formed by each contraction. In the majority of healthy animals, the pulse rate and heart rate should be equal.

The pulse rate is taken by placing one or two fingers over an artery and feeling for the pulse. Each pulse felt is counted as one beat. Pulse or heart rates should be recorded as beats per minute, abbreviated as bpm (e.g., 120 beats per min = 120 bpm). It is often easier to count the number of beats over a shorter period of time, such as 10 or 15 seconds, and multiply that number by the number of units of time per minute. For example, if 30 beats are counted in 15 seconds, the 30 beats can be multiplied by 4 to produce the number of beats per minute (30 beats × 4 = 120 bpm).

There are several major arteries and veins where the pulse can be taken in the dog or cat. The most commonly utilized is the femoral artery (Figures 9.1 and 9.2).

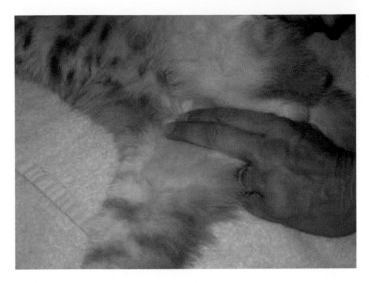

Figure 9.1 Taking pulse in the femoral artery of a cat. Source: Courtesy of Dr Lori Renda-Francis, LVT.

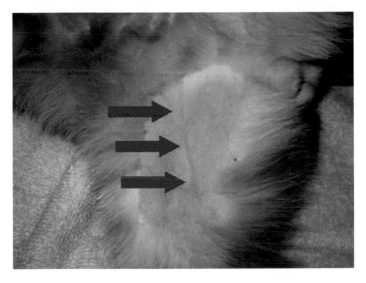

Figure 9.2 Arrows pointing to the femoral artery of a cat. Source: Courtesy of Dr Lori Renda-Francis, LVT.

In fact, the pulse quality in both the femoral artery and the dorsal pedal artery should be palpated. Variations in the strength of the pulse between these areas may indicate an abnormality in perfusion (the ability of blood to get to the periphery of the animal). Alternatively, the pulse may be taken at the *palmar aspect of the carpus* (metacarpal artery) and/or the ventral aspect of the tail base (caudal artery) in cats and dogs. If anesthetized, the lingual (glossal or tongue) pulse may be used. In horses, the heart rate can be auscultated behind the elbow (left or right). The facial pulse can be palpated on the medial side of the ramus of the mandible, forward of the muscular portion of the cheek. The health-care team usually will auscultate the heart while palpating the pulse. This will aid in determining a pulse deficit, which may indicate an *arrhythmia*. A pulse deficit is a difference in the number of heartbeats and pulse beats.

In contrast to the pulse rate, the heart rate is obtained by listening to the thoracic (chest) cavity with a stethoscope and counting each beat of the heart. As with the pulse rate, the heart rate is recorded as beats per minute.

Dogs have two normal heart rhythms. Normal sinus rhythm is defined as a regular heartbeat coupled with a normal heart rate. Sinus arrhythmia is characteristic of dogs and is defined as the heart and pulse rates increasing with inspiration and decreasing upon expiration.

While auscultating the heart, cardiac murmurs may be heard. These may be positional, so it is important for the health-care team to place the patient in sternal or standing position. Turbulence that disturbs the normal *laminar flow* of blood causes what is known as a heart murmur. Typically, murmurs are secondary to dysfunctional valves or *septal defect*s.

Table 9.2 gives the minimum and maximum pulse rates for different species and ages.

Pulses may be described as one of the following:

- normal
- absent
- weak
- thready
- bounding
- irregular.

The veterinary health-care team should also evaluate the pulse pressure and character. Systemic hypotension, or a drop in blood pressure, may be indicated by decreased pulse pressure. The health-care team needs to assist the veterinarian in determining the cause of this hypotension to rule out serious cardiac conditions. Blood pressure readings should be taken on all patients. It is best to wait to take a reading until the pet has acclimated to the hospital setting as much as possible. This will help to avoid false high blood pressure readings. Normal systolic blood pressure in the dog and cat is less than 170 mmHg and normal diastolic blood pressure is less than 120 mmHg.

Table 9.2 Normal pulse rates.

Animal type	Minimum pulse rate	Maximum pulse rate
Adult dog	70 bpm	160 bpm
Large/giant breed adult dog	60 bpm	140 bpm
Toy breed dog		180 bpm
Puppy		220 bpm
Adult cat	120 bpm	240 bpm
Kitten	120 bpm	240 bpm
Adult horse	32 bpm	40 bpm
Neonatal foal	80 bpm	120 bpm

Respiration

Respiratory rate is another vital assessment that should be performed on every patient. The animal's breaths should be counted when the animal is at rest or as relaxed as possible.

Respiration rate is the number of breaths an animal takes per unit of time. As with pulse and heart rates, the respiration rate is totaled and recorded as breaths per minute. The number of breaths can be observed by watching the animal inhale or exhale. However, some breaths may be missed by the observer and thus the number of breaths recorded may be artificially low. A better method for recording the number of respirations is through the use of a stethoscope. Just like recording heart rate, the respiration rate can be counted by placing the stethoscope on the thoracic cavity and counting each breath heard for the specified amount of time.

The normal respiration rate for a dog is 18–34 breaths per minute and for the cat the normal is 16–40 breaths per minutes.

The use of a stethoscope to auscultate the lungs is very important when determining the respiratory rate. The depth of the breath in addition to the rate of breaths should be evaluated. Respiration includes an *inspiration* and an *expiration* phase. Ideally, the feline or canine patient is in sternal recumbency during the measurement, and the pediatric head of the stethoscope should be used. The health-care team members should auscultate both sides of the chest, ventrally and dorsally, and pay close attention to the respiratory pattern. Also important to note is the respiratory effort of the patient. In horses, the health-care team members will auscultate the trachea and lungs to listen to and evaluate breath sounds.

To describe respiratory function, the health-care team should be familiar with the following terms:

- tachypnea – very rapid breathing
- hyperpnea – breathing that is deeper and more rapid than normal
- depth of respiration – volume of air inspired with each breath:
    - increased depth of respiration conveys a greater demand for oxygen
    - shallow respiration is indicative of metabolic issues or mechanical injuries
- dyspnea – respiratory difficulty or distress based on subjective observation
- labored breathing – breathing difficulty typically indicated through abdominal movements (increased abdominal muscle involvement) happening at the same time
- hyperventilation – shallow, rapid respiration typically observed in conjunction with severe *metabolic acidosis* and severe respiratory distress.

Pain assessment

The veterinary health-care team is responsible for assessing the pain level of every patient. Since veterinary patients do not talk or understand human language, this is a difficult task as pets cannot

Box 9.3 Signs of pain.

- Behavior and disposition changes – hiding; inappetence; changes in posture, voiding, abnormal gait, not wanting to move
- Protecting painful area – not wanting to be touched, threatening behavior
- Increase in frequency of vocalization
- Licking/biting affected area
- Scratching/shaking affected area
- Restlessness – pacing
- Sweating in certain species
- Increased heart rate, muscle tension, hypertension

say or point to where it hurts. There are similarities in anatomical and chemical pain perception pathways between humans and animals, and therefore it is prudent to believe that veterinary patients would experience pain in similar scenarios that human patients feel pain. The recognition of pain and management of pain in animals is considered today to be good medicine.

The relief of pain in animals can help improve the patient's wellbeing and shorten recovery time. Recognizing pain in veterinary patients and managing that pain can help to prevent the patient from harming itself or the caretaker, improve patient health, and decrease the length of hospitalization (Box 9.3).

Pain is defined as an unpleasant sensory or emotional experience that the individual associates with actual or potential injury. Nociceptors (nerve endings that conduct pain responses) are found throughout the tissues, and when these are stimulated, physiological pain results. Pain can be classified into the following:

- peripheral
- neuropathic
- clinical
- idiopathic.

Pain can also cause many harmful effects on the body and result in *immunosuppression*, an increase in tissue breakdown, reduction in healing, an increase in autonomic nerve activity, and emotional stress.

Animals, like humans, react differently to pain. Pain signs can be masked in a patient lying still in a cage giving the impression that the patient is not in pain when in fact the patient may be trying to avoid pain caused by movement. It can be very difficult to recognize pain in patients. Taking the history and discussing the typical behavior of the patient with the owner will help when assessing the patient for pain, as will a complete physical examination.

It is important for health-care team members to be familiar with the more obvious signs of pain seen in veterinary patients. These signs should be documented in the medical record and brought to the attention of the veterinarian and veterinary technician when observed.

During the physical exam, you may observe that a patient is experiencing pain in a certain area of its body. Ideally, you should be able to assess the severity of the pain. Cats can be difficult to assess since they tend to hide signs of pain and disease. The following pain scales are generally accepted as the standard of pain assessment.

Scale 1: Noninteractive behavior scoring

Grade 0 — no pain or discomfort

Grade 1 — seems to be in a comfortable position

Grade 2 — shifting positions but quiet

Grade 3 — restless, anxious, and unsettled

Grade 4 — vocalizing, becomes stiff, guards with body parts or thrashing

Scale 2: Interactive behavior scoring

Grade 0 — shows greeting behavior, wagging tail

Grade 1 — curious, approaches but hesitates with movement

Grade 2 — hesitates to approach, restricted interaction, not moving comfortably

Grade 3 — wary, slow movement usually away from person, guarding

Grade 4 — unaware of surroundings, not moving, vocalizing

Scale 3: Palpation

Grade 0 — can palpate or touch

Grade 1 — can palpate or touch, no resistance, may look at or sniff area

Grade 2 — may slightly object to gentle palpation, may lick lips or affected area, holds body still

Grade 3 — withdraws immediately, mild vocalization, tense or guarding/stiffness

Grade 4 — tries to escape, bites, grinds teeth or grimaces, ears are back, hides affected area, loud vocalization

Nutritional assessment

The nutritional status of patients needs to be assessed every time they come to the hospital. If the patient is hospitalized, the health-care team should monitor the patient's nutritional status a minimum of once a day, depending upon the disease condition and reason for hospitalization. Nutritional assessment of patients will help to determine whether or not they are at risk for malnutrition.

As discussed in Chapter 6, the nutritional management of pets is an ongoing, cyclical process. The nutritional evaluation of patients includes assessment of the patient, the food, and the feeding method. Patient assessment is the first step and allows the determination of the patient's key nutritional factors and their

levels. The key nutritional factors of the patient, as determined by the veterinarian and veterinary technician, become the basis for the second step, known as the feeding plan. The feeding plan consists of recommendations for food and feeding methods. The veterinarian will make the recommendation for the patient (in wellness nutrition, a nutrition technician may make the recommendation). The assessment of the current food and feeding method will determine whether the current feeding plan is appropriate. The veterinary assistant plays an important role in this ongoing process. Weighing patients when they enter the hospital and documenting all discussions with the owner as they pertain to the pet's nutritional status in the medical record are important responsibilities of the veterinary assistant.

The five vital assessments described above need to be determined and all information pertaining to these assessments needs to be documented in the medical record.

Age and Gender

The final two items that may be part of your physical exam or requested by the owner are to determine the age and gender of the pet. The best way to estimate a pet's age is to evaluate its teeth. Dogs and cats have deciduous (baby) teeth and permanent (adult) teeth (Table 9.3). Each tooth has a specific eruption time for the deciduous (baby) teeth and replacement time for the adult teeth (Table 9.4). With these eruption times you should be able to estimate a pet's age. Determining an actual date of birth is impossible.

General nursing care

General care of animal patients includes attending to the medical, physical, and emotional needs of these patients and oftentimes their owners. In addition to the above material, there are several other areas that contribute to excellent general care for all patients.

Table 9.3 Number of deciduous and permanent teeth in dogs and cats.

Species	Deciduous	Permanent
Dog	28	42
Cat	26	30

Table 9.4 Timeframe of tooth eruption in dogs and cats.

	Deciduous Puppies	Kittens	Permanent Dogs	Cats
Incisors	4–6 weeks	3–4 weeks	12–16 weeks	11–16 weeks
Canines	3–5 weeks	3–4 weeks	12–16 weeks	12–20 weeks
Premolars	5–6 weeks	5–6 weeks	16–20 weeks	16–20 weeks
Molars	—		16–24 weeks	20–24 weeks

Weight

A patient's weight is measured in one of two units of measurement: pounds (lb) or kilograms (kg). To obtain an accurate weight, the animal must stay as still as possible to allow the scale to record the weight. This may be difficult with active or fractious animals.

Care must be taken when reading the units of measurement on the scale. Some scales record the weight with a decimal while others record the weight in pounds and ounces. These are not interchangeable (5.8 lb does not equal 5 lb 8 oz but rather 5.5 lb as there are 16 ounces in a pound).

If needed, the patient's weight can be converted from one unit of measurement to another with the following equivalency:

1 kg = 2.2 lb

Example: 22 lb is how many kilograms?

22 lb × 1 kg/2.2 lb = 10 kg

Note that the unwanted units cancel out.

Capillary refill time

The patient's capillary refill time is often used as an indicator of blood volume and circulatory status. To measure capillary refill time, the veterinary assistant lifts the lip of the patient, places his or her finger on the patient's gums, and applies a small amount of pressure so the gum area beneath the finger blanches. The assistant times how long the gum takes to return to normal color. Capillary refill time for cats, dogs, and horses should be less than 2 seconds. Observing the color of the patient's mucous membranes is another method to determine the circulatory status of the patient. For example, in patients suffering from shock, the mucous membrane color appears pale due to the fact that blood has been redirected to the body's vital organs.

Husbandry and care

Clean, well-groomed animals are believed to feel better and recover from illnesses more rapidly; are less likely to develop *contact dermatitis* from urine scalding or feces soiling; and are more likely to have limited or more readily managed dermatological problems.

Patients should be kept in clean, comfortable, and secure housing with the health-care team focused on decreasing and ideally eliminating stress from the environment. As discussed in an earlier chapter, all animals should have proper identification on them and on their cage. When a pet urinates or defecates in its environment the health-care team should clean the area as quickly as possible.

If the patient is recumbent, prevention and management of decubital sores (bedsores) and scalding from urine is a key component to proper nursing. Some patients may have neurological or orthopedic conditions or may be critically ill, thus causing them to be recumbent for long periods of time. Patients soiling themselves and their cage with feces and urine can cause serious and long-term problems, and can delay and complicate recovery. Decubital sores may also result in *sepsis*. The best policy for decubital sores is to prevent them from occurring. Decubital sores result from continuous pressure and damage to the overlying skin above bony prominences. Air and water mattresses, foam padding, synthetic fleece, straw, and grids/gates have all been suggested as bedding types to help reduce the frequency and severity of decubital ulcers. It is best that the bedding be disposable or have a surface that does not retain water. If water remains in contact with the skin it can worsen the problem. Another nursing skill that will decrease the prevalence and severity of decubital ulcers is frequent turning of a recumbent patient. This involves turning the patient from side to side to relieve the constant pressure on one side. Ideally, the patient should be turned every 2–4 hours. If decubital sores develop, they should be cleaned with a surgical scrub preparation. The area must be completely dried following the cleaning.

Exercise should be permitted and encouraged, as long as it is not detrimental to the health or healing of a patient. Care should be taken to exercise in a safe, secure, and controlled environment so the animal is not injured or lost. Walking the patient on a leash is also a basic form of physical therapy. Walking provides exercise, environmental stimulation, and a means to reduce *peripheral edema* and improve muscle tone and strength.

Intravenous fluid administration

Administering fluids intravenously (IV) is the route of choice when treating animals that are critically ill, severely dehydrated, *hypovolemic*, or experiencing an electrolyte or metabolic disorder. Fluid administered IV has the most rapid effect on blood volume because vascular access supplies the most direct route to plasma volume. If fluid loss is severe, the deficits must be replaced quickly. Fluid losses which occur over time allow for the body to adjust; consequently, slow fluid replacement is usually all that is necessary. Intravenous delivery allows for changes in fluid rate to meet patient requirements. Complications (e.g., infection, *phlebitis*, *hematoma* formation, *thrombosis*) are more numerous with IV administration due to direct access to the venous system.

The size of the catheter should be considered in veterinary patients. Catheter flow rate is controlled by the following three factors: patient's blood pressure, level of resistance in the administration system (e.g., catheter size and placement), and the pressure or height of the fluid source. The catheter's flow resistance depends on its length and diameter. If rapid fluid administration is warranted, the largest gauge, shortest length catheter is best. It is important to remember that the maximal rate of fluid flow increases as the radius of the catheter *lumen* is increased. The smallest gauge catheter that provides adequate flow should be utilized for routine maintenance.

Catheter placement and maintenance

Veterinary hospitals should create a standard operating procedure for IV catheter placement and its maintenance and ensure all team members understand and implement the protocol. Information specifying frequency of patient evaluation and catheter inspection, bandage care and maintenance, length of time a catheter can remain in a patient, and catheter replacement guidelines should be part of the protocol. It is important that a routine fluid check for animals receiving IV fluid therapy includes verification of proper IV fluids being administered to the patient at the correct rate, in addition to ensuring the proper workings of the catheter.

Fluids can be administered using a fluid pump or by gravity flow. Regardless of the method used, the fluid bag should be labeled with a scale showing the level of the starting fluid along with anticipated fluid levels by the hour. This aids in monitoring the volume of fluid administered. If a fluid infusion pump is to be used, the administration set is placed in the pump and the pump is set to deliver the prescribed rate in mL/hr and total volume to be infused. Most pumps have an alarm and will stop if an obstruction or air bubble is detected in the line.

Personal protective equipment

The veterinary hospital owner or hospital manager is obligated to provide veterinary team members with personal protective equipment (PPE). There are a wide variety of hazards to which team members may be exposed in the veterinary hospital and in which PPE is required. All team members must be aware of the PPE needed in each instance. In addition, there are tools and equipment which make potentially hazardous events less hazardous. For example, make sure team members are using capture/restraint equipment: cages, snares, cat bags, and poles. Wear protective leather gloves when handling a fractious animal. Ensure latex examination gloves and a surgical mask are worn when handling a stray, wild, or unvaccinated animal. Be sure to maintain an appropriate distance from the work area or animal (where applicable) and be cognizant of proper restraint techniques to ensure no harm comes to the team member or the patient.

Zoonotic diseases

Zoonotic diseases are infectious diseases that can be passed from animals to humans, with some being more readily spread in this way than others. Exposure to the organisms that cause disease can occur in any of the following ways:

- inhalation
- ingestion
- through broken skin contact
- through mucous membranes and contact with eyes
- accidental inoculation by a needle.

Veterinary team members must be aware of a wide variety of zoonotic diseases. The following are just a few of the many zoonotic diseases to which team members may be exposed.

Rabies is a viral disease that is nearly always fatal. Rabies can affect any warm-blooded animal. The virus is spread through contact with an infected animal's saliva. Often, rabies is transmitted through a bite of the infected animal. It has also been shown to be transmitted when virus-rich saliva comes into contact with open wounds or mucous membranes. It is important for team members to remember and discuss with pet owners that rabies is always present in wild animals such as bats, raccoons, and skunks. More recently, states throughout the US have confirmed record high numbers of rabies cases in companion animals. Therefore, members of the veterinary team have the potential to come across a rabid pet at the veterinary hospital.

The prevalence of rabies varies across the country so it is important to know the prevalence data for the region or community in which you work. Veterinary teams must remember to wear PPE when handling an unvaccinated, wild, or stray animal. PPE, such as gloves (rubber or latex), gowns, and goggles, is necessary in cases where the vaccination history of the pet is unknown, or if helping treat a wild animal.

Bacterial infections

Veterinary medicine professionals have the potential to be exposed to a variety of pathogenic and nonpathogenic bacteria. Pathogenic bacteria examples include *Salmonella* spp., *Pasteurella* spp., *Escherichia coli*, *Pseudomonas* spp., and resistant *Staphylococcus* spp. Additionally, methicillin-resistant *S. pseudointermedius* (MRSP) is becoming more prevalent. Bacteria can be transmitted through direct contact with animals and/or their **exudates**. PPE should be worn if team members have cuts or open lesions. Bacteria can also be aerosolized and subsequently inhaled or absorbed through mucous membranes. Good personal hygiene protects against exposure to bacteria.

Fungal infections

One of the most common fungal infections in veterinary medicine is ringworm. It is important to know that ringworm is not a worm but rather an infection of the skin caused by a fungus known as *Microsporum*. It is important to educate owners that ringworm is passed between animals and humans. Especially susceptible species are cats and horses. Again, wearing PPE and practicing good personal hygiene are the most effective protections against ringworm infection. Fungal spores of *Microsporum* spp. can also be carried to other locations (e.g., your home) on clothing and can infect other animals or other people.

Internal parasites

Although the eggs of common internal parasites, such as roundworms, can infect humans, they usually do not mature into adult parasites; however, they can lead to other issues. The larvae of roundworms can migrate into organs in the human body.

Typically, they then develop into visceral larval migrans, which resembles a cyst-like growth. Unless they develop in a vital organ, the "cysts" generally are not noticeable but if they develop in a vital organ, they can cause significant and permanent damage. For example, if they develop in a human's eye, permanent damage to the retina and blindness may result. Puppies almost always have some level of roundworm infestation as worms are passed from the bitch to the fetus through the placenta and through lactation. Thus, when the infected puppy defecates, roundworm eggs can survive for long periods of time (even outside) where there is a high probability of the eggs being picked up and ingested by another mammal. Cutaneous larval migrans is especially prevalent in the southern United States, where winters are warm and humid.

Another common internal parasite, hookworms, can also cause problems in humans. Children who play barefoot where pets defecate frequently may be affected, as well as people who lie on the ground where dogs have defecated. Unlike the visceral cysts from roundworms, cutaneous larval migrans are relatively easy to spot and appear as small, red lines in the regions where the parasite has burrowed into the skin from the soil. These marks are often itchy and lengthen as the parasite moves subcutaneously from one part of the body to another.

Protozoal infections

Toxoplasma gondii is a protozoan. An infestation can result in toxoplasmosis which, while not harmful to most humans, can have devastating effects on the development of a human fetus by causing hydrocephalus and intellectual disability. Veterinary team members must educate pregnant women in an attempt to reduce potential exposure to *Toxoplasma*. Additionally, women in the veterinary profession are urged, if possible, to have *Toxoplasma* titers assessed before becoming pregnant.

Giardia and coccidia are also zoonotic protozoal agents, which typically lead to diarrhea and gastrointestinal issues in humans. Contact with infected animals (particularly puppies and kittens) is the typical route for spread, but they can also be spread by drinking contaminated water.

External parasites

Sarcoptic mange is a mite that causes itching and can readily spread to humans from animals. Always wear PPE when treating veterinary patients with mange, including gloves and a gown. Also, ensure that hands are washed thoroughly with disinfecting soap immediately after the procedure.

Hazardous waste

In veterinary medicine, team members must be aware of various hazardous materials, how they affect people and animals, and where to dispose of them (Table 9.5). There are numerous potential hazards, particularly from sharp objects which may cause physical trauma and potential exposure to the medication or substance caused by a puncture or laceration. It is imperative that we try to prevent accidents, and thus individuals should always keep sharps, needles, scalpel blades, etc. capped or sheathed until ready for use. After using a needle, do not attempt to recap it, as the risk for puncture is high. Also, it is recommended to not remove the needle from the syringe for disposal as this often results in injury. The hospital must have designated sharps containers in relevant areas and the entire needle and syringe should be disposed of in the designated sharps containers immediately after use. Do not try to overfill a sharps container as again this can lead to lacerations and punctures. When the sharps container is full, seal it and replace it with a new one.

Table 9.5 Disposing of hazardous materials.

Material	Medical waste	Normal trash
Sharps (any device with the potential to puncture, lacerate, or penetrate skin)	Any and all used needles and scalpel blades. Glass or plastic that is contaminated with a human disease-causing agent	Glass or hard plastic that is not contaminated with human disease-causing agents can be disposed of as normal waste
Medical devices (e.g., blood tubes, vials, catheters, intravenous tubes, etc.)	Biomedical waste if it contains *human* pathogens or was used for chemotherapy	Any/all devices containing/contaminated with animal blood (except from primates)
Animal tissue/animal blood	Dead animals or animal parts infected with zoonotic diseases	Tissues from routine surgical procedures (castration, ovariohysterectomy, etc.)
Laboratory cultures	Microbiological cultures (bacterial, fungal, or viral) of *human* pathogens; considered biomedical waste	All laboratory cultures = biomedical waste
Bandages/sponges	Used absorbent materials, saturated with blood/body fluids which contain *human* pathogens	Sponges or bandages used on animals not infected with zoonotic disease
Animal waste	Waste from patients infected with a zoonotic disease transmitted by means of the waste. Waste from chemotherapy patients for up to 48 h after the last treatment	Waste from animals not infected with a zoonotic disease

Do not open a sharps container that has been sealed or stick your fingers into one for any reason. Never throw needles or sharps directly into regular trash containers, regardless of whether or not they are capped.

Hazardous drugs

Medicines are created to prevent, manage, and sometimes cure disease. Thus, it can be easy to forget that all medicines are chemicals, and chemicals can be dangerous. Within the pharmacy in the veterinary hospital, you can be exposed to all kinds of drugs. Liquids can splash in eyes, vapors can be accidently released and thus inhaled. Handling, crushing, or breaking tablets can leave powder residue on hands, with the potential for ingestion the next time the team member puts their hands near their mouth or eyes.

Cytotoxic drugs (CDs) are prescribed to treat patients with cancer and are so potent that even small exposures can cause harm. Veterinary team members involved with administering cytotoxic drugs must wear PPE that is not used for any other purpose, such as powder-free chemotherapy gloves, disposable aprons or gowns, surgical masks, and eye protection, when preparing CDs. The preparation of chemotherapy drugs should always occur inside a biological safety cabinet. To ensure the safety of all team members, follow all instructions on the safety data sheet (SDS), on the package insert, and in the hospital's chemotherapy safety plan.

Common diseases

Respiratory disease

Respiratory tract diseases typically result in inflammation, irritation, and obstruction or restriction of the airway, each of which can cause an assortment of clinical indicators. Discharge from the nose of an animal results from inflammation or irritation of the mucosa and can be serous (clear liquid), mucoid (opaque and sticky), mucopurulent (green-yellow and mucoid), or hemorrhagic (bloody). It is important for the team member to note whether the discharge is occurring on one side or both sides of the nose.

Nasal discharge and edema can compromise the patient's airflow, leading to open-mouth breathing in some patients and potentially a diminished sense of smell. This may lead to anorexia, especially in cats, and this is a serious result. The following signs and symptoms should be noted.

- *Sneezing*: frequent, rapid bouts of sneezing are abnormal.
  - In dogs, sneezing is observed most often with inhalation of foreign material.
  - In cats, sneezing is often associated with viral infection of the upper respiratory tract.
- *Facial swelling*: a patient with nasal discharge, congestion, and/or sneezing should be examined for facial swelling which may accompany the causative disease.

- *Stertor/stridor*: obstruction of the **pharynx** or larynx can cause:
  - stertor, a loud snoring/snorting sound
  - stridor, a high-pitched inspiratory wheeze.
- *Cough*: a cough is a forceful expulsion of air from the lungs through the mouth. It may be a reflexive or conscious action resulting from irritation or inflammation to the pharynx, larynx, trachea, **bronchi**, or **pleura**.
- *Pleural effusion* is the build-up of excessive fluid within the thoracic cavity.
- *Dyspnea*: also known as respiratory distress, this is difficulty breathing typified by increased respiratory rate or effort, often with an abdominal component to the breath.

Cardiovascular disease

An abnormality which affects the **myocardium**, valves, rhythm conduction, pericardium (sheath covering the heart), or the overall make-up of the heart (shunts) is known as heart disease. In cats, myocardial disease accounts for the majority of heart disease; in dogs, valvular disease accounts for the bulk of cardiac disease cases. Many patients are asymptomatic at home or owners may miss subtle clinical signs, such as mild exercise intolerance, lethargy, or tachypnea. Early detection of heart disease depends on thorough annual physical examinations and, for susceptible breeds, screening echocardiography. A patient with heart disease may exhibit **tachycardia**; a weak, bounding, or asynchronous femoral pulse; a heart murmur; and/or an arrhythmia. Diagnosis of heart disease relies on diagnostic imaging of the heart – radiography and **echocardiography** – and **electrocardiography**.

Gastrointestinal tract

Diseases of the gastrointestinal (GI) tract result in local inflammation or infection, and potentially obstruction. Knowing and understanding the signs and symptoms help to focus the medical history questions, identify the anatomical location of the problem, and direct diagnostic and therapeutic approaches.

- *Regurgitation* is the passive expulsion of material from the mouth, pharynx, or esophagus. Nausea and abdominal contractions are not present. Patients may exhibit difficulty eating, hypersalivation, and gagging. The material that is regurgitated usually consists of undigested or partially digested food.
- *Vomiting* is the expulsion of contents from the stomach and upper small intestine. Vomiting is an active process that requires abdominal contraction known as retching. Nausea often precedes vomiting, with patients exhibiting anxiety, hypersalivation, vocalization, and lip smacking. Vomitus can comprise any combination of undigested or digested food, hair, mucus, bile, and gastric secretions. Some patients may vomit intestinal parasites (e.g., roundworms) or pieces

of foreign material that they ingested (yarn, ribbon, tennis balls, plastic bags, etc.). Remember that vomiting patients may become dehydrated and have an imbalance of electrolytes.

- *Diarrhea* is the frequent passage of loose, often watery, and unformed stool. When a medical history of a patient with diarrhea is taken, it is important to ask the owner about the duration, severity, frequency, amount, and quality of the patient's stools. Although the owner may be uncomfortable with this discussion, it is important to educate them that this information can assist in localizing diarrhea to the small or large bowel. In addition, knowing the duration of the signs helps to determine the right diagnostic testing approach. Patients with diarrhea are also at risk for dehydration.

- *Constipation* is the infrequent and often difficult passage of hard stool. When taking a history, the team member must question the owner regarding when the last normal bowel movement was observed. Constipation can be a primary GI problem caused by bowel obstruction or diminished bowel motility. It may also occur secondary to orthopedic pain (cannot posture to defecate), environmental stressors (e.g., poor litter box management), and dehydration. It is essential to complete a full systems review when obtaining a medical history, to evaluate all potential causes.

Urinary diseases

Diseases of the urinary tract are common in cats and dogs and may originate from anywhere in the entire urinary tract – upper and lower.

Urolithiasis

A urolith is a stone which forms from mineral salts in the urinary tract. Formation depends upon urine pH, urine concentration, and urine saturation. Clinical signs are dependent upon the location, number, size, and shape of the urolith as well as concurrent presence of urinary tract infection. Classification of urolithiasis is centered on the main mineral component, such as struvite, calcium oxalate, or urate. Clinical signs are dependent on the location of the urolith. If the urolith is located in the bladder, no clinical signs may be present but more commonly, stranguria (straining to urinate), pollakiuria (abnormally frequent urination), and hematuria (blood in urine) are seen. If the urolith is in the urethra, frequent attempts may be made to urinate, and dribbling of urine may be noted; complete obstruction represents a medical emergency.

Treatment of uroliths consists of surgical or procedural removal and/or medical dissolution (often with therapeutic diets), depending on the anatomical location and composition of the stone. In the case of uroliths causing urethral obstruction, immediate relief of the obstruction via urinary catheterization and correction of electrolyte imbalances that result from the obstruction are required.

Feline lower urinary tract disease

Feline lower urinary tract disease (FLUTD) refers to the group of signs indicating irritation of the bladder and urethra in the cat, such as stranguria, dysuria, hematuria, pollakiuria, and inappropriate urination. FLUTD is most common in adult cats between 2 and 6 years of age. It may be classified as nonobstructive or obstructive. In more than half the patients with nonobstructive FLUTD, the underlying cause is feline idiopathic cystitis (FIC). The other common cause of nonobstructive FLUTD is the presence of uroliths. The most common causes of obstructive FLUTD are urethral plugs and uroliths. Urethral plugs comprise a mucoprotein matrix and crystalline material, commonly struvite crystals. Urethral obstructions are a medical emergency. Signs are abdominal pain, vomiting, altered mental status, and the inability to pass a normal stream of urine. Immediate relief of the obstruction and correction of electrolyte imbalances that result from the obstruction are required.

Chronic kidney disease

Chronic kidney disease (CKD) is an irreversible, progressive loss of functioning **renal** tissue. There are a variety of causes of CKD. Some cases may even be idiopathic, meaning the cause is not known. Clinical signs relate to impairment of fluid homeostasis, uremia or the build-up of toxins in the bloodstream, and electrolyte abnormalities which result from the kidney(s) no longer able to function properly. Azotemia occurs in CKD patients. Azotemia refers to serum elevations of the protein metabolites creatinine and blood urea nitrogen. Urine specific gravity (USG) measures the concentration of urine and reflects the hydration status and kidney function of the patient.

Endocrine disease

The endocrine system in dogs and cats consists of a number of organ systems which can give rise to a variety of disease conditions, depending upon which system is affected.

Hyperthyroidism is a disease that most commonly affects cats. Here the thyroid gland is overactive and produces large amounts of the thyroid hormones thyroxine (T_4) and triiodothyronine (T_3). This increased production results in an increased basal metabolic rate (BMR). In 98% of patients, hyperthyroidism is caused by a unilateral or bilateral benign functional thyroid adenoma; 2% of patients have malignant thyroid **carcinoma**. Clinical signs are related to the increased BMR and include weight loss, increased appetite, increased activity level, **polyuria** and **polydipsia**, vomiting, and diarrhea. Potential findings in hyperthyroid cat histories and examinations include tachycardia, a heart murmur, an enlarged thyroid gland, behavioral changes, weight loss, and hypertension. Elevated serum T_4 concentration confirms the diagnosis of hyperthyroidism in most patients.

Hypothyroidism is a disease seen predominantly in dogs. Dogs with this disease have an underactive thyroid, which results in below normal circulating levels of thyroid hormones. Consequently, a decrease in BMR is seen. The most common causes of hypothyroidism include immune-mediated destruction and idiopathic *atrophy* of the gland. There are many clinical signs but the most common are weight gain, exercise intolerance, altered mentation, and lethargy caused by the decreased BMR. On physical examination, hypothermia, *bradycardia*, *truncal alopecia*, and *seborrhea* may be noted. Diagnostic confirmation includes documenting low serum T_4 and free T_4 levels and elevated thyroid-stimulating hormone levels, as well as evaluating complete blood count (CBC) and a full serum chemistry panel.

Diabetes mellitus

Diabetes mellitus (DM) is another prevalent disease condition in dogs and cats. There are two types of DM. Type 1 or insulin-dependent DM results from insufficient production of insulin by pancreatic beta cells. Type 1 is more common in dogs. Type 2 or noninsulin-dependent DM is a result of insulin resistance characterized by the body's inability to respond properly to *endogenous* insulin. Cats are more prone to type 2 DM. Clinical signs for both types include *polyphagia*, weight loss (generally in a previously obese patient), polyuria, and polydipsia. Cats with advanced DM frequently present to the veterinary hospital with a *plantigrade stance*. Dogs with DM may present with cataracts. Diagnosis by the veterinarian consists of documenting elevated blood glucose with concurrent glucose in urine. Cats are particularly prone to stress-induced *hyperglycemia*; as a result, elevated *fructosamine* levels may be used to confirm DM in cats.

It is important for all members of the veterinary team to understand the two forms of DM and how the disease is managed in cats and dogs. If DM is not controlled, it can progress to a condition called diabetic ketoacidosis (DKA). This also may occur in patients that have yet to be diagnosed. DKA occurs when the patient's body continues its inability to use glucose, thus resulting in an alternative pathway for carbohydrate metabolism. By-products of this pathway are ketones, which are toxic metabolites. The presence of ketones in urine (ketonuria) is a hallmark finding of DKA, as is the fruity odor of the breath that ketones impart. Patients with DKA are critically ill and can present with anorexia, depression, polyuria, polydipsia, weight loss, and vomiting. DKA is an emergency. When the pet presents to the hospital in DKA, they are often dehydrated and hypothermic, have altered mental status, and may have cardiac arrhythmias.

Immune-mediated disease

Immune-mediated diseases occur when the immune system of an animal fails to recognize its own tissues and cells. As a result, the immune system labels cells and tissues with antigen, thus triggering an immune response against these parts of the animal's own body. *Autoimmunity* may be idiopathic or may result from an underlying disease process. Secondary immune-mediated disease can be a result of infection, cancer, vaccine administration, or exposure to certain drugs or toxins.

Infectious disease

Infectious disease is caused by *pathogenic* microorganisms which invade the host/patient and take over the tissues and fluids. There are numerous infectious diseases that affect the cat and dog. These include a variety of pathogens, such as viruses, bacteria, fungi, and *rickettsiae*. Infectious diseases can be transmissible, such as kennel cough, or nontransmissible, such as a cat bite abscess. The steps of infection and related terms are as follows.

1. The pathogen must avoid the host's defense systems, reproduce in the host, and cause disease.

2. The reservoir can be an animal, insect, or fomite (inanimate objects – bowls, cages, clipper blades, towels, scrubs, etc.) in which the pathogen can survive.

3. Portal of exit includes where/how the pathogen leaves the reservoir and is often seen by team members as clinical signs of the disease process (e.g., sneezing).

4. The mode of transmission is the path the pathogen travels to the next host.

   a. Direct transmission – immediate; requires direct contact of skin or mucous membranes with infected animal or its secretions or excretions, ingestion of virus, inhalation of virus.

   b. Indirect transmission = delayed; involves contact with a contaminated *fomite* or is transmitted via a biological vector such as an insect.

   c. *Transplacental* transmission.

5. Portal of entry or the route of infection relates to where/how the pathogen gains entry into the host.

6. Host susceptibility means that exposure to a pathogen does not guarantee infection and disease. Rather, the animal must be susceptible to the pathogen, meaning the host has an immature, suppressed, or deficient immune system and cannot fight and kill the pathogen.

Contagious infectious diseases are those that are transmitted directly between animals or indirectly through fomites contaminated with animal secretions. Vector-borne infectious diseases are those that require a *biological vector* for transmission. As mentioned above, zoonotic diseases are infectious diseases transmitted directly from animals to humans. Shared-vector zoonoses are infectious agents that can infect a human or an animal via a common vector such as fleas and ticks. Infectious diseases transmitted from humans to animals (e.g., dermatophytosis) are termed reverse zoonoses.

It is of the utmost importance that all veterinary team members understand how to control transmissible infectious diseases and are able to educate pet owners. The following steps are crucial in interrupting the infection process.

1. Kill the pathogen while it is in the host or animate reservoir using antibiotics, antiviral, or antiparasitic medication.

2. Kill the pathogen while it is living on a fomite by sanitizing, disinfecting, or sterilizing.

3. Kill the pathogen while it is living in/on a vector. This can be achieved using preventive antiparasitic medication, environmental pesticide, and soap and water.

4. Strengthen host defense systems by:
   a. administering vaccination
   b. maintaining proper health and nutrition.

5. Decrease host exposure through:
   a. limiting exposure of immunodeficient and immunosuppressed individuals
   b. adhering to proper isolation protocols for contagious animals to prevent spread of disease.

Veterinary patients are not able to provide care for themselves, so the veterinary health-care team must provide the services that will prevent and manage illness. This responsibility often is assigned to the veterinary technician and the veterinary assistant.

References

Barr, B.S., Brooks, D., Javsica, L., Zimmel, D. 2009. Nursing care. In: *Equine Manual for Veterinary Technicians*. Reeder, D. et al. (eds). Wiley-Blackwell, Ames, IA.

Burns, K.M. 2006. Managing overweight or obese pets. *Veterinary Technician*, June, 385–389.

Burns, K.M. 2011. Owner education and adherence. In: *Practical Weight Management in Dogs and Cats*. Towell, T. (ed.). Wiley-Blackwell, Ames, IA.

Liss, D. 2018. Small animal medical nursing. In: *Clinical Textbook for Veterinary Technicians*, 9th edition. Bassert, J.M., Beal, A.D., Samples, O.M. (eds). Elsevier Saunders, St Louis, MO.

Maugham, J., Cave, C. 2016. The essentials of patient care. In: *The Complete Textbook of Veterinary Nursing*. Ackerman, N., Aspinall, V. (eds). Elsevier Butterworth Heinemann, London.

Sirois, M. (ed.). 2017. Nursing care of dogs and cats. In: *Principles and Practice of Veterinary Technology*, 4th edition. Elsevier, St Louis, MO.

Sirois, M. (ed.) 2017. Veterinary anesthesia, analgesia, and anesthetic nursing. In: *Principles and Practice of Veterinary Technology*, 4th edition. Elsevier, St Louis, MO.

Thomas, J.A., Lerche, P. 2011. *Anesthesia for Veterinary Technicians*, 4th edition. Mosby, St Louis, MO.

www.wiley.com/go/burns/textbookvetassistant2

Please go to the companion website for assignments and a PowerPoint relating to the material in this chapter.

Chapter 10 Exam Room Procedures

As an assistant, there are several exam room procedures that you may perform or help the technician perform. You must feel comfortable performing these procedures because they often take place in front of the owner and with nervous or potentially aggressive patients.

Recognizing ectoparasites

Frequently you will need to identify *ectoparasites*. These are parasites found on the animal, usually within the coat. You will frequently observe them while performing a routine physical exam. Three of the four most common ectoparasites are shown in Figures 10.1–10.3.

The fourth ectoparasite frequently seen on dogs and cats is *mites*. These are not visible to the naked eye. A sample must be taken from the patient and viewed under a microscope. Collecting the sample will be the job of the technician or veterinarian. It should be noted that several species of mites are contagious to humans.

When looking for ectoparasites, you may not find the actual insects, but you may see other tell-tale signs they are present on the patient. Fleas feed on the animal's blood. After digesting the patient's blood, the flea will excrete the remains. This is known as flea dirt (Figure 10.4). Lice will lay eggs on an animal's hair shafts. These are called *nits*.

You may also be required to perform grooming. Grooming procedures include toenail trimming, ear cleaning, anal gland expression, bathing, and general grooming.

Nail trimming

Many owners do not routinely examine their pets' toenails. This can lead to serious overgrowth problems. Some dogs will naturally wear down their nails by running or walking on hard surfaces. Dogs that spend the majority of their time indoors fail to wear down their nails. When this occurs, the nail will continue to grow, become very long, and may even curl under and grow into the foot pad. This can be a painful condition that leads to lameness and possibly infection of the foot and nail. A normal, well-worn nail should be even with the bottom of the paw pads. When the dog walks, the nail should not touch the ground.

In cats, we tend to see less of an overgrowth problem because of their natural tendency to sharpen their claws. Also, many cats have been declawed by their owners to prevent this tendency. Cats that do have nail overgrowth problems tend to be overweight or older and less active.

Once overgrowth has occurred, it is up to a veterinary professional to trim the nails. Before you can trim an animal's nails, you must be familiar with the anatomy.

Nail anatomy

Dog and cat nails are somewhat similar to human nails (Figures 10.5 and 10.6). Human nails are essentially a flat layer of **keratin** with a hidden blood supply. Dog and cat nails are appendages with a blood supply as well as associated nerve endings. This blood supply runs down the center of the nail and is referred to as the "*quick*."

The outer surface of the nail is hardened keratin. No nerve endings or blood vessels are found in this outer surface. Dog nails will be either white or black while cat nails tend to be entirely white. The white nails tend to be easier to trim since the quick can be seen within the nail.

The goal of trimming a nail is to cut approximately one-eighth of an inch in front of the quick. If the nail is cut too close and the quick is cut, the dog or cat will react in pain, and bleeding will occur. This

Textbook for the Veterinary Assistant, Second Edition. Kara M. Burns and Lori Renda-Francis.
© 2022 John Wiley & Sons, Inc. Published 2022 by John Wiley & Sons, Inc.
Companion website: www.wiley.com/go/burns/textbookvetassistant2

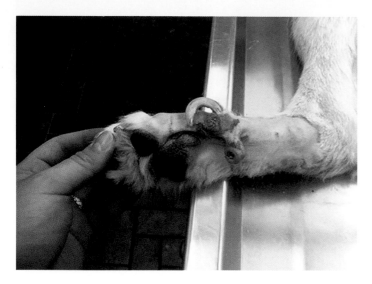

Figure 10.1 Overgrown nails. Credit: https://www.flickr.com/photos/cyborgsuzy/5695129174.

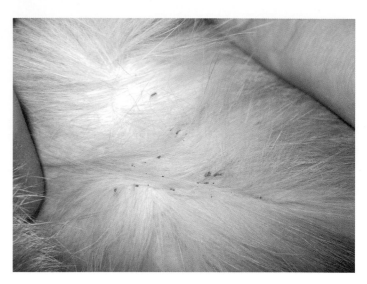

Figure 10.4 Flea dirt. Source: Courtesy of Dr Lori Renda-Francis, LVT.

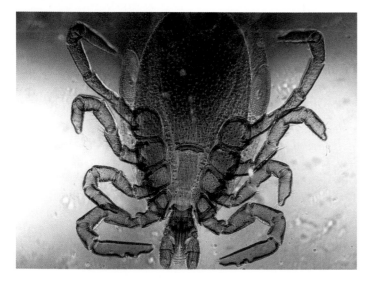

Figure 10.2 Tick. Source: Courtesy of Dr Lori Renda-Francis, LVT.

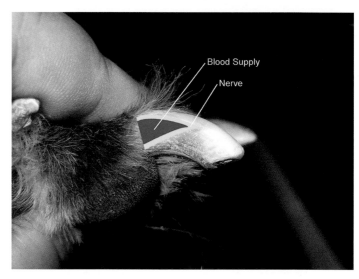

Figure 10.5 Dog nail anatomy. Source: Courtesy of Dr Lori Renda-Francis, LVT.

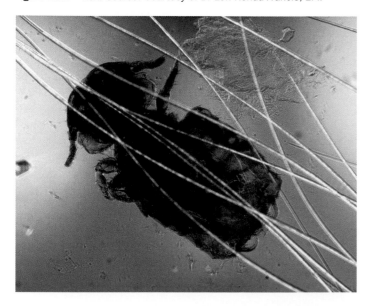

Figure 10.3 Louse. Source: Courtesy of Dr Lori Renda-Francis, LVT.

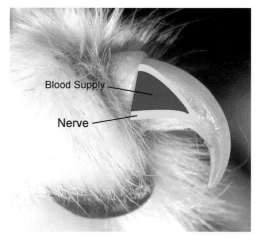

Figure 10.6 Cat nail anatomy. Source: Courtesy of Dr Lori Renda-Francis, LVT.

tends to occur more frequently in dogs, especially in those with black nails. We will address how to stop the bleeding later.

There are two main types of nail trimmers: guillotine and scissor-like (Figures 10.7–10.10).

Which tool to use is often a question of personal preference. Many people find the guillotine type easier for dog nails. The scissor type is frequently used for cats or nails that have grown into the foot pad. Human toenail clippers are most often used for puppy and kitten nail trims.

The guillotine-type trimmer has a ring through which the nail is placed. Make sure the side with the screws is facing the nail and that the blade moves up toward the bottom of the nail. Squeezing the handle causes the blade to move forward to slice off the portion of the nail within the ring. Scissor-type trimmers are used in the same fashion as scissors. They will cut the nail at the location the blades are placed.

You will not be able to see the quick in dark-colored nails. This makes it much more difficult to avoid the quick when trimming.

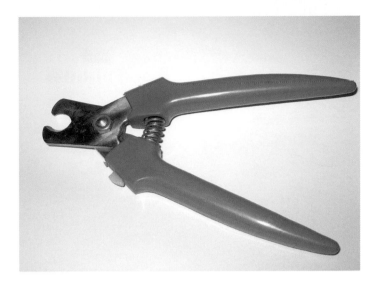

Figure 10.9   Scissor trimmers. Source: Courtesy of Dr Lori Renda-Francis, LVT.

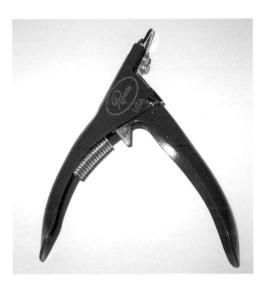

Figure 10.7   Resco. Source: Courtesy of Dr Lori Renda-Francis, LVT.

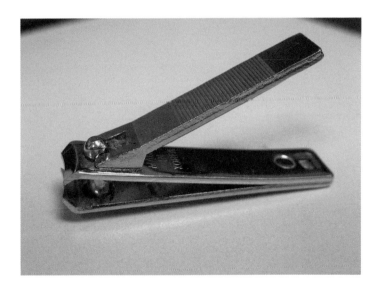

Figure 10.10   Human nail trimmer. Source: Courtesy of Dr Lori Renda-Francis, LVT.

The best way to avoid the quick is to trim the nail in several small cuts.

As you trim the nail, look at the cut edge. The color of the nail will change. Initially there will be two distinct layers, lighter colored tissue on the curved, lower part of the nail and darker colored tissue on the top. As you continue to trim the nail, the two tissue layers will become *homogenous* in color. This change in color indicates you are close to the quick. If you notice a gray or pink oval shape, stop cutting. The quick is just past that portion of the nail.

If you do cut the quick, it will bleed. To stop the bleeding, first apply pressure to the cut nail. Occasionally this will be sufficient to stop the bleeding. If the bleeding does not stop quickly, you will need to use one of the available cautery agents. The two most common agents used to stop the quick from bleeding are styptic powder (sold under the brand name Kwik-Stop®; see Figure 10.11) or silver nitrate ($AgNO_3$) sticks (Figure 10.12). Both of these agents are very effective at stopping bleeding from the quick.

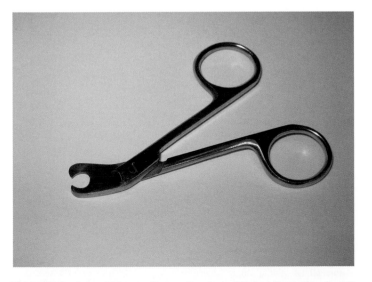

Figure 10.8   Cat nail trimmer. Source: Courtesy of Dr Lori Renda-Francis, LVT.

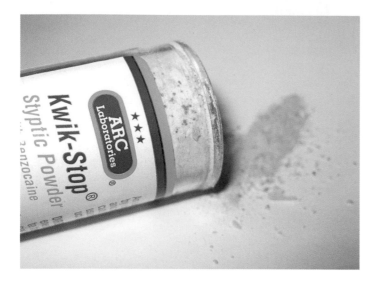

Figure 10.11   Kwik Stop. Source: Courtesy of Dr Lori Renda-Francis, LVT.

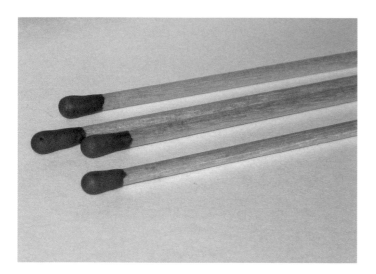

Figure 10.12   Silver nitrate sticks. Source: Courtesy of Dr Lori Renda-Francis, LVT.

To use styptic powder, apply a moderate amount to the bleeding quick. Apply pressure to the area for several seconds. Check the area for continued bleeding. If present, repeat application until the bleeding has subsided.

With the silver nitrate stick, you will need to apply pressure to the quick with the silver nitrate end of the stick. Many dogs find this uncomfortable and will briefly struggle. As with the styptic powder, check the area for continued bleeding, repeating the steps as necessary. It should be noted that silver nitrate tends to stain skin, clothing, and countertops.

Often you may find nails overgrown and curled into the foot pads. This occurs frequently in **dewclaws**. Overgrown nails are often painful. Use scissor-type trimmers to remove the overgrown portion of the nail. Be aware that the quick will continue to grow with these nails and therefore increase the likelihood of bleeding. If this occurs, use the methods described above to control the bleeding. After trimming the overgrown nails, alert the veterinarian so he or she can check for signs of infection.

Antibiotics and pain medications are often prescribed, depending on the severity of the injury or infection.

Ear cleaning

To assist the health-care team in keeping the external ear canal clean and free of disease, the ear canal should first be examined. A visual assessment occurs first, in which the assistant notes any debris, cerumen (wax), **foreign bodies**, etc. It is imperative that the external ear canal be examined prior to applying cleaning or medicated agents, as damage to the ear may result in loss of hearing, vestibular dysfunction, or facial nerve paralysis. Some breeds may have a build-up of hair/fur in their external ear canal, which can trap debris and lead to infection. The team member should also note any odor – this may or may not be related to the external ear canal (vs the inner ear), but it is important to note and document. A thickened **pinna** may indicate an **aural hematoma**. It is also important to note if the patient experiences any pain during the exam. All findings should be documented and brought to the attention of the veterinarian. The veterinarian will examine the entire ear to determine whether the ear requires cleaning. He or she will also determine whether there is anything preventing the patient's ear from being safely cleaned.

Routine ear cleaning is a common exam room procedure. Many breeds of dogs are prone to ear infections known as otitis. Before you start cleaning a patient's ear, you should be familiar with the basic anatomy (Figure 10.13). The ear has three major sections: outer ear, middle ear, and inner ear. The outer ear refers to the ear flap (pinna) and ear canal. Depending on the breed, the pinna can be erect or floppy. Unlike the human ear canal, which is straight, the dog and cat ear canals bend at approximately 90° as they enter the deeper portion of the ear.

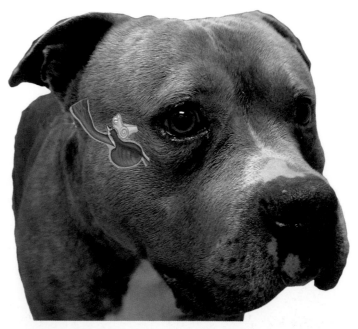

Figure 10.13   Ear anatomy. Source: Courtesy of Dr Lori Renda-Francis, LVT.

The outer ear is separated from the middle ear by the tympanic membrane, commonly referred to as the ear drum. The tympanic membrane must be intact before ear cleaning can occur. The veterinarian will determine this. Note that the tympanic membrane is fragile, especially when disease is present, and can be damaged during the ear cleaning procedure. The utmost care must be taken to avoid damaging this structure. On the other side of the tympanic membrane lie the three small bones of the ear, the Eustachian tube, and an air-filled structure known as the bulla.

The inner ear consists of the cochlea, the vestibule, and the semicircular canals which are membrane-lined bony structures within the temporal bone of the skull. For routine ear cleaning, the section of the ear you will be concerned with is the outer ear.

In general, dogs tend to have more ear problems than cats. Variations exist within dogs as well. Dogs with floppy pinnae are more prone to ear infections than those with erect pinnae. Also, dogs with excessive hair within their ear canals may have more build-up of debris.

When evaluating the ear prior to cleaning, you may note the following signs of disease: redness, odor, discharge, or debris. The discharge or debris may range from black (yeast), yellow or tan (waxy secretions), green (infection, pus) or coffee grounds (ear mites). There may be varying degrees of the debris categories. Small amounts of debris can be normal in a healthy ear canal.

Several items will be required for routine ear cleaning: ear wash solution, cotton balls, hemostats, and cotton tip applicators. Ask the veterinarian what type of ear cleaning solution should be used based on the patient's condition. Ear cleaning solutions contain several chemicals, each with its own purpose. Some solutions may contain drying agents or alcohol which may irritate an already damaged ear canal.

Most dogs and cats do not like having their ears cleaned and will require some sort of restraint. This means someone will need to restrain the dog for you or, in the case of small breed dogs or cats, you can wrap them in a towel or place them in a restraint bag.

Inspect the ear canal for excessive amounts of hair. If present, it can be removed by gently plucking it out using hemostats. Ask the veterinarian before removing the hair because this may increase the amount of inflammation in the ear canal, thus worsening the condition.

Ear wash can be placed directly into the ear canal. Avoid making contact with the infected tissue within the ear; this can transfer infectious agents to the tip of the bottle which can potentially be transferred to another patient. Make sure the cleaning solution gets on the ear flap as well. There are several grooves on the ear flap where debris can collect. Most animals will shake their heads after having cleaning solution in their ears.

Next, massage the base of the ear to distribute the cleaning solution and to help break up some of the debris. Many dogs will make groaning noises when this is being done. After massaging the ear, use a cotton ball to remove the excess cleaning solution and debris. Cotton tip applicators can be used to remove debris from the grooves on the pinna. Avoid inserting applicators into the ear canal. This can damage the tympanic membrane and pack waxy debris further into the canal. These cleaning steps can be repeated until the ear canal is clean. Repeat with the other ear if

needed. Overcleaning the ear can lead to further irritation of the ear canal (Figure 10.14).

After the ears are clean, you may be asked to apply medication prescribed to the patient. This medication should be placed into the ear canal in the same manner in which the cleaning solution was. Avoid coming in contact with the affected tissue. Be sure to massage the base of the ear to distribute the medication. Repeat if needed.

Eye medications

Administering eye medications is another common exam room procedure. While the veterinarian or veterinary technician will conduct the examination of the eye along with any necessary testing, the veterinary assistant may assist with the application of medications to the eye.

Eye medications can be either an ointment or drops. When applying eye medications, it is important to make sure that the tip of the tube or bottle does not come in contact with the patient's eye. It is also important to make sure the animal is being properly restrained.

The first step is to have the restrainer slightly elevate the animal's nose. With one hand, use your thumb and finger to gently hold open the upper and lower eyelids. With the other hand, hold the bottle of drops or the tube of ointment. Hold the bottle or tube at least 1 inch away from the eye. You will want to rest the palm of your hand on top of the animal's head to help stabilize it. This is a very important step because if the animal moves, you want to make sure your hand moves with it so that the tip does not inadvertently injure the eye.

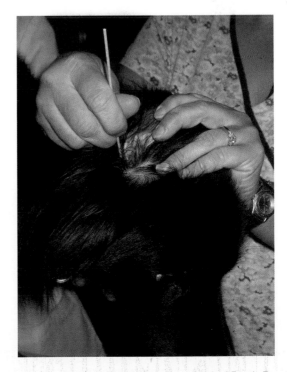

Figure 10.14   Ear cleaning. Source: Courtesy of Dr Lori Renda-Francis, LVT.

If you are administering drops, you would squeeze the bottle so that 1–2 drops of liquid drip on to the eye, making sure you do not touch the eye's surface with the tip. Then close the eye lid and gently massage (Figure 10.15).

If you are administering an ointment, you would then squeeze the ointment into the eye, making sure you do not touch the eye's surface with the tip. Typically, you will administer about ¼–½ inch strip of ointment for most ophthalmic medications. Close the eyelid and gently massage it to allow the ointment to spread over the eye (Figure 10.16).

Anal glands

Clients may indicate that their dog has been "scooting" along the ground or licking its anal area. Many clients misinterpret this as meaning their dogs has worms. Most often this behavior indicates that the dog's anal glands are full and may need to be expressed.

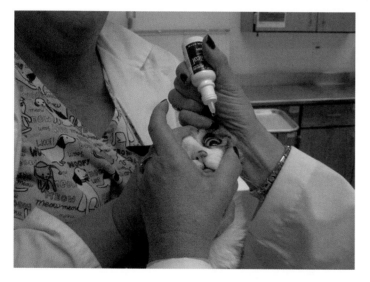

Figure 10.15 Eye drops. Source: Courtesy of Dr Lori Renda-Francis, LVT.

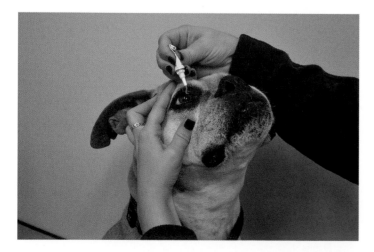

Figure 10.16 Eye ointment. Source: Courtesy of Dr Lori Renda-Francis, LVT.

Anal glands, or sacs as they are sometimes called, are two normal anatomical structures found just inside the rectum of both dogs and cats. These are used as scent glands and are normally expressed when an animal defecates or is frightened. The glands are located at approximately 4–5 o'clock and 7–8 o'clock (Figure 10.17). Normal material within these glands is a tan to yellow fluid which can have a skunk or fish-like odor. This odor is usually what owners describe smelling after their dog has been scooting. Many animals are unable to express these glands due to thickening of the material within the glands, infection, inflammation, or impaction.

There are two ways to express the anal sacs. The first way is external anal sac expression. This method can be performed by the veterinary assistant or veterinary technician. With the dog restrained in a standing position, use a gloved hand and a gauze sponge or paper towel to cover the anus while applying gentle, consistent pressure around the glands. Push inward and toward the opening of the anus at the 4 o'clock and 8 o'clock positions to express both glands at the same time. This should cause the gland to express its contents onto the paper towel or gauze square. You may need to repeat this motion until the gland is completely expressed. You should no longer be able to feel the anal gland once it is emptied. Repeat with the other gland. If the material is too thick to easily express, inform the veterinarian.

The second way to express the anal sacs is through internal anal sac expression. This method should be performed by the veterinary technician. With a gloved hand or the use of a finger cot (Figure 10.18), the veterinary technician will place KY® Jelly or another lubricant on the index finger and insert it into the rectum until the sac can be palpitated with the index finger on the inside

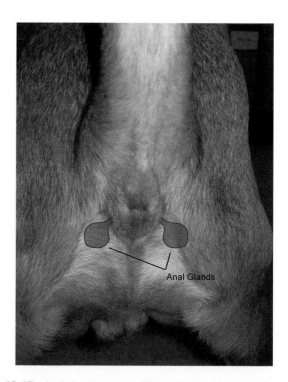

Figure 10.17 Anal gland anatomy. Source: Courtesy of Dr Lori Renda-Francis, LVT.

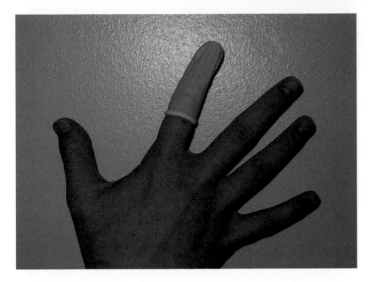

Figure 10.18 Finger cot. Source: Courtesy of Dr Lori Renda-Francis, LVT.

and the thumb on the outside. When the technician feels the entire sac, he or she will gently squeeze and milk the material out of the duct.

Once the glands are expressed, you should clean the *perianal* area with warm water or waterless shampoo. After the area is cleaned, application of an odor minimizing spray is recommended.

The best time to express an animal's anal glands is just prior to bathing. This way the animal can be thoroughly cleaned afterward.

Bathing animals

Bathing an animal is frequently the job of a veterinary assistant. There are a few rules you should follow to ensure a thorough bathing is performed.

Just like humans, dogs do not like to be bathed in water that is too hot or too cold. Aim for water temperature around 70–72 °F. Before starting a bath, apply eye lubricant into the animal's eyes to prevent water or shampoo from running into them and causing irritation. Place cotton balls into the ear canals to prevent water from entering.

It is best to work from the head back when bathing. This will ensure that the entire animal is bathed and no areas are missed. This will also increase your chance of finding fleas if they are present on the animal. Make sure the shampoo you choose is safe for dogs and cats (or puppies and kittens if bathing younger animals). You may be asked by the veterinarian to bathe patient using a medicated shampoo. Make sure you read the shampoo bottle to determine if there are special instructions. Many medicated shampoos must remain on the animal for several minutes before being rinsed.

One of the most important components in bathing an animal is the process of rinsing. To avoid leaving residual shampoo on the patient, it is important to rinse thoroughly. Residual shampoo on the pet may cause itching and dry skin, which may lead to longer-term *dermatological* problems. When rinsing the animal, again work in a head-to-tail direction to ensure all areas are thor-

oughly rinsed. Avoid getting water into the eyes and avoid over-saturating the ear area.

Once the animal is rinsed, you may or may not be asked to apply a cream rinse. If so, follow the above described method for bathing. Once finished, make sure to remove the cotton balls from the ear canals.

When drying the animal, remove as much water as possible using a dry, absorbent towel. Many veterinary hospitals have electric drying fans that can be used to dry the patient quickly. Care must be taken when using these fans. Check on the animal frequently to prevent overheating or burning.

Administering oral medications

When you are ready to administer oral medications, make sure you have all your supplies ready. Also remember to double-check the medication prior to administration to make sure it is the correct medication and the proper dose. Once the medication is given, you will want to immediately record it in the animal's record or chart.

Giving oral medications to a dog

When administering a pill or capsule, have your restrainer gently tilt the animal's chin upward. This causes the jaw muscles to relax and makes it easier to open. It also allows gravity to help keep the pill from falling out. Next wrap your fingers around the top part of the muzzle and press the dog's lips into his teeth, wrapping his lips over the teeth as he opens his mouth. Hold the pill between your thumb and first finger of the hand that is not holding the dog's nose. Drop the pill straight down along the center of the tongue to the very back of the mouth. Quickly close his mouth and hold his head until he has swallowed the medication (Figure 10.19). Be sure to reward with a treat. If he will not swallow the pill, you can try rubbing his throat or tapping on his nose

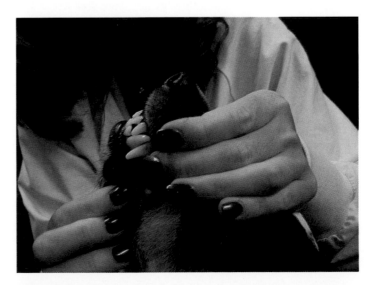

Figure 10.19 Giving oral medication to a dog, Source: Courtesy of Dr Lori Renda-Francis, LVT.

to help facilitate swallowing. It is a good idea to check the dog's mouth after you think that he has swallowed it to ensure that the pill has indeed been swallowed.

If you are giving a liquid medication, you can start off the same way with the head tilted slightly upward. Then place the tip of the syringe in the corner of the dog's mouth, pull at the lip commissure to create a small pocket, and squirt the medication into the space between the cheek and gums (the "cheek pouch"). Insert the liquid medication at the same rate at which he is swallowing. Care should be taken to not squirt the liquid directly into his mouth because we would not want him to inhale it into his lungs (Figure 10.20).

Giving oral medications to a cat

When administering either a pill or liquid, place the cat on a flat surface, and have your restrainer hold onto the body of the cat. If he is wriggly, a towel may be needed to wrap the cat and keep him quiet and comfortable. Use one hand to hold the cat's head. Place your hand over the top of his head. Your thumb and fingers should wrap around the sturdy cheek bones – the cat's head is a triangle or wedge shape, so holding the widest part in your hand allows the greatest amount of control.

If you are giving a liquid medication, place the tip of syringe in the corner of their cat's mouth, and squirt the medication into the space between the cheek and gums (the "cheek pouch"). Hold onto the cat's head until he swallows the medication. Be careful not to squirt the medication in without allowing them to swallow (Figure 10.21).

If you are giving a pill or capsule, hold the pill between the thumb and first finger of the hand that is not holding the cat's head. Use your middle finger to open the cat's mouth by pressing downward on the front of his jaw and then drop the pill straight down along the center of the tongue to the very back of the mouth (Figure 10.22). Close his mouth, and hold his head until he has

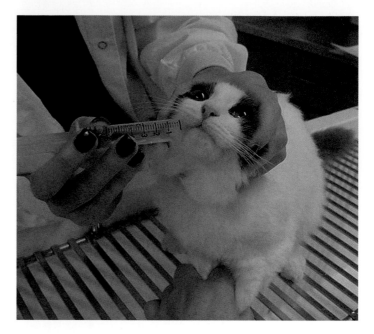

Figure 10.21 Administering liquid medication to a cat. Source: Courtesy of Dr Lori Renda-Francis, LVT.

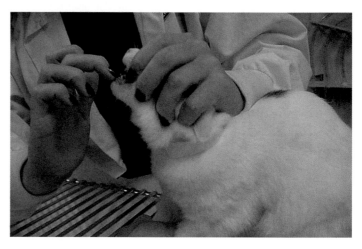

Figure 10.22 Administering a pill or capsule to a cat. Source: Courtesy of Dr Lori Renda-Francis, LVT.

swallowed the medication. If he will not swallow the pill, you can try rubbing his throat or tapping on his nose to help facilitate swallowing. It is a good idea to check the cat's mouth after you think that he has swallowed it to ensure that the pill has actually been swallowed.

Maintaining exam room equipment

Part of the veterinary assistant's responsibility will be to properly care for and maintain commonly used tools and equipment in the exam room. It is important to always follow the manufacturer's instructions for proper care and maintenance. Proper care and maintenance will help insure longevity as well as protecting patients from potential cross-contaminations.

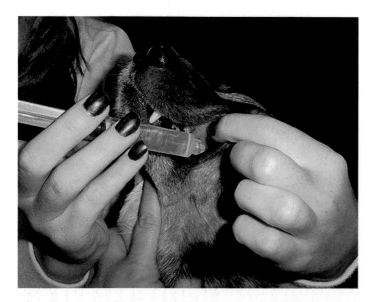

Figure 10.20 Administering liquid medication to a dog. Source: Courtesy of Dr Lori Renda-Francis, LVT.

Ophthalmoscopes and otoscopes

Two common instruments utilized in the exam room are the ophthalmoscope (Figure 10.23) and the otoscope (Figure 10.24). These instruments are usually interchangeable on a single, rechargeable handle (Figure 10.25).

The rechargeable handle should be kept in the instrument case when not in use. It should be stored in the "OFF" position – there will be a single "click" sound as you rotate the ring at the top of the handle, as the small button located there shifts into the raised, "OFF" position. Handles are usually either charged in a charging stand or plugged into the wall. If you are using a charging stand, the flat end

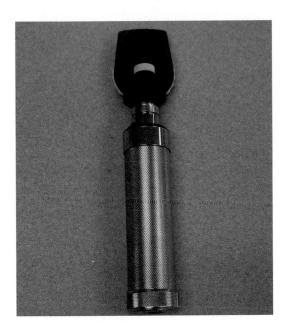

Figure 10.23 Ophthalmoscope. Source: Courtesy of Dr Lori Renda-Francis, LVT.

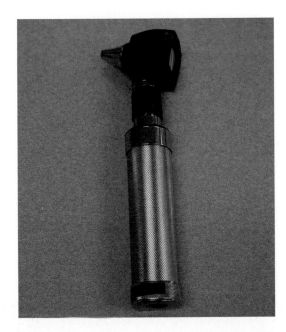

Figure 10.24 Otoscope. Source: Courtesy of Dr Lori Renda-Francis, LVT.

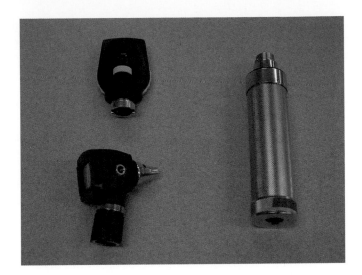

Figure 10.25 Interchangeable handle. Source: Courtesy of Dr Lori Renda-Francis, LVT.

of the handle should be set into the charger and pressed down until the light comes on to indicate that charging has started. If you have a plug-in handle, the top one-third of the handle will unscrew, and beneath, you will find a standard plug. Inert the prongs of the plug into a wall socket, as normal. Handles should be placed in the charging position at the end of each working day. If the instrument is not going to be used for a long period of time, then the battery should be removed to preserve it and prevent leakage. Periodically check the batteries for corrosion or oxidation (rust). The external surface of the handle should be cleaned after each use with a lint-free cloth and 70% alcohol. Check the fit of both the ophthalmoscope head and the otoscope head on the handle to be sure that they snap into place firmly and do not feel loose or wiggle.

The ophthalmoscope head contains the system of condensing apertures and focusing lenses for the eye exam, and a light bulb. When storing the ophthalmic head, the lens disc should be set to the "0" setting, which is just an empty hole, no lens. This protects all the lenses within the head and prevents dust and debris from accumulating on them. Dust should be wiped from the instrument daily. The head should be wiped down after each use with a lint-free cloth and 70% alcohol or 1:10 bleach solution, and thoroughly dried to prevent liquid from entering the head apparatus or drying and leaving a residue on any of the lenses. The lenses should each be wiped with a lint-free cloth or lens paper. Lenses should be routinely checked for cracks or other damage, and the lens selection disc on the side of the head should be checked to ensure that it does not stick or move too freely. This head cannot be repaired so if one lens becomes damaged, the whole head must be replaced. There is a light bulb located in the base of the head that needs periodic replacement. Check to ensure light quality routinely and if the light emitted is dim or flickers, the bulb should be replaced. To replace it, pull the base of the bulb straight out, and press the new bulb straight in. Check to ensure that the light quality is acceptable before putting the ophthalmoscope head back into use.

The otoscope head consists of a light source, a magnification lens, and a variety of removable specula ("ear cones") so that the otoscope can be fitted appropriately to the size of the patient being examined.

The used speculum should be removed from the otoscope head for cleaning. There are several acceptable ways to clean an otoscope speculum; check with your hospital to see what method they prefer. Some will have you wipe down all surfaces with a cotton-tipped applicator, soaked in 70% alcohol. You can push the applicator through the hole in the speculum to remove any debris. This is acceptable cleaning between patients unless an ear infection is present. Another acceptable method is washing thoroughly in hot water to remove visible debris, then soak for 20 minutes in a sterilizing solution, such as chlorhexidine or bleach. Rinse in fresh water and dry thoroughly. Some hospitals have a speculum cleaning instrument which contains several brushes to scrub the specula, and is filled with a disinfectant. If used, this instrument should be cleaned and have the disinfectant solution replaced regularly. For all methods, visually examine the speculum after cleaning to ensure that no debris remains, especially within the small end of the speculum that is placed in the ear.

The exterior of the otoscope head should be cleaned with a lint-free cloth and 70% alcohol or 1:10 bleach solution. The head should be dried thoroughly to prevent excess liquid from damaging or leaving residue on the lens or light source, which can decrease the visibility. The lens should be cleaned with a lint-free cloth or a lens wipe. Ensure that there are no dents in the ring that holds the speculum. There is a light bulb located in the base of the head that needs periodic replacement. Check to ensure light quality routinely and if the light emitted is dim or flickers, the bulb should be replaced. To replace it, pull the base of the bulb straight out and press the new bulb straight in. Check to ensure that the light quality is acceptable before putting the otoscope head back into use.

Thermometer

There are several types of thermometers used in veterinary practice (Figures 10.26 and 10.27). After each use you need to wipe down the probe end of the thermometer with a cotton ball and 70% alcohol. Inspect the probe end to ensure that no fecal material remains. Wipe down the digital end of the thermometer, too. Rinse the probe end in fresh, cool water to remove the alcohol. Air dry the thermometer before storing.

Nail trimmers

Inspect your clippers for signs of rust. Inspect the motion of the clippers for wobbling, stiffness, squeaking, or other signs of poor function. To clean them, wash with soap and water to remove dirt

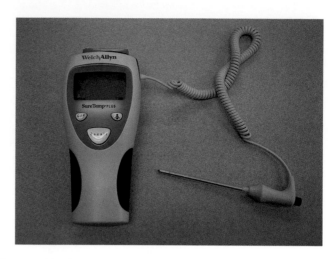
Figure 10.26 Thermometer. Source: Courtesy of Dr Lori Renda-Francis, LVT.

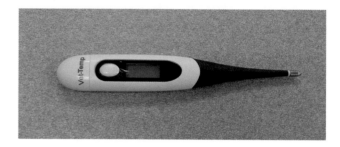
Figure 10.27 Thermometer. Source: Courtesy of Dr Lori Renda-Francis, LVT.

and debris, then wipe down the surface with 70% alcohol and a paper towel. Pay particular attention to the cutting surfaces or blades. This should be done after every use.

Scale

Check the scale for damage, wear and tear on a daily basis, including batteries or AC cord for corrosion, oxidation or bent prongs. Make sure that all four corners of the scale are solidly on the floor and the scale is not right up against the wall. Ensure that the scale reads "0.0" before each use. Clean all surfaces with a clean damp cloth or paper towel to remove debris. Do not immerse the scale in water or liquid cleaning solution. Check your scale's manual as to whether the surface should be cleaned with a disinfectant solution or with mild antimicrobial soap and water only. Some scales require annual professional calibration.

www.wiley.com/go/burns/textbookvetassistant2

Please go to the companion website for assignments and a PowerPoint relating to the material in this chapter.

Chapter 11 Immunology

All veterinary health-care team members should have an understanding of immunology, but this understanding will differ widely among the roles of the veterinary team. It is important for veterinary assistants to have a general understanding of immunology.

The role of the immune system in the body is to eliminate pathogenic agents. Thus, immunity can be described as protection against a certain pathogen. The immune system is composed of cells, tissues, organs, and organ systems functioning as the body's mechanism of defense. This system is viewed as two separate lines of defense – nonspecific and specific (or innate and acquired). There are other terms that can be used interchangeably, but for the purpose of this discussion we will use innate and acquired.

The nonspecific/innate line of defense refers to immunity that the animal is born with and does not possess specific antigen recognition. This includes maternal antibodies from *colostrum* as well as physicochemical barriers (e.g., skin, mucous membranes). The specific/acquired line of defense possesses more definitive specificity of antigen recognition. It is developed or acquired in the body. It should also be stated that innate and acquired immunity interact.

Innate immunity

As explained above, innate immunity (nonspecific) is hereditary or present at birth. Animals are innately immune to certain diseases that affect some species but not others. A number of factors play a role in the ability of the animal to resist pathogens (Box 11.1). These factors respond in the same way each time regardless of the type of pathogen. The first of these factors is the genetic factor which is a result of the animal's species, breed, or strain. The second factor is physical. Certain physical components of the animal's body, providing they are not damaged, will help to create a barrier (external and internal) to prevent an assault on the body. The physical barrier can be broken down into four parts.

- *Skin* – the skin is the largest organ in the body. Sebum is produced by the sebaceous glands, creating an acidic surface pH, which prevents reproduction of pathogenic bacteria and creates a sustainable environment for normal bacteria. Sweat containing antibacterial enzymes is released from the sweat glands.

- *Mucous membranes* – animals produce secretions from their mucous membranes. These secretions act to wash away foreign materials. Tears are produced by the conjunctiva to keep it clear while the respiratory tract produces mucus. Antibacterial enzymes are found in the saliva.

- *Hair* – cilia (microscopic, moving hairs) can be found on the surfaces of epithelial tissues within the body, specifically in the respiratory system. These ciliated mucous epithelia snare bacteria and foreign particles and sweep them away from vulnerable organs.

- *Secretions* – in addition to those secretions discussed above, stomach acids provide an unreceptive environment for ingested pathogens.

The third factor affecting innate immunity is the inflammatory response. Wounds to the body or an infection provoke inflammatory cells in the skin to produce substances that cause the *capillaries* to dilate. Dilated capillaries allow fluid to leak out, resulting

Textbook for the Veterinary Assistant, Second Edition. Kara M. Burns and Lori Renda-Francis.
© 2022 John Wiley & Sons, Inc. Published 2022 by John Wiley & Sons, Inc.
Companion website: www.wiley.com/go/burns/textbookvetassistant2

Box 11.1 Four subclassifications of immunity.

1. Natural active immunity occurs when antibodies are produced by lymphocytes in response to the animal having experienced a certain disease process. Natural active immunity is important for combating viruses. Antibodies produced during the disease process and the subsequent destruction of the antigen allow for lifelong protection.
2. Artificial active immunity occurs when an inactivated form of the disease is introduced into the animal's body. This encourages lymphocytes to produce specific antibodies without causing clinical signs and symptoms. This is the theory behind vaccination. An inactive form of the disease is introduced in the hope that the animal's lymphocytes will produce antibodies to combat the disease, should the animal contract it in the future.
3. Artificial passive immunity occurs when an antiserum (antibodies from another animal) is given to produce immunity to a specific disease. The antiserum is produced within a donor animal and the serum is given to the recipient animal. This is very important for animals with poor immune systems. Animals that have had no prior exposure to disease by infection or vaccination must receive artifi-cial passive immunity in the form of antisera to provide instant protection. These antibodies are foreign to the animal and are subsequently broken down by the animal's immune defense system. If an artificial passive immunity is given to an adult animal (antiserum), protection may last only a few days.
4. Natural passive immunity can be described as the innate ability to respond to some antigens, as is seen in neonates (very young animals). In young animals, the response is slower and weaker compared to older animals because older animals have been exposed to many different antigens and have developed many antibodies. Until a neonate develops the ability to produce antibodies, it is at greater risk of contracting a disease. Neonates get antibodies through the colostrum from the mother which provides protection for approximately 12 weeks. Neonates must ingest the mother's milk soon after birth because they do not have digestive enzymes. This enables the large antibody protein molecules to pass undigested through the intestinal wall and into the bloodstream.

in swelling and redness of the area. Other substances call white blood cells (especially neutrophils) to the area to fight the infection. Thus the inflammatory response is crucial to the eradication of the initial injury or infection.

Acquired immunity

Acquired immunity is, as the name implies, immunity acquired throughout the life of an animal. It is also known as specific immunity and plays a role in combating specific infectious diseases. Specific antibodies must be developed in response to an attack by specific antigens. Antigens are substances that the body recognizes as foreign invaders.

The initial encounter that an animal has with a specific antigen will cause the primary response – production of antibodies to that antigen within 7–10 days. The animal may develop symptoms of the disease, but if the immune system interacts with that pathogen again, the antibodies will be produced within 24 hours, killing the disease prior to symptoms developing. This is known as the secondary response.

Cell-mediated immunity

Cell-mediated immunity relies on cells, specifically lymphocytes. As with antibodies, lymphocytes recognize certain antigens (e.g., fungi, parasites, intracellular bacteria, or tumor cells). Lymphocytes assist in destroying these by **lysing** the infected or cancerous cell or organism.

Vaccination

Veterinary health-care team members base vaccinations of animals on the principles of immunity – passive and active – discussed above (Table 11.1). Vaccinations provide immunity to susceptible animals by introducing a disrupted and harmless version of the pathogen into the body. This causes an immune

Table 11.1 Vaccine terminology.

Antiserum	Serum from an individual previously immunized against an antigen that contains antibodies specific for that antigen.
Active immunity	This refers to an animal's production of antibody as a result of infection with an antigen or immunization.
Passive immunity	This refers to the immunity that is the result of the animal's receiving antibodies from colostrum or synthesized antibodies.
Inactivated vaccine	A vaccine that consists of a noninfectious agent, such as whole killed pathogens or selected antigenic subunits in sufficient amount to induce immunity.
Recombinant vaccine	A vaccine that consists of a live, nonpathogenic virus into which the gene for a pathogen-related antigen has been inserted.
Toxoid	Inactivated antigenic toxin molecules that stimulate development of the animal's own antibodies.
Vaccine	A biological product representing a pathogenic organism that stimulates immunity toward the pathogen.

response without the development of clinical signs. The theory is that vaccination of the animal will protect it from developing clinical symptoms when it is naturally exposed to the disease.

The veterinary team has vaccines available to protect companion animal and equine patients against common infectious diseases. Currently, veterinary teams protect patients with three types of vaccines: live attenuated vaccine, killed vaccine, or recombinant vaccine. The live attenuated (modified-live) vaccine uses live organisms that have been attenuated (weakened) by culturing the pathogen in controlled conditions. The result is a stimulation of the immune response. Live attenuated vaccines can cause the disease but typically only mild clinical signs will be observed.

Killed vaccines contain dead organisms that have been killed by ultraviolet, heat, or sublethal chemicals. The dead organisms cannot divide within the body so repeated doses are needed to produce sufficient levels of antibodies within the animal. A recombinant vaccine can be made up of a live nonpathogenic virus into which the gene for a pathogen-related antigen has been inserted. The virus is injected into the animal and the viral genes, including the inserted gene for the antigen of concern, are expressed. The animal produces antibodies to the specific pathogen without ever having been exposed.

Young animals with an underdeveloped immune system may require 2–3 injections before a vaccination can provide protection. Typically, vaccinations for young animals follow this schedule.

1. The vaccine should be given as maternal antibody levels begin to decrease, resulting in antibodies forming in the young animal. The first vaccine should be administered to puppies at 6 weeks of age and to kittens at 8 weeks of age.

2. A second vaccine dose should be administered 2–3 weeks later. This will result in the production of antibodies in a shorter time frame, typically within 12–24 hours.

3. One year later, a booster vaccine should be administered to increase the production of antibodies to the vaccination.

Vaccine administration routes

Vaccinations are given to animals by one of the following routes: *subcutaneous*, *intranasal*, or oral. The subcutaneous route is the most common, and the American Animal Hospital Association (AAHA) guidelines for subcutaneous injection routes should be followed. Sterile equipment must be used when vaccinating an animal. The nasal route of vaccination involves placing drops into the external nares (nostrils) using a modified syringe. These vaccinations create local antibody and cell-mediated immunity, especially in respiratory diseases. This type of vaccination may be difficult to administer in *brachycephalic* breeds due to their shorter nose and muzzle. Proper handling and restraint of these animals must be undertaken by the veterinary health-care team member. The oral route of vaccination is rare, but has been used with some vaccines in Europe.

Vaccines must be stored in the refrigerator and shipped on ice at 2–4 °C or 35.6–39.2 °F. The microorganisms within a live vaccine will be killed by warm temperatures.

Veterinary assistants should be familiar with potential causes of vaccination failure. These causes include but are not limited to:

- expiry date of vaccine has passed
- improper storage
- incorrectly administered vaccine
- inaccurate timing of the vaccination schedule
- excessive use of alcohol or disinfectant on the skin prior to vaccination.

All health-care team members must be aware of the risk of an allergic reaction, potentially leading to *anaphylaxis*, when any foreign substance is introduced. Veterinary health-care team members must also educate the pet owner on the signs of an adverse reaction and give complete instructions, including an emergency phone number to call, should any adverse reactions and/or questions arise following a vaccination. Symptoms the veterinary health-care team and the owner should be looking for are as follows:

- swelling
- redness
- rash or hives
- gastrointestinal signs – vomiting, diarrhea
- depression
- lethargy
- ataxia
- shock
- respiratory distress.

There is also a concern regarding the apparent association between vaccines and a particular type of cancer (sarcoma) at the injection site in cats. As this concern has increased and more research has been conducted, the American Association of Feline Practitioners has issued a recommendation that different vaccines be given at different locations on the feline body. The current recommendation is that feline leukemia virus vaccine (FeLV) be given in the left hindlimb as distally as possible and rabies vaccine given in the right hindlimb as distally as possible. Vaccines used to be given in the scruff but this is no longer recommended. The new guidelines will help the team and manufacturer to track the vaccine type, vaccination date, and vaccine location, so if an injection site tumor develops the team and manufacturer can trace it back to the vaccine itself.

Vaccinations help to prevent certain diseases through the regular administration of the vaccine and owner education about the disease. All veterinary health-care team members should be familiar with the guidelines and protocols of the administration of vaccinations to pets.

- AAHA canine vaccination guidelines: www.aaha.org/aaha-guidelines/vaccination-canine-configuration/vaccination-recommendations-for-general-practice/
- AAHA feline vaccination guidelines: www.aaha.org/globalassets/02-guidelines/feline-vaccination-guidlines/resource-center/2020-aahaa-afp-feline-vaccination-guidelines.pdf

References

Centonze, V. 2011. Pathology, response to disease, and preventive medicine. In: *Principles and Practice of Veterinary Technology*, 3rd edition. Sirois, M. (ed.). Elsevier, St Louis, MO.

Dingle, H., Rock, A. 2006. Prevention of the spread of infectious disease. In: *The Complete Textbook of Veterinary Nursing*, Aspinal, V. (ed.). Elsevier Butterworth Heinemann, London.

Kennedy, M.A. 2010. Review of basics of immunology: the innate and adaptive response. *Veterinary Clinics of North America Small Animal Practice*, 40, 369–380.

McVey, S., Shi, I. 2010. Vaccines in veterinary medicine: a brief review of history and technology. *Veterinary Clinics of North America Small Animal Practice*, 40, 381–392.

Sirois, M. 2011. Clinical chemistry and serology. In: *Principles and Practice of Veterinary Technology*, 3rd edition. Sirois, M. (ed.). Elsevier, St Louis, MO.

www.wiley.com/go/burns/textbookvetassistant2

Please go to the companion website for assignments and a PowerPoint relating to the material in this chapter.

Chapter 12 Laboratory Procedures

Laboratory considerations

Many of the daily tasks that are the responsibility of veterinary technicians and veterinary assistants fall within the laboratory setting. Whether the laboratory testing is done in house or is sent to a reference laboratory, the veterinary assistant plays a role. Many factors influence the variety of procedures performed in an in-house laboratory: equipment, team member expertise, financial restrictions, and amount of time available, to name a few.

The veterinary assistant works with the credentialed veterinary technician to obtain and prepare samples, perform tests, and record results. An additional duty would be to assist in the preparation of samples when utilizing a commercial reference laboratory. Furthermore, an increased awareness of the significance of the results is expected, which can have an impact on the nursing care provided to the patient.

Laboratory diagnostic testing provides invaluable tools for the care and wellbeing of the veterinary patient in the following aspects.

- *Assists with accurate diagnosis* – diagnostic procedures/laboratory tests help the veterinarian to make a definitive diagnosis.
- *Assess the severity of a condition* – this assessment may influence the choice of treatment and the ensuing recovery of the patient.
- *Assess response to treatment* – this assessment provides understanding in regard to the patient's progress.

Additionally, the veterinary hospital's laboratory is an area where significant revenue may be generated, so it is recommended to perform as many diagnostic tests as possible in house. To do this, the veterinary assistant must have knowledge of procedures, equipment, and the tests being performed. Most diagnostic tests can be performed in house by well-trained veterinary support staff. Today's in-house laboratories have become increasingly advanced with affordable analytic instruments.

Safety

The veterinary hospital laboratory has many potential hazards of which the veterinary assistant needs to be aware. Some of these potential hazards include, but are not limited, to the following.

- Biological agents
- Chemicals, with the potential to be toxic or corrosive
- Sharp objects
- Toxic fumes
- Eye contaminants
- Zoonoses
- Fire

Hazard warning signs should be used as they give clear indications of potential dangers in the laboratory.

A safety program for the in-house laboratory is vital to ensure the safety of the veterinary healthcare team. Systematic laboratory practices which are required to be integrated into the hospital laboratory safety policy are mandated by the Occupational Safety and Health Administration (OSHA; www.osha.gov/laws-regs). The hospital safety policy must include procedures and precautions for the use and preservation of equipment. Safety equipment and supplies such as the following must be available:

- eyewash stations
- fire extinguishers
- spill clean-up kits

Textbook for the Veterinary Assistant, Second Edition. Kara M. Burns and Lori Renda-Francis.
© 2022 John Wiley & Sons, Inc. Published 2022 by John Wiley & Sons, Inc.
Companion website: www.wiley.com/go/burns/textbookvetassistant2

- hazardous and biohazard waste disposal containers
- proper PPE.

Health-care team members working in the laboratory need to know the location of the items and must be trained in their proper use. The veterinary hospital must have laboratory safety policies in writing and the policy manual must be located in an accessible spot in the laboratory area. In addition, employees must be notified that eating, drinking, applying cosmetics, and adjusting contact lenses in the laboratory are prohibited. Signage to this effect should be visible.

Observe safety guidelines

It is important to observe safety guidelines when working in the laboratory to ensure the hospital teams' health and safety.

- Wear a long-sleeved laboratory coat, gloves, mask (where necessary), and eye protection at all times.
- Wear minimum jewelry.
- Ensure a wash basin/sink reserved for hand washing is available along with antibacterial soap and disposable paper towels.
- Wash hands when entering or departing the laboratory.
- All work surfaces should be cleaned and disinfected daily and after every hazardous procedure.
- As soon as you have finished with equipment, clean it and store it away to avoid accidents.
- Samples and contaminated equipment should be disposed of safely and properly.
- Sharps containers and clinical waste bags must be available in the laboratory at all times.
- If hazardous chemicals are used, take note of warning labels and act accordingly.
- Many bacteria are potential pathogens and should be handled in a contained environment such as a safety cabinet.
- Know where the first aid kit is stored, what action to take in an emergency, and be familiar with the incident protocols.
- List all procedures in a laboratory manual so that all team members use the same methodologies.

Equipment

The diagnostic tests which are routinely performed in the hospital laboratory will frequently dictate which equipment is needed. At a minimum, the following will be needed:

- glassware
- microscope
- clinical centrifuge
- microhematocrit centrifuge
- refractometer
- blood chemistry analyzer
- cell counters.

Glassware

Glassware is commonly found in veterinary laboratories. Glassware is used to measure and hold reagents and samples. The type of glassware that is most common is borosilicate glass (Pyrex®) as it is harder than ordinary glass.

It is important that all glassware is thoroughly cleaned to remove any contaminated material that might interfere with the accuracy of the tests. New glassware should always be washed before use.

Cleaning glassware

- Rubber gloves should be worn.
- Contaminated glassware should be soaked in an approved disinfectant for 24 hours prior to cleaning.
- Any residues should be removed with the aid of a soft bristle brush. The glassware should then be washed in commercial laboratory detergent, following the manufacturer's instructions, or in an ultrasonic bath.
- The glassware should then be rinsed thoroughly two or three times in distilled/deionized water to remove all traces of the cleaning solution, which could affect the accuracy of results.
- The glassware should be allowed to drain and then dried in a drying cabinet. Bottles should not be dried with their stoppers in place, as the water will not evaporate.
- Once dry, the glassware should be stored in a cupboard or drawer to protect it from dust, grease, and possible damage.
- The same method should be adopted to clean plasticware, although cooler water should be used. Organic solvents should be avoided as they could cause damage.
- Pipettes can prove difficult to clean, especially if left, but must be thoroughly cleaned.

Microscope

A binocular compound light microscope is a key piece of laboratory equipment. Microscopes are used to examine a variety of specimens: blood, urine, semen, exudates, transudates, other body fluids, feces, etc. Microscopes are also utilized in identifying internal and external parasites and initially to characterize bacteria.

A compound light microscope produces an image by using a combination of lenses. Compound light microscopes are made up of many interacting pieces (Figure 12.1) along with a light path. The stage and slide holder keep the glass slide to be evaluated in place. Depending on user preferences, left- or right-handed stages are obtainable. Focus knobs, both coarse and fine focus, are used for just that – focusing the image of the glass slide being viewed.

The ocular system and the objective system make up the two systems of the compound light microscope. The ocular lenses are found in the eyepieces. Typically they have a magnification of 10×,

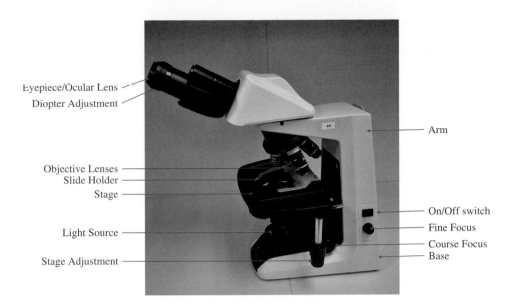

Eyepiece/Ocular Lens
Diopter Adjustment

Arm

Objective Lenses
Slide Holder
Stage

On/Off switch
Fine Focus

Light Source

Course Focus
Base

Stage Adjustment

Figure 12.1 Binocular microscope. Courtesy of Lori Renda-Francis, LVT, PhD

which means the ocular lens provides 10 times the magnification of an object. A monocular microscope has one eyepiece; a binocular microscope has two eyepieces. The binocular microscope is the most commonly used type of microscope. The binocular head is necessary for many routine laboratory evaluations. The majority of compound light microscopes also include three or four objective lenses providing different magnification power. Typically the veterinary laboratory microscope includes the following objective lenses: 4× (scanning), 10× (low power), 40× (high dry), and 100× (oil immersion).

Total magnification of the object being viewed is calculated by multiplying the ocular magnification power by the objective magnification power.

It is important for the veterinary team member to acclimate themselves to the "reverse" views obtained when using a compound light microscope. The object in view appears upside down and reversed. Additionally, the actual right side of an image is viewed as its left side, and the actual left side is viewed as its right side. Mechanical stage movement (and thus movement of the slide) is also reversed.

Microscope care

All team members should follow the manufacturer's recommendations for use and routine maintenance of the microscope. Important care tips include the following.

- Use high-quality lens tissue to clean the lenses.
- Wipe the microscope clean after every use.
- Keep microscope covered when not in use.
- Clean the eyepiece with lens paper.
- Cleaning and adjustment by a microscope professional should be performed at least annually.
- Always have extra light bulbs available.

Centrifuge

A centrifuge is a machine with a rapidly rotating container that applies **centrifugal force** to its contents, to separate fluids of different densities or liquids from solids.

As a rotor spins in a centrifuge, a centrifugal force is applied to each particle in the sample; the particle will then sediment at the rate proportional to the centrifugal force applied to it. The **viscosity** of the sample solution and the physical properties of the particles also affect the sedimentation rate of each particle.

If the sample is made up of solid and liquid parts, the liquid portion is known as the supernatant and the solid component is known as the sediment. The supernatant, such as plasma or serum from a blood sample, can be removed from the sediment and stored, shipped, or analyzed.

Veterinary practice laboratories often have more than one type of centrifuge. The microhematocrit centrifuge is designed to hold capillary tubes, whereas a clinical centrifuge accommodates test tubes of varying sizes.

Clinical centrifuges typically used in the veterinary laboratory are differentiated by the head of the centrifuge. Most often, the veterinary team will use either a centrifuge with a horizontal centrifuge head (swinging arm) or an angled centrifuge head.

Samples/specimens are centrifuged at a precise speed for a certain time for maximal accuracy. Care must be taken to not run a centrifuge too fast or too long. Doing so risks rupturing cells and destroying the morphological features of cells in the sediment. Conversely, a centrifuge that runs too slowly or does not run long enough may result in the specimen not completely separating or concentrating the sediment. Information regarding speed and time of centrifugation should be developed for all laboratory procedures and followed for maximal accuracy.

Refractometer

A refractometer measures the refractive index of a solution. Light rays bend as they pass from one medium into another medium with a different optical density; this is known as refraction. The degree of refraction results from the concentration of solid material in the medium. Refractometers are calibrated to a zero reading (zero refractive index) with distilled water at a temperature between 60°F and 100°F (15.6°C and 37.8°C). Refractometers are used in the veterinary hospital most often to determine the specific gravity of urine or other fluids along with the protein concentration of plasma or other fluids. It is important for veterinary assistants to remember that refractometers are delicate optical instruments which need to have proper care to ensure precise results.

Refractometers must be cleaned after each use. This involves wiping dry the prism cover glass and cover plate. Lens tissue must be utilized to protect the optical surfaces from scratches. Always consult the manufacturer's cleaning instructions.

Quality control

Cleaning and maintenance of instruments and equipment are essential in order to extend the life of the instrument/equipment and to avoid downtime, which is not economical. All equipment comes with a manual listing all components which require inspection and regular maintenance. The veterinary hospital should keep a notebook scheduling the maintenance required for each piece of equipment. Ensure each instrument has its own page and includes the following information.

- Instrument name
- Serial number
- Model number
- Purchase date
- Points to be checked
- Frequency of checks
- Record of test readings
- Changes made to restore accuracy and precision of readings
- Cost and time associated with necessary repairs and restoration
- Name or initials of the person performing the maintenance

Results obtained from this maintenance should be recorded in the notebook *and* kept in a permanent record.

Sample collection

Blood

Examining blood samples aids the veterinary team by providing invaluable understanding regarding the health status of a patient. In addition, blood samples aid in diagnosis, monitoring response to treatment, and gauging the severity of disease conditions.

Venipuncture is used to collect blood samples and involves the use of a syringe and needle. The veterinary assistant helps in this process by assembling the proper equipment prior to the team member taking the blood sample. The correct needle gauge should be selected with the following in mind: use the largest gauge with the shortest length possible. This allows for the sample to be taken promptly and reduces potential damage to the red blood cells. Clippers and an appropriate disinfectant swab/wipe to clean the site, along with the appropriate blood collection tube, should be close at hand.

The following steps allow for proper collection technique and handling.

1. Handling and restraint for venipuncture are dependent upon the species and sampling site. Manual restraint is usually adequate for restraining dogs and cats. If the patient is fearful or aggressive, we should employ Fear Free® handling techniques to ensure the safety of the team member and patient. In some instances, sedation may be required, especially if working with exotic species.

2. All equipment should be assembled prior to collection, and the sample tube labeled with the correct information for identifying the sample and patient.

3. Once the animal is properly restrained by the veterinary assistant, the venipuncture site should be clipped and cleaned with an appropriate medium to ensure asepsis.

4. The **proximal** part of the vein needs to be **occluded**, thus making the vein easier to visualize and prevent the blood from returning to the heart. "Raising the vein" occurs when the vein is "held off" typically by the individual restraining.

5. While tensing the skin over the venipuncture site, the needle should be inserted at a shallow angle. Once in the vein, pull back slowly on the syringe plunger to ensure the blood is not subjected to excessive pressure. Excessive pressure could damage red blood cells and lead to collapse of the vein.

6. Once the required volume has been obtained, the needle is carefully removed from the vein. The assistant should then apply pressure on the injection site to prevent bleeding.

7. Transfer the blood sample quickly to the previously selected sample tube.

8. If the sample is transferred to a sample tube containing **anticoagulant**, ensure the blood is gently squirted into the tube to the fill line to ensure proper dilution of the anticoagulant; the bottle should then be inverted or rolled to mix the contents. Avoid violent shaking as this can damage the red blood cells.

9. The time of the sample should be written on the prelabeled sample tube.

10. Dispose of any waste properly.

Following this protocol helps to ensure the red blood cells will not be damaged and release their hemoglobin and potassium into the

Table 12.1 Anticoagulants and cap colors.

Anticoagulant	Test	Tube cap color
Ethylenediaminetetraacetic acid (EDTA)	Routine hematology	Purple
Heparin	Biochemistry	Green
Sodium citrate	Coagulation profiles	Blue
No anticoagulant	Biochemistry	Red

plasma. The rupture of red blood cells is known as hemolysis. You will know if hemolysis occurs as the plasma or serum will be pink in color. Hemolysis will ruin all the tests used in hematology with the exception of total white blood cell counts and hemoglobin levels. The presence of free hemoglobin also interferes with biochemical tests. Thus, it is essential to avoid hemolysis.

Hematology is the study of the physical characteristics and the number of cells per unit volume in blood. To perform hematology, the blood sample must not be allowed to clot. To prevent the blood from clotting, the clotting process must be halted by the addition of chemicals immediately on collection of the blood sample.

Anticoagulants fall into two categories.

- Those that block calcium – ethylenediaminetetraacetic acid (EDTA), oxalates, citrates, and fluorides.
- Those that interfere with the enzyme systems – heparin and fluorides.

Table 12.1 lists the anticoagulants and their assigned tube cap colors.

Urine

Urine can be a potentially hazardous substance and thus, PPE in the form of protective disposable gloves should be worn when collecting urine and analyzing patient urine. Preferably, the urine sample should be sterile, but this can only be achieved through cystocentesis.

Techniques used to collect urine are as follows.

Voided, free flow
- Midstream overnight sample.
  - Best for routine urinalysis.
  - Best indicator of the true composition of urine.
- First stream of urine.
  - Best sample to collect for lesions low in the urethral tract.
  - Most likely to be contaminated.
- End stream.
  - Best to collect for examination for prostatic disease, hemorrhage, or sediment that might have collected on the floor of the bladder.

- Use a well-cleaned container to collect the sample and then transfer to a sterile container.
- Commercial sterile collection kits are available.

Manual expression
- Convenient if bladder contains enough urine to be isolated manually on palpation of the abdomen.
- Take care to prevent undue pressure rupturing the bladder.

Catheterization
- *Aseptic* passage of a tube into the urethra to collect urine directly from the bladder.
- Potential for introduction of bacteria from the urethra into the bladder and nosocomial infections.

Cystocentesis
- Passage of a needle through the abdominal wall and into the bladder.
- Delivers the best sample for culture of bacterial growth and antibiotic sensitivity.

Preservation
It is best to examine the urine sample as soon after collection as possible. Immediate examination is ideal and it should definitely be performed within an hour after collection. Not doing so results in the growth of bacteria which will cause decomposition of the urea and the production of ammonia. This, being alkaline, will elevate the pH of the sample. This will then enable the development of phosphates, which interferes with subsequent testing. If testing of the urine sample cannot be performed quickly, it is recommended to refrigerate the sample. Do not freeze the sample.

If refrigeration is not possible, chemical preservatives may be used. Formalin or thymol are two preservatives used but the most common chemical preservative used in the veterinary hospital is boric acid. This will preserve and inhibit bacteria growth for ~4 days. In addition, it helps to maintain cells and urinary casts. It is commercially available in red-capped specimen containers.

Urine physical properties
The physical properties, including color, odor, turbidity, pH, and specific gravit,y should be observed at the beginning.

Urochrome is the pigment responsible for the color of normal urine. Typically, it is yellow and the depth of color is indicative of the urine's concentration. There is variation in the depth of color with the spectrum going from almost colorless to a darkish brown. This variation is a result of a number of factors: urine concentration, diet, species, breed, and exercise regimen.

Abnormal colors may be the result of:

- presence of blood, hemoglobin or myoglobin – reveal a red/pink urine color
- bile pigments – result is orange urine

- drugs
- food.

The odor of normal urine typically is sour. In stale urine ammonia may be smelt. If the urine is fresh, ammonia may be due to the presence of urease-producing bacteria (commonly involved in cystitis). Male animals, as opposed to females, often produce very strong-smelling urine – this is especially true in cats. This is important in territorial scent marking. Animals with diabetes mellitus may produce a sweet and fruity urine that smells of pear drops. This is due to the presence of ketone bodies and occurs in unstable DM patients. This can also be smelt on the breath of ketoacidotic animals.

Urine is usually clear. The presence of mucus, pus, and vaginal or prostatic secretions can make the urine turbidity appear abnormal.

pH is the expression of the hydrogen ion concentration in a volume of liquid. A pH above 7.0 is alkaline while a pH below 7.0 is acidic. False pH results may occur if the urine sample is not kept cool and covered. Veterinary team members should remember that urine pH is affected by diet in that carnivorous animals have acid urine, while herbivorous animals have alkaline urine.

Normal pH:

- dog 5.2–6.8
- cat 6.0–7.0.

Acidic urine = *pyrexia*, *acidosis*, high-protein diets, starvation, diabetes mellitus, and muscle *catabolism*.

Alkaline urine = urinary retention or infection, *alkalosis*, a diet with high vegetable content, or certain medications.

Urine pH can be determined by pH papers, multireagent dipsticks, or electrode pH meters.

Specific gravity is the density of a known volume of a fluid compared with an equal volume of distilled water. Distilled water has a specific gravity of 1.000.

Normal specific gravity:

- dog 1.015–1.045
- cat 1.020–1.040.

A single measurement of specific gravity should not be taken as conclusive, as the specific gravity of urine varies considerably, even within the same individual. A finding of elevated specific gravity may be the result of dehydration or lack of fluid intake. Lower levels of specific gravity are seen in conditions such as *diabetes insipidus*, chronic renal failure, or different causes of polydipsia.

Feces

Fecal samples provide excellent insight into the health and functioning of the gastrointestinal system. Fecal samples aid in a diagnosis of endoparasites, viral disease, and gastrointestinal disease.

Fecal samples can be collected in two ways: directly from the rectum, or feces that have been passed. A prelabeled sample container should be used. Also, there are specific fecal sample containers which may be used. These contain a spatula-like tool

attached to the inside of the lid to aid in collection. Some bacteria and viruses can be intermittently "shed" into the feces of the animal. If this is suspected, the veterinary team member should collect a 3-day pooled sample. To do this, a small portion of feces should be collected for 3 consecutive days and placed in the sample container. Then the collection of feces samples is thoroughly mixed together before any tests are performed.

Feces content will be a direct result of the diet that the animal consumes. Thus it is important, when submitting a fecal sample for analysis, to mention the patient's diet on the laboratory submission form.

Fecal sample evaluation can be divided into gross or macroscopic examination, which entails assessment of the overall appearance (consistency, odor, color, mucus, and parasites), and microscopic examination which helps to detect parasites, bacterial or yeast infections, and assessment of impaired digestion or absorption of the digestive system.

Analysis of feces

Most endoparasites produce eggs or larvae which pass out of the body in the host's feces. It is important for the veterinary assistant to be familiar with fecal flotation and how to perform this method of parasite determination.

Fecal flotation

When performing a fecal floatation, be sure to mix stool material with a solution (often sodium nitrate) that is more dense than the eggs of the worms. This allows for the parasite eggs to float to the surface. The eggs are collected from the surface using a glass slide. The slide is examined under a microscope, and the appearance of the eggs identifies what type of adult parasite is present (Figures 12.2–12.4).

All that is needed is about a 1-inch piece of fresh stool. Preferably, the sample should be as fresh as possible and not more than 24 hours old. Additionally, it should be as free as possible of grass, gravel, kitty litter, etc.

Recording samples and test reports

It is crucial that the sample taken be correctly linked with the patient from which it was taken. It is also important that the tests required are linked with the sample provided and the results of the tests performed linked with those requested and the sample itself. If each stage of the process is recorded accurately immediately upon completion, this should not be a problem.

Protocol

Collect the sample and place in a prelabeled container. This container should be labeled with the owner's name and address and the patient's name or, if computerized, labeled with a reference number identifying the patient, specimen, and pet owner. Ensure the type of sample tube or container to be used is verified prior to the sample being collected, as different tests will require different preservatives.

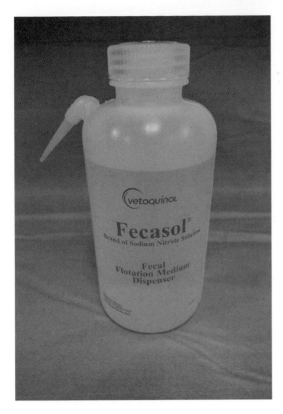

Figure 12.2   When performing a fecal floatation, be sure to mix stool material with a solution (often sodium nitrate) that is denser than the eggs of the worms

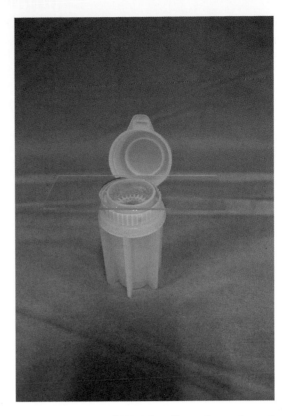

Figure 12.4   The eggs are collected from the surface using a glass slide. The slide is examined under a microscope, and the appearance of the eggs identifies what type of adult parasite is present.

- Age and gender (including neuter status) of the patient
- A description of the sample(s)
- A clinical history and provisional diagnosis from the veterinarian
- Details of any medication the patient is currently prescribed
- The tests required
- The date the sample was taken
- Additional information beneficial to the interpretation of the results (e.g., fasted sample, time medications were last given, etc.).

Note that histology samples should be accompanied by a chart indicating the sample sites.

Upon receipt of the sample at the laboratory, a reference number should be assigned (if not already given earlier in the process) and this number should be placed on the form and all equipment, e.g., microscope slides, tubes, etc. This ensures the laboratory request form accompanying the sample is clearly marked to decrease any confusion regarding the samples and to whom they belong. This is especially important when tests are undertaken on multiple samples. Many veterinary hospitals link the laboratory equipment to the practice management system, thus allowing for automatic download of the results to the patient's medical record.

Test results should then be reported to the veterinarian. This can be in the form of the laboratory report form or printout, or a communication to say that the results are available in the patient's

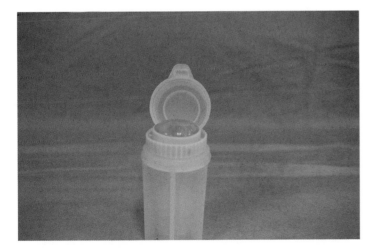

Figure 12.3   This allows for the parasite eggs to float to the surface

It is important to remember that laboratory request forms should be completed, regardless of whether the tests are to be performed in house or sent to a laboratory. Typically, the request form includes the following.

- Vet hospital name and address
- The name of the veterinarian who ordered the laboratory diagnostic and to whom the results should be returned
- Pet owner's name and address
- Name, species, and breed of the patient

medical record. Commercial reference laboratories can also email or fax the interpretation of the results. In the case of email, generally these will automatically attach to the patient's clinical history via the practice management system.

Again, notification that the results have been returned should be given to the veterinarian and any other appropriate team members and also recorded on the patient's records immediately on receipt if sent by fax. Communicating the results to the client is usually undertaken by the veterinarian or credentialed veterinary technician if so directed.

References

Allan, L., Ackerman, N. 2016. Laboratory diagnostic aids. In: *Aspinall's Complete Textbook of Veterinary Nursing*, 3rd edition. Ackerman, N., Aspinall, A. (eds). Elsevier, London, pp. 637–664.

Fisher, M. 2016. Parasitology. In: *Aspinall's Complete Textbook of Veterinary Nursing*, 3rd edition. Ackerman, N., Aspinall, A. (eds). Elsevier, London, pp. 595–623.

Sirois, M. 2020. Laboratory procedures. In: *Elsevier's Veterinary Assisting Textbook*, 3rd edition. Elsevier, St Louis, MO.

www.wiley.com/go/burns/textbookvetassistant2

Please go to the companion website for assignments and a PowerPoint relating to the material in this chapter.

Chapter 13 Pharmacology

The study of drugs and their effect on living organisms is known as pharmacology. Clinical pharmacology is concerned with the effects of drugs in treating disease. Simply put, the term "drug" describes any chemical agent that has a specific effect on the body. Although the veterinary assistant typically does not play a role in administering drugs to a patient, it is important for all members of the health-care team to understand the types and actions of drugs used in the veterinary patient.

Drugs are prescribed for use in the diagnosis, treatment, or prevention of disease in humans or animals. A **veterinary drug** has been approved for the diagnosis, treatment, or prevention of disease in animals. The majority of drugs utilized in veterinary medicine are actually human drugs that have been found to be effective in managing veterinary patients as well.

It is of the utmost importance for veterinary assistants to review the chapter on restraint, as restraining patients is a very important responsibility for veterinary assistants, especially when the health-care team is administering medications to a patient. Some administration of medications may startle (injection) or elicit pain in the patient. Therefore, proper restraint and technique are imperative.

All health-care team members should grasp the terms used in pharmacology and administration of medications to patients. Table 13.1 defines the terms.

Plants and minerals are traditional sources of drugs. The active components in plants are useful as drugs. These components are alkaloids, glycosides, gums, oils, and resins. Alkaloids typically end in –ine, with glycoside names ending in –in. Some of the more commonly known alkaloids are caffeine and atropine. Glycoside examples are digoxin and digitoxin. Bacteria and molds are utilized when producing many antibiotics and anthelmintics (dewormers). Electrolytes make up the mineral sources of drugs in addition to such minerals as iron and selenium.

For the drug to have the desired effect, it must reach the target tissue. If the proper route of administration is not used, the amount of drug reaching the target tissue may be extremely altered. The administration route refers to how a drug enters the body. Drugs with systemic actions whose route of administration is oral (per os or PO) must cross the gastrointestinal lining of the stomach or small intestine. Drugs given through an injection are known as parenterally administered drugs. Parenteral administration can be intravenous (IV), where the drug is injected into a vein, or intraarterial, where the drug is injected into an artery. IV injection allows the blood containing the drug to pass through the heart and mix with the blood in circulation before being delivered to the body tissues. Intraarterial injections allow for fast, high concentrations of the drug in tissues supplied by that specific artery. Intramuscular injections (IM) allow for the administration of drugs directly into the muscle mass. Subcutaneous injections (SQ, SC) are given beneath the skin, into the subcutis. Intraperitoneal injections (IP) are given in the abdominal cavity. These are typically used when IV or IM injections do not suffice or when a large volume of solution needs to be given to insure rapid absorption.

Drugs go through a development and testing process before being approved for use by the appropriate government agency. This process is lengthy and time intensive and the results are typically sent for approval to the US Food and Drug Administration (FDA). Upon approval, a drug will be designated as either an over-the-counter (OTC) drug or a prescription drug. OTC drugs are those medicines that do not need a prescription. OTC drugs are considered safe for use without the supervision of a veterinarian or physi-

Textbook for the Veterinary Assistant, Second Edition. Kara M. Burns and Lori Renda-Francis.
© 2022 John Wiley & Sons, Inc. Published 2022 by John Wiley & Sons, Inc.
Companion website: www.wiley.com/go/burns/textbookvetassistant2

Table 13.1 Pharmacology terms and definitions.

Term	Definition
Indication	Reason for using a drug
Contraindication	Reasons to not use a drug
Pharmacokinetics	Physiological response and movement of a drug in the body
Pharmacodynamics	How drugs exert their effect
Toxicity	Manifestations of adverse drug reactions

cian. The caveat is that the OTC drug is safe if the directions on the label are followed. Prescription drugs are to be used under the supervision of a veterinarian – these require a prescription. However, before a veterinarian can prescribe a drug for a patient, a valid veterinarian–client–patient–relationship (VCPR) must be in place.

The FDA Code of Federal Regulations Title 21 CFR 530.3(i) defines the components of a valid VCPR as follows.

1. A licensed veterinarian has accepted the responsibility for making medical judgments regarding the health of an animal and the need for medical treatment. Additionally, the pet owner has agreed to follow the directions of the veterinarian.

2. There is sufficient knowledge of the animal by the veterinarian to initiate a general or preliminary diagnosis of said animal's medical condition.

3. The veterinarian is readily available for follow-up in the event of an adverse reaction or should the therapy regimen not be successful.

This relationship can exist only when the veterinarian has recently seen and is familiar with the keeping and care of the animal through examination and/or by medically appropriate and timely visits to where the animal is kept.

Drugs typically have three different names: chemical, general (or nonproprietary), and trade (or proprietary) name. The chemical name is given to describe the drug's chemical make-up. The generic name is given to the specific chemical compound. In today's society, a popular generic name is ibuprofen. The proprietary name is a name given to a drug that is unique to the company and its particular brand of drug. A proprietary or trade name of ibuprofen is Advil®. It is not unusual for one generic name drug to be sold under many various trade names (e.g., Advil, Motrin®, etc.).

The potential for harm exists in every drug, especially when it is given to the wrong patient or not according to the protocol. The utmost care and attention must be paid when working with medications and patients. If a drug has the potential for toxic effects or if it must be given by specific, trained personnel, the FDA states that drug cannot be approved for use in animals unless under the supervision of a licensed veterinarian. This is referred to as a prescription drug. Prescription drugs under FDA guidelines must have a label stating the following: "Caution: Federal law restricts the use of this drug to use by or on the order of a licensed veterinarian." However, the statements "for veterinary use only" or "only sold to veterinarians" on some drugs are not prescription

drug designations. Veterinarians also have some freedom to use a drug in ways not defined on the label, as long as they take responsibility for the outcome. Again, documentation is crucial. Use of drugs in this way is termed "extralabel" or "off label use." OTC drugs are those that do not require a prescription. Many OTC drugs are used "extralabel" in a veterinary practice.

Controlled substances are drugs that have the potential for abuse dependence by humans. With controlled substances, careful and meticulous records must be kept, and certain controlled substances must be kept in a locked, secured area with exact record keeping regarding their use. Many of these drugs are used during anesthesia or for pain relief and pain management in veterinary medicine. Use of controlled substances is restricted to a defined group of individuals registered with the Drug Enforcement Agency (DEA), which includes manufacturers, distributors, pharmacists, and licensed practitioners. Controlled substances are categorized into five schedules (I, II, III, IV, and V) by the DEA on the basis of their potential for abuse (Table 13.2).

As discussed previously, a VCPR must exist when prescribing a drug or medication for a patient. There are specific guidelines to which veterinarians must adhere when writing a prescription.

- Veterinary prescription drugs must only be used by or on the order of a licensed veterinarian.

- A binding VCPR must exist.

- The drug prescribed must meet proper requirements for labeling.

- The drug must be dispensed in quantities necessary for treatment of the animal. Most states have a requirement that the animal (or herd) must be seen within a specified time period to be considered a valid VCPR. Unlimited refills should never be written.

- Documentation of all prescriptions must be accurate and current.

- Prescription drugs must be appropriately handled and stored safely.

The prescription label tells the owner what medication is in the container and gives directions for the use of the medication. There are many abbreviations that are commonly used when writing a prescription. These abbreviations can be found in Table 13.3. Prescription containers should be childproof, unless requested otherwise by the owner. This is typically the case for elderly owners or owners who have a disability or weakened state that makes opening the container difficult. If nonchildproof containers are requested, this must be documented in the patient's medical record. Requirements for prescription labeling may vary slightly from state to state, but the following are typically included on a prescription label:

- name, address, telephone number of the veterinarian and hospital writing the prescription

- date of prescription

- owner's name and address

- animal's name and species

Table 13.2 Controlled substances categories.

Schedule	Abuse potential	Substances	Comments
I	High	Heroin, LSD, marijuana, mescaline, methaqualone	Use not accepted in a hospital setting in the United States Research use only
II	High	Opium, morphine, hydromorphone, cocaine, methadone, meperidine, fentanyl	Risk for severe psychic or physical dependence in humans Require a written prescription; no refills permitted
III	Moderate	Anabolic steroids, opioids, barbiturates, nonnarcotic drugs	Risk for moderate to low physical dependence but high psychological dependence in humans Oral or written prescription permitted with a maximum of five refills in 6 months
IV	Low	Barbital, phenobarbital, butorphanol, tramadol, diazepam, midazolam	Risk for limited physical or psychological dependence in humans Oral or written prescription permitted with a maximum of five refills in 6 months
V	Low	Codeine, dihydrocodeine, diphenoxylate	No DEA limit on prescriptions

DEA, Drug Enforcement Agency; LSD, lysergic acid diethyamide.

Table 13.3 Common abbreviations used in prescriptions.

Abbreviation	Meaning
BID	twice a day
cc	cubic centimeter
disp	dispense
g or gm	gram
gr	grain
h	hour
kg	kilogram
lb	pound
mg	milligram
mL	milliliter
od	right eye
os	left eye
PO	by mouth
prn	as needed
q	every
q8h	every 8 hours
qd	every day
QID	four times a day
QOD	every other day
SID	once a day
TID	three times a day
tsp	teaspoon
tbs	tablespoon

- Rx symbol
- drug name
- drug concentration
- quantity dispensed
- directions for properly dispensing the medication
- expiry date of the drug
- number of refills allowed
- signature of the person writing the prescription
- DEA registration number (if the drug is a controlled substance).

Drugs may be identified by various names. The **chemical name** of a drug depicts its chemical structure and typically is determined when the drug compound is being developed. Additionally, during development, a drug's generic name will be established by the developing company and the FDA. The generic name is the official identifying name of the drug which is then used by manufacturers. When a particular manufacturer produces and markets a drug, it will be assigned a trade name. This is also known as the **brand name**. Since multiple manufacturers may produce the same drug, one generically named drug may be known by multiple trade names. The trade name can be identified by a ® (registered) or ™ (trademark) symbol following it and is often capitalized. On a drug label, the generic name is typically listed after the trade name and is not usually capitalized.

Drug classifications

A large class of drugs which include antibacterial and antifungal compounds are known as antimicrobials. They are used to kill or inhibit the growth of microorganisms.

Antibacterial drugs

Antibacterial drugs refer to substances which kill or inhibit the growth of bacteria. "Antibacterial" and "antibiotic" are terms which are often used interchangeably although antibiotics are actually antibacterial compounds produced naturally by microorganisms.

Antibacterial drugs are classified according to their mechanism of action, their spectrum of activity (Gram-positive, Gram-negative, or anaerobic organisms), and whether they are bactericidal (kill bacteria) or bacteriostatic (inhibit bacterial replication).

In antibacterial therapy, the goal is to assist the body's natural defenses in the removal of bacterial pathogens while reducing the risk for *toxicity* to the patient.

Antifungal compounds

Fungal infections are a result of various fungal organisms, yeasts, and *dermatophytes*. Antifungals are toxic to specific fungal organisms. Antifungals bind to or inhibit production of *ergosterol* in the cell membrane. This in turn leads to the death of the cell. Managing systemic fungal infection can take weeks to months of antifungal treatment. Throughout antifungal therapy, patients must be watched closely for side-effects, such as decreased appetite, anorexia, and vomiting. Specific antifungal therapies have the potential for development of significant organ toxicities, and therefore routine monitoring of liver and/or kidney chemistries is recommended.

Antiparasitic drugs

Endoparasitic drugs

Endoparasites are parasites that live in the tissues and organs of their host (Table 13.4).

Through a variety of mechanisms of action, antiparasitic drugs focus on these different classes of parasites. In an effort to expand the spectrum of activity, antiparasitic compounds are frequently used in combination.

Ectoparasitic drugs

Ectoparasites are parasites that live outside the host. Examples include insects such as flies, lice, and fleas, as well as ascarines such as ticks and mites. Controlling ectoparasites involves preventing host–parasite interaction. This is achieved through the use of contact insecticides, such as organophosphates and pyrethrums (pyrethrins or pyrethroids). Another approach to controlling ectoparasitic infestation involves the use of insecticides or adulticide therapy. The most common means of drug delivery for ectoparasite control is topical application.

Table 13.4 Endoparasites.

Endoparasite	
Nematodes	Roundworms, hookworms, whipworms, lungworms, heartworms
Cestodes	Tapeworms
Trematodes	Flukes
Protozoa	*Giardia*, coccidia

Similar to endoparasiticides, ectoparasiticides have a variety of mechanisms of action. These include ectoparasiticides which function as repellents, those that target the parasite's nervous system, or those that target growth and development of the parasite. It is imperative that veterinary team members understand the risk for toxicity when using ectoparasiticides. The veterinary team must be cognizant of and monitor for signs of toxicity during use. Pet owners must be educated regarding these dangers as well.

Veterinary medicine has safe and effective ectoparasiticides that favorably target the nervous system of invertebrates or their growth and development. Therefore, the use of more toxic repellents (e.g., pyrethrums in cats, organophosphates, and carbamates) is relatively infrequent in veterinary medicine.

Endocrine drugs

Insulin

Diabetes mellitus (DM) is a disease of impaired carbohydrate, protein, and fat metabolism coupled with insulin deficiency. Insulin is a hormone which is generated in the beta cells of the pancreas and is responsible for cellular uptake of glucose.

Diabetes mellitus occurs in many species including humans, dogs, and cats. The cause of DM in dogs typically differs from the cause in cats. It is important to remember that dog and cat DM patients have lost significant beta cell mass and are insulin deficient at the time of diagnosis. Consequently, insulin is necessary to treat DM in both species. Insulin is administered by injection.

The make-up of insulin is a series of linked amino acids (AAs) specific to each species, but with little variation. Insulin is well conserved across species so therapeutic insulin products may be animal derived (porcine or bovine), human derived, genetically engineered (human recombinant), or synthetic. In the veterinary hospital, the veterinarian can best match the source of insulin to the species being treated based upon AA sequence similarities.

It is also important for veterinary team members to understand additional differences between insulin products. These include the action of the insulin, in addition to the insulin's ability to decrease blood glucose, also known as biological activity. The biological activity of insulin is expressed as units of activity per milliliter (U/mL). It is important for every member of the veterinary team to understand that the activity determined for each type of insulin corresponds to the type of syringe needed to administer the appropriate dose. In other words, insulin with a bioactivity of 40 U/mL requires a U-40 insulin syringe, and insulin with a bioactivity of 100 U/mL requires a U-100 insulin syringe.

Gastrointestinal drugs

Gastrointestinal (GI) drugs include antiemetics which are used to stop or control vomiting. Conversely, GI drugs also include emetics, which are given to induce vomiting in the case of certain toxin ingestion. Antidiarrheals are used to control diarrhea, and laxatives are used to increase the fluid content of stool and/or increase GI movement to promote defecation. Prokinetic drugs can be used to increase GI movement in cases of constipation. To manage mucosal ulcers in the stomach or intestines, antiulcer drugs are often indicated. To stimulate the appetite in an anorexic patient or supplement digestive enzymes, specific drugs may be used.

Cardiovascular drugs

Heart disease may result from damaged cardiac muscle, disease of the valves, **pericardial** disease, abnormalities in heart rhythm, or altered coronary circulation. Heart disease can progress to congestive heart failure (CHF), which often results in fluid accumulation in the lungs, body cavities, and tissues. Managing CHF relies on the nature of the primary problem. Often managing CHF includes the use of multiple drugs, such as:

- diuretics to reduce fluid accumulation
- inotropic agents to improve the contractility of cardiac muscle
- antihypertensives to modulate blood pressure
- antiarrhythmics to control heart rhythm abnormalities.

Anticonvulsants

Anticonvulsants are used for long term control of epileptic seizures in veterinary patients. The common ones of which veterinary team members should be aware are phenobarbital, potassium bromide (KBr), and levatiracetam. These drugs influence the release of **neurotransmitters** and decrease seizure-associated neuronal activity. It is important to recognize and be familiar with the side-effects of these anticonvulsant drugs and be ready to educate pet owners regarding signs to watch out for. Side-effects may include dose-dependent drowsiness and/or ataxia, with possible increased water intake, increased urination, increased food intake, and potential weight gain.

Both **status epilepticus** and **cluster seizures** require immediate treatment. Diazepam is a drug that can be used in this instance. Diazepm is a benzodiazepine tranquilizer and is typically administered intravenously in the hospital setting to stop seizure activity. Alternatively, levatiracetam may be administered intravenously or subcutaneously for treatment of status epilepticus or cluster seizures.

Anti-inflammatory drugs

Injuries to tissue result in inflammation. Inflammatory mediators lead to the recognized signs of inflammation: redness, heat, swelling, and pain. Both glucocorticoids (steroids) and nonsteroidal antiinflammatory drugs (NSAIDs) are used to treat inflammation. However, using NSAIDs and glucocorticoids at the same time is not recommended because of the significant risk of ulceration and/or perforation in the GI tract.

Glucocorticoids are available in many forms (i.e., tablets, suspensions, solutions, and topical forms). They reduce inflammation by blocking the action of phospholipase. Glucocorticoids are very strong anti-inflammatories. However, long-term use or high doses may result in considerable side-effects, such as **immunosuppression**, delayed wound healing, **polyuria/polydipsia**, and DM.

As mentioned, NSAIDs also reduce inflammation. The most significant side-effect to be aware of with NSAID use is GI upset and ulcer formation. Additionally, veterinary team members must also watch for acute kidney injury and **hepatotoxicity** in patients being managed on NSAIDS.

Vaccines

Vaccinations are given to provide protection to the vulnerable young animal whose immune system is underdeveloped or to an animal that has not previously had vaccinations. Typically, the process involves an initial vaccination followed by 2–3 additional vaccinations. The first vaccination is given in young patients as maternal antibody levels begin to fall; antibodies will be formed within 7–10 days. A second dose is given 2–3 weeks later, stimulating the production of yet more antibodies with a quicker response time of 12–24 hours. This initial course provides antibodies for several months and should be bolstered 1 year later with a "booster" vaccine to strengthen the acquired immunity. Failure to present the animal for the initial booster may result in a two-dose vaccine plan similar to the initial course.

Vaccines can be administered by the following routes.

- *Subcutaneous* – this is the most common route and is typically administered in the scruff. Subcutaneous injection sites need to be altered to prevent skin irritation if using this route for a course of injections.
- *Intranasal* – drops are placed into the external nares via a modified syringe. Local antibody and cell-mediated immunity are created via this route for respiratory diseases such as *Bordetella bronchiseptica*.
- *Oral* – not a common route, especially in North America. It is used in some European vaccines.

For vaccines to remain effective, they must be stored in a refrigerator at 2–4 °C (35.6–39.2 °F) and remain cold. Warm temperatures will kill the microorganisms within a live vaccine. The veterinarian or veterinary nurse/technician should understand how to reconstitute vaccines and know which, if any, vaccines can be mixed to reduce the number of injections given.

Storage and disposal of drugs

The drug manufacturer defines storage recommendations for a specific drug based on the results of stability studies conducted on the finished product. Storage recommendations must be followed to prevent premature degradation. This will help to ensure the safety and effectiveness of a drug for the lifetime of the product. All health-care team members should be aware of the storage recommendations for a particular drug. These recommendations can be found in the package insert accompanying the product.

Additionally, to ensure the purity and potency of the final dosage form based on controlled stability studies, the manufacturer should also provide product expiry dates. This ensures the purity and potency of the product as long as the product is stored following the manufacturer's recommendations. All approved drug products are required to have standard expiry dates (month, day, year) as mandated by the FDA.

As a reminder, controlled substances are drugs that have the potential for abuse dependence by humans. With controlled substances, careful and meticulous records must be kept, and certain controlled substances must be stored in a locked, secured area with exact record keeping regarding their use.

The Department of Environmental Quality, the Environmental Protection Agency, the FDA, and local boards of pharmacy are all responsible for overseeing drug disposal. Disposal of controlled substances is regulated by the DEA. When removing expired and/or unused drugs, do not dump them down the drain, flush them down the toilet, throw them in the trash, or discard them in the ground.

It is advised that the veterinary hospital return expired drugs to the manufacturer or the distribution company for credit, or send to a reverse distribution company (RDC). Here, the RDC functions as the intermediary between the drug purchaser and drug vendor. The RDC provides credit to the drug purchaser for a returned drug; when credit is not acceptable, the RDC discards or destroys a returned drug on a per-pound cost basis. Approved disposal of a controlled substance is provided only through an RDC.

Prescriptions are packaged in a variety of containers. Plastic vials are available in numerous sizes, which are measured in drams. Typically the vials are light brown or blue in color to help protect the medication from deterioration due to sun exposure. The dispensing of liquids is in bottles with either a twist cap or dropper top. Certain medications begin as a powder and must be reconstituted with a specific amount of water to form a liquid medication. Both of these are typically accompanied by a syringe or dropper to draw up the correct amount. It is imperative that the proper amount and technique for drawing up the medication are discussed with the owner in detail and documented. The owner should demonstrate that he or she knows how to dispense the medication to insure understanding and compliance.

References

Beal, A.D., Viviano, K.R. 2018. Pharmacology and pharmacy. In: *Clinical Textbook for Veterinary Technicians*, 9th edition. Bassert, J.M., Samples O., Beal, A.D. (eds). Elsevier Saunders, St Louis, MO.

Bill, R.L. 2017. *Clinical Pharmacology and Therapeutics for Veterinary Technicians*, 4th edition. Elsevier, St Louis, MO.

Bowden, S. 2016. Fundamental pharmacology. In: *Aspinall's Complete Textbook of Veterinary Nursing*, 3rd edition. Ackerman, N., Aspinall, V. (eds). Elsevier Butterworth Heinemann, London.

Harris, H., Rock, A. 2016. Prevention of the spread of infectious diseases. In: *Aspinall's Complete Textbook of Veterinary Nursing*, 3rd edition. Ackerman, N., Aspinall, V. (eds). Elsevier Butterworth Heinemann, London.

Romich, J.A. 2010. *Fundamentals of Pharmacology for Veterinary Technicians*, 2nd edition. Cengage Learning, Boston, MA.

Samuelson, K. 2011. Pharmacology and pharmacy. In: *Principles and Practice of Veterinary Technology*, 3rd edition. Sirois, M. (ed.). Elsevier, St Louis, MO.

Sonsthagen, T. 2020. *Tasks for the Veterinary Assistant*, 4th edition. Wiley Blackwell, Ames, IA

Wanamaker, B.P., Massey, K.L. 2015. *Applied Pharmacology for Veterinary Technicians*, 5th edition. Saunders, St Louis, MO.

www.wiley.com/go/burns/textbookvetassistant2

Please go to the companion website for assignments and a PowerPoint relating to the material in this chapter.

Chapter 14 Radiology

As a veterinary assistant, you will have many exciting duties on the veterinary health-care team. One area in which you will assist is radiology. Radiology is a vital area as quality radiographs are an essential tool in veterinary diagnostics and treatment. However, radiation can be hazardous. There are several safety measures of which the veterinary assistant needs to be aware. Following these safety procedures allows for the safety of the veterinary health-care team and your patients. These procedures will help keep you safe and enhance your role as a valued veterinary team member.

All health-care team members should have a basic understanding of radiographs. X-rays are a type of *electromagnetic radiation*. X-rays are similar to visible light with the exception that x-rays have a shorter wavelength, higher frequency, and higher energy. The higher energy leads to x-rays' potential danger.

The production of x-rays occurs when fast-moving electrons from the cathode, a negatively charged electrode, collide with the anode, or the positively charged electrode. When charged particles (electrons) are slowed down or stopped by the *atoms* of a target area, an x-ray results. This process occurs inside the x-ray tube to create an x-ray beam. An x-ray beam is composed of bundles of energy that travel in a wave. These bundles are known as quanta and are referred to as photons. Photons have no mass or electrical charge and are made up of pure energy which is transported, or "carried," by the wave. The x-rays are then captured on a photographic plate. The image created is called a radiograph.

The energy in electromagnetic radiation is highly variable, with the energy of the radiation proportional to the wavelength. For example, the shorter the wavelength, the greater the energy. Therefore in radiography, x-rays that have a shorter wavelength penetrate farther than rays that have longer wavelengths.

Radiology safety measures and guidelines

1. *You must be 18 years of age or older* to assist in radiographic procedures. Pregnant women should never assist in radiographic procedures because radiation damages all living cells, especially rapidly developing cells such as fetuses. *Somatic damage* is damage to the body over a period of time. You may not have any symptoms from overexposure for a long time, but damage may have occurred. Somatic damage can take the form of cancer, cataracts, and sterility. *Genetic damage* occurs to your reproductive genes (DNA). This can result in birth defects in future generations.

2. *Wear a dosimeter badge* every time you work in radiology. The dosimeter badge is a personnel x-ray monitoring badge that holds a small piece of radiographic film. It is pinned to the outside of your clothing. These badges are a very effective way to evaluate radiation exposure. Someone in your clinic will periodically collect all the dosimeter badges and send them to a federally regulated testing laboratory where they will be analyzed. The dosage information collected will then be issued to the clinic in a report. You will always have a replacement badge because it is very important that your exposure is always monitored. As a veterinary assistant, you should be issued a dosimeter badge. It is very important that this badge be worn at all times if you are assigned to help out in radiology. Wearing the badge every time will accurately monitor your radiation exposure levels and help maintain a healthy workplace.

3. *Wear protective apparel and protective eye coverings.* When you are assisting the licensed veterinary technician or veterinarian

Textbook for the Veterinary Assistant, Second Edition. Kara M. Burns and Lori Renda-Francis.
© 2022 John Wiley & Sons, Inc. Published 2022 by John Wiley & Sons, Inc.
Companion website: www.wiley.com/go/burns/textbookvetassistant2

taking radiographs, it is very important to protect yourself from harmful rays by wearing protective garments and eye coverings. These garments are lined with lead and are essential for maximum protection. Proper protective garments will include a lead apron, lead gloves, a lead thyroid shield, and lead glasses or goggles. To help maintain the effectiveness and longevity of protective garments and equipment, it is important to store them correctly. Hang aprons – do not fold them. Folding can create creases which can lead to damage. Gloves and thyroid shields should be stored flat. Eyewear should be returned to protective cases when not in use. It is very important to inspect all protective wear regularly and report any defects to your hospital manager. As a veterinary assistant, this may be one of your important responsibilities.

4. *Maintain a radiographic log book.* This will be a place for you to record the patient, type of radiograph being taken, exposure measurements, and the result. Keeping a log book is a good way to help your clinic reduce radiation exposure. Using the log as a guide to previous diagnostic radiographs will help you avoid retakes in the future.

5. *Collimation is important.* The collimator is part of the x-ray machine. It is an adjustable narrow tube that can be used to direct or narrow the primary beam. Collimating the beam is an effective way to help reduce scatter radiation and an aid in obtaining a quality diagnostic radiograph. Remember to never aim the collimator toward any person or open door.

6. *Look away from the **primary beam** during exposure.* While assisting in radiographic procedures, it is important to turn your head, close your eyes, and look away from the primary beam while a picture is being taken. This small action will help protect your eyes by limiting radiation exposure.

7. *Utilize proper restraint during a radiographic procedure.* As a restrainer, you never want to be exposed to the primary beam. To help reduce exposure to **scatter radiation**, you should stand at the end of the table and try not to lean into your patient. It is very important to remember to never sit on the x-ray table! When possible, utilize sandbags and other restraint tools instead of humans. Also, to help minimize exposure it's a good idea to take turns with other veterinary assistants for restraining during radiographs.

Cleaning screens

The quality of a radiograph is determined by the amount of diagnostic information it contains. This is called radiographic quality. As a veterinary assistant, one of your jobs may be to maintain your clinic's radiographic screens. Screens get dusty and collect fur, which can show up as unwanted artifacts on the radiographic image. The screens are very susceptible to damage, which can contribute to a poor-quality radiograph. To ensure the image is as pristine as possible, it is very important to regularly examine and clean all your clinic's screens.

1. *Remove all debris from screens.* This can be done by using a pressurized air can to blow the debris off. If you do not have

this, a soft brush can be substituted. Be very gentle if using a brush, and avoid applying pressure. Screens are expensive and very sensitive.

2. *Clean the protective screen surface.* Use a commercial screen cleaner and carefully follow all manufacturer directions. Cautiously pour cleaning solution on a dampened gauze square and gently clean the screen surface. If you do not have a commercial screen cleaner, it is acceptable to use mild soap and water.

3. *Dry the cassette.* After you have finished cleaning, leave the cassette open to dry. Make sure the cassette is placed vertically so that no new debris settles on the clean surfaces. It is very important that the screen as well as the entire cassette be completely dry before you place a new film in it. Please remember that cassettes should be stored completely *closed* when dry after cleaning.

4. *Reload with film.* When the screen and cassette are completely dry, you should reload with film so it will be ready for use. As a veterinary assistant, you will probably do this routinely, so remember to take care when loading or removing film. Do not touch the screen or write on the film while it is in the cassette as this will cause scratches. The screen surface is very delicate, and any scratches sustained are permanent.

Labeling, filing, and storage of radiographs

Labeling

Radiograph labels are very important and essential to proper patient care. Also, if a legal situation should arise you need to be prepared with accurate information. When you are working in a veterinary clinic or hospital you will be required to follow its protocol. Usually the following information is required when labeling a patient's radiograph: identification of the patient, including name, age, breed, and gender as well as owner's last name and address of veterinary clinic or hospital, date, and left or right marker.

There are several ways to label a radiograph.

- *Photoimprinting.* This label system is quite common. It consists of a lead blocker on the outside of the cassette. Many cassettes have this built right in. You will write the accurate patient information on an identification label (usually a card) which is placed in the photoimprinter in the dark room. When you are ready to develop your radiograph in the dark room, you will remove the exposed film from the cassette and place it on the ID label card (which was previously placed on the photoimprinter) and press down on the photoimprinter. A small light indicates that the information from the label has been imprinted on your film. The film is now ready to be processed. Within minutes, you will have a properly labeled radiograph to present to your veterinarian.

- *Lead markers.* This is also a common method of labeling. Small lead letters and numbers are put in a holder (also made of lead) which is placed on the cassette before taking the radiograph. It is a very simple and effective labeling method but as you can imagine, it takes time, which can be a problem when your doctor needs the radiograph ASAP!

- *Lead tape.* This is a type of labeling tape that has been lined with lead. The advantage is that you can write the patient's information on the tape using a pen or pencil. Then the tape is either put in a special lead holder or just placed on the cassette before exposure.

Filing

One of the many responsibilities you may have as a veterinary assistant is filing radiographs. It is a good idea to have an organized efficient system that will be easy to use. To start with, each film (no matter what size) must be stored in its own envelope, and all the envelopes should be the same size and accurately labeled with the following information:

- patient's name
- owner's last name
- date
- type of radiograph.

An organized filing system could be based on many factors. Quite often, an alphabetic, numeric, or color-coded system will be in place. It is your responsibility to make sure you are trained and understand the filing system used in your hospital.

Proper storage of radiographic film

Every state has its own laws regarding how long veterinarians are legally required to store radiographs. Usually it ranges from 3 to 5 years after the patient's last visit or treatment. Your clinic or hospital may have additional requirements that go beyond the state law. It is important that you learn and adhere to all your practice guidelines.

Your clinic will likely have a designated storage area for radiographs. Ideally, radiographs should be stored vertically, not horizontally. As in any organized filing system, it helps to have dividers in place to help separate the films as well as ensuring they remain upright. Make sure you understand the radiographic storage system in place at your hospital so you can easily retrieve a requested radiograph when needed.

Radiographic positioning

Proper patient positioning is one of the most important parts to insuring a good radiograph. Inaccurate positioning and improper restraint can lead the veterinarian to misread a radiograph. Therefore it is imperative that the veterinary health-care team be familiar with proper restraint and positioning of patients (Figure 14.1). We have discussed terminology in prior chapters, but it is useful to review these for proper radiograph technique.

- Ventral (V): body area situated toward the underside of quadrupeds.

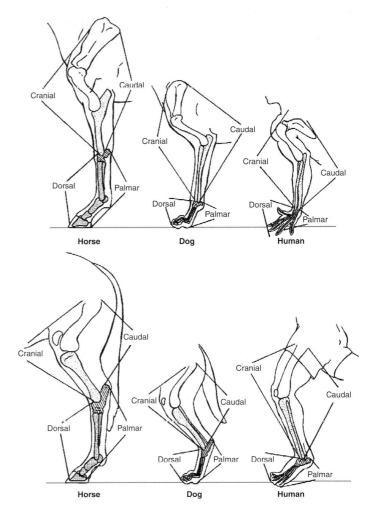

Figure 14.1 Radiographic positions. Source: Reproduced from Lavin, L.M. 2007. *Radiography in Veterinary Technology*, 4th edition. Elsevier, St Louis, MO.

- Dorsal (D): body area situated toward the back or topline of quadrupeds. Opposite of ventral.
- Medial (M): body area situated toward the median plane or midline.
- Lateral (L): body area situated away from the median plane or midline.
- Cranial (Cr): structures or areas situated toward the head (formerly anterior).
- Caudal (Cd): structures or areas situated toward the tail (formerly posterior).
- Rostral (R): areas on the head situated toward the nose.
- Palmar (Pa): situated on the caudal aspect of the front limb, distal to the carpal joint.
- Plantar (Pl): situated on the caudal aspect of the rear limb, distal to the hock or tarsus joint.
- Proximal (Pr): situated closer to the point of attachment or origin.
- Distal (Di): situated away from the point of attachment or origin.

The veterinary health-care team must recognize that certain radiographic positions may warrant sedation and possibly general anesthesia. It is also understood that certain positional devices may assist in obtaining a quality radiograph. For example, sandbags, foam blocks and wedges, wood blocks, and a radiolucent trough may be used to keep a patient in a desired position for a radiograph. Additionally, tape, gauze, rope, and compression bands are commonly used in veterinary practices. The utilization of positional devices, and sedation if necessary, will reduce the amount of manual restraint needed. Restraint by health-care team members should be utilized as little as possible for the protection of the team member and the patient. Manual restraint should be considered when sedation might cause further harm to the patient.

When positioning patients for a radiograph, the health-care team must include all crucial anatomical regions in the primary beam. Finding the most suitable pose in an attempt to produce a precise reproduction of the anatomical area is the main goal in positioning. The following are important points to consider when attempting to position the patient for an accurate radiograph.

- Patient's wellbeing.
- Restraint and immobilization of the patient.
- Minimal trauma to the area being radiographed.
- Least risk of exposing health-care team members assisting with the radiograph.

The patient's wellbeing should be considered throughout the radiographic examination. Health-care team members must be patient with the process as it may be difficult to get the animal positioned perfectly the first time. Keep in mind that taking a radiograph may be scary to an animal, and the team is trying to keep the animal in a specific, unnatural, and oftentimes painful position. Refer back to when we talked about proper handling procedures and work with the animal in a slow manner using a quiet and soothing voice. The quickest way to lose a potential position and frighten the animal is to restrain the patient too strongly and speak loudly. The spinning of the rotating anode produces a noise that often frightens animals. Patients that exhibit signs of anxiety will often benefit if the rotor is started prior to the radiograph to let the patient become familiar with the new noise.

You are taking a two-dimensional picture of a three-dimensional anatomical structure. Therefore two views of each anatomical area should be taken at right angles to each other. It is also important to position the area to be examined closest to the film, as this will help to reduce distortion of the area to be examined. When radiographing a patient's limb, the veterinarian will often ask that the opposite corresponding limb also be radiographed to compare normal against the potentially abnormal physical appearance.

Processing

Film processing in radiology is comparable to the processing of any other type of photograph. Processing of veterinary films occurs either manually, with the use of wet tanks and hangers, or through an automatic processor. It is during the imaging process that 95% of imaging artifacts occur.

Developer components

The developer is an alkaline solution with a pH of 9.8–11.0. Phenidone and hydroquinone are the two main components in the developer.

Fixer components

The fixer's chief component is sodium thiosulfate. Sulfur is another component. Should the fixer fail for any reason, the sulfur precipitates and a "rotten egg" smell permeates the area. This is known as sulfiding.

Another important component is the hardener whose function is to ensure that the emulsion stays attached to the base. The chemicals in a manual tank must be stirred with an up-and-down motion or the hardener will remain at the bottom of the tank. Then, if the film is left in the wash for a prolonged period, the emulsion will slide off the base.

Over the years, the developer and fixer components have changed dramatically. Chemical manufacturers have developed products that mix together and meet most municipal hazardous waste standards. Consequently, in most areas it is safe to dispose of the chemicals down the drain with the other waste products from the facility, as long as they are in small discharge quantities.

Every veterinary hospital should review the chemical waste guidelines with its municipality. Additionally, the component sheets from the chemical manufacturer must always be accessible. The hazardous waste sheets for most chemicals are available online and are always available from the manufacturer.

It is important to note that clear water makes up 98–99% of the liquid in the chemical bottles that are then diluted again when mixed for use.

Manual (nonautomatic) processing

Most veterinary hospitals have moved to automatic processing of radiographs. However, there are a few hospitals which are still processing film manually. The chemicals used in manual processing are the same as for automatic processing but the temperature and time are quite different (Table 14.1).

Table 14.1   Manual processing of radiographs.

Process	Time	Temperature
Developer	4 minutes with agitation	68 °F (20 °C)
Rinse	15–30 sec with agitation	68 °F (20 °C)
Fixing	8 minutes with agitation	68 °F (20 °C)
Washing	12 minutes with agitation	68 °F (20 °C)

A 14 × 17 inch (35 × 43 cm) film is lifted almost parallel with the team member's eyes when the hangers are moved from tank to tank. Therefore, it is extremely important that the team member does not splash chemicals during this procedure.

The wet tanks are always checked for the correct temperature (68 °F/20 °C), and the chemicals are agitated immediately before processing the films. This is the only time the chemicals are agitated. Agitating the chemicals before radiography is premature, and the chemicals will have settled by the time the film is introduced into the tanks.

Cleanliness is essential during film processing because it is very easy to splash chemicals onto the cassettes and screens. In the manual processing area, the cassettes must never be left open on the counter.

Chemical fumes can be irritating, and the chemicals are dangerous to ingest or splash into one's eyes. It is required that safety glasses and gloves be worn whenever chemicals are handled. This requirement comes from the the Workplace Hazardous Materials Information System (WHMIS) and the Occupational Safety and Health Administration (OSHA).

Remember, the developer is highly alkaline and the fixer is highly acidic and so both chemicals must be treated with respect. It only takes a couple of seconds for one drop of fixer concentrate to melt the lens of the eye. An eyewash station must be positioned close to the processing area and must be checked regularly by the clinic's quality assurance officer. When handling chemicals, it is essential that personnel are equipped with protective safety goggles and rubber gloves.

Developing the image

The first step in processing the film is developing the image. The developer's purpose is to cause the underlying image to become visible. This is achieved by immersing the film in a chemical solution.

Areas of the film that are unexposed typically are not affected, unless the film is left in the developer for too long. If this does happen, the unexposed areas will start to react to the developer, resulting in the film density increasing. This is known as developer fog.

The hanger is held by the top and the film is introduced into the chemicals slowly and steadily. Once the film is completely immersed, it is agitated slowly in an up-and-down movement, several times. This is done to ensure that any air bubbles that may have entered with the film are removed. The timer is set for *4 minutes*. At 2 minutes, the film is agitated up and down once again. This moves away the used chemicals directly next to the film and places fresher chemicals against the film.

At 4 minutes, the film is agitated up and down 2–4 times followed by being moved to the intermediary wash tank. Again, it is agitated 2–4 times in the wash tank to stop the development and remove some of the developer. The next step is to place it in the fixer tank.

Fixing the image to the film is the third step in manual processing. All of the emulsion not affected by radiation and developing is removed and the image becomes visible.

The film is then placed into the fixer tank using the same method: introduced slowly and steadily and then agitated up and down. This agitation removes air bubbles that have been carried into the fixer and remain on the film.

This step requires the timer to be set for *8 minutes*. After 2 minutes, the light may be turned on and the film checked. If there is still unexposed emulsion on the film, the fixer is no longer fresh and should be changed once the films are processed. At 4 minutes, the film should have cleared completely and may be viewed momentarily on an illuminator by the veterinary team.

Following the review of the film, it is placed back into the fixer to complete the fixing process. It is essential that the fixing process be completed to ensure the archival quality of the image.

Next, the film is removed from the fixer and lowered into the wash tank. The entire film, including the hangers, must be submerged in each solution. The fixer will clean the developer out of the clips of the hangers, and the wash will remove the fixer from the hangers, thus leaving them clean for the next film.

It is critically important that the films are removed from the wash water and placed on the drying rack within 2–3 hours (at most) of washing.

If the processing is completed correctly, no artifacts will be seen on the films. It is important for all team members to remember that the drying process may take several hours. Even if the films feel dry to the touch, the emulsion will take longer to dry completely. Thus, placing the films in the envelope before completely drying results in them sticking together and being impossible to separate.

The film must be dried either by hanging the films in a dryer cabinet or by allowing them to dry naturally in the air. Drying removes 85–90% of the moisture in the film emulsion. If too much moisture is removed, the emulsion will crack, compromising the quality of the image.

The film is now ready to be reviewed and stored permanently.

Automatic processing

The automatic processor enables the procedure of producing a visible image on the film. The process is fast, efficient, and will not imprint an artifact or scratch the emulsion off the film during the process. Most automatic processors now are sold as "90-second" processors. This means what is says – the film enters the processor and exits within 90 seconds

The feed tray is located at the entrance of the processor. The film is placed either horizontally or vertically on this tray, and a motor drive accepts and propels the film into the processor. The film must be placed squarely on the tray. When a film enters the feed tray, it is within 1–2 inches (2.5–5 cm) of the developer. Once the film enters the processor, *do not* draw it back onto the tray.

Think of the processor as an assembly line which is pulling the film across a series of rollers through the developer, fixer, and wash tanks.

The film is affected by several systems once it enters the processor. Each system is vital to the production of the final image

Every time a roller touches the film, there is the possibility of an artifact or damage to the fragile emulsion. The main drive motor must be high quality to ensure that it runs evenly and consistently for many years.

The chemistry used in automatic processing is the same as that used in manual processing. The typical temperature is 34 °C (93 °F). The time the film is in the developer solution is set dependent upon the individual processor and programmed so the chemicals have time to react sufficiently to optimize the image. The rates of replenishment are also preset to preserve the correct concentrations of developer and fixer.

The image is in the formation stage while in the developer; however, many problems can occur during this process. Approximately 80% of processing artifacts occur during the development stage. The image may be deleted in places where the latent image undergoes pressure from a swollen roller, or it may acquire density from other factors.

The film travels through the fixer and into the wash tank. This is an important part of the process as it must be thoroughly washed to preserve its archival quality. If the film is not washed with flowing water, staining or sulfiding may result.

The dryer temperature should be set to ensure that the films are not tacky or sticky. Roughly 85–95% of the moisture should be removed from the films as they travel through the dryer. Additionally, the film base may become fragile and crack if the films are overly hot when they come out.

Digital imaging and processing

Digital radiography is steadily replacing analog systems in the veterinary practice as digital radiography becomes progressively more available and increasingly affordable. The process by which images are obtained and presented on computer monitors in a gray-scale digital display is known as digital radiography. Currently, three main types of digital systems exist: computed radiography (CR), digital radiography (DR), and charge coupled device (CCD) technologies. An advantage with digital radiography is that the digitized image can be viewed with computer software which enables contrast, brightness, zoom, and pan adjustments. In addition, it allows for the measurement of anatomical structures.

Additional advantages of digital radiography include the following.

- The need for film is eliminated.
- Processing chemicals are not needed.
- Elimination of screens.
- Current x-ray machines can be retrofitted to use DR.
- Standard CR systems are accepted without changes needing to be made to the grid cabinet or Bucky mechanism.

With CCD systems, the veterinary hospital will need to purchase a radiology generator and table. Currently, CCD systems are competitively priced when compared to CR and DR. Another advantage with DR systems is they might slash the quantity of repeat radiographs needed. Another factor is a hard copy film can still be produced from digital radiography.

Computed radiography

Computed radiography uses a cassette system similar to conventional film screen systems. With CR, there is an imaging plate (IP) which contains a *photostimulable phosphor*. This is able to store the radiation level received at each point on the plate. Thus the need for film to view radiographs is removed. Additionally, the cassette goes through a computer scanner using a scanning laser beam, as opposed to chemical processing. Electrons then relax to a lower energy level, and light is produced. The light dimensions are relative to the amount of radiation reaching the IP and being absorbed by the IP. The light is measured, and the result is the generation of the digital image. Next, the fluorescent light in the reader is erased by the imaging plate, with the IP reloaded into the cassette for reuse. This allows for the imaging plate to be reused numerous times.

Digital radiography

Digital radiography employs an imaging plate consisting of an array of detectors. The detectors are responsible for converting the x-rays into an electrical signal which in turn is digitized to an image by the computer. The imaging plate is linked to a computer dedicated to that function. This eliminates the need for a cassette. The imaging plate can be permanently positioned in an x-ray table or be portable according to the needs of the veterinary team member.

Ultrasound

A noninvasive method of imaging soft tissues is known as ultrasonography. In this method a *transducer* transmits low-intensity, high-frequency sound waves into the soft tissues. These sound waves interact with tissue interfaces. Some of the sound waves are reflected back to the transducer; some are transmitted into deeper tissues. Sound waves reflected back to the transducer (echoes) are computer analyzed to produce a gray-scale image.

The use of ultrasound and radiography gives the veterinarian an excellent diagnostic tool. While radiographs reveal the size, shape, and position of the patient's organs, ultrasound reinforces these findings while providing the soft tissue textures and dynamics.

Quality control

Quality control (QC) is a process by which individuals review the quality of all factors involved in production. It is important to not only identify the actions that are necessary to ensure equipment performance, but also to verify the performance of equipment. QC is part of quality assurance (QA). QA is the documentation of all factors which relate to a certain policy or protocol. QA documents quality control and ensures that a facility, system, or administrative component performs safely and satisfactorily in service to a patient. Scheduling, preparation, and efficiency during an examination or treatment are all part of QA, as is reporting the results and conducting quality control.

Quality assurance involves the entire hospital, whereas QC is the testing of each of the factors, especially the equipment within the hospital. To ensure QC of the equipment in radiology, it is important to understand and follow the information presented above.

Conclusion

As a veterinary assistant, you will be called into action in almost every department of your clinic or hospital. Radiology is an exciting part of your job. Assisting the veterinarian or credentialed veterinary technician in obtaining diagnostic radiographs is very rewarding. Understanding safety measures and positional techniques will not only protect you and your teammates but also the animals you love. Being a vital veterinary team member is your goal. You will be amazed how successful your career will be if you learn, review, and stay current with the radiology protocols in place at your veterinary hospital. The more accurate you are, the better a veterinary assistant you will be and the more valuable a veterinary team member you will become!

References

American Veterinary Medical Association. State Legislative Resources. Available at: www.avma.org

Brown, M., Brown, L.C. 2018. *Lavin's Radiography for Veterinary Technicians*, 6th edition. Elsevier, St Louis, MO.

Prendergast, H. 2020. *Front Office Management for the Veterinary Team*, 3rd edition. Elsevier, St Louis, MO.

Sirois, M. (ed.). 2017. Diagnostic imaging. In: *Principles and Practice of Veterinary Technology*, 4th edition. Elsevier, St Louis, MO.

www.wiley.com/go/burns/textbookvetassistant2

Please go to the companion website for assignments and a PowerPoint relating to the material in this chapter.

Chapter 15 Surgical Assisting

Asepsis is a term used to describe a condition of sterility where there are no living organisms present. ***Aseptic technique*** is a method used to prevent contamination of wounds or other susceptible sites by organisms that have the ability to cause infection. It is important for all veterinary personnel to have a thorough understanding of aseptic technique to ensure that all surgical equipment is properly cleaned and sterilized.

It is nearly impossible to eliminate 100% of potentially harmful bacteria from the surgery. Therefore, techniques have been developed to help separate the sterile area (items free from bacteria) from the nonsterile area (areas where bacteria may be present). The ultimate goal is to have a sterile, germ-free environment.

The sterilization process

As a veterinary assistant, you will be responsible for preparing surgical equipment and supplies and sterilizing items by use of an autoclave (Figure 15.1).

An autoclave is an instrument used to sterilize equipment and supplies used in the surgery room. This is accomplished by subjecting them to high-pressure, saturated steam. Items are placed in the autoclave and sterilized at 250 °F at 15 pounds per square inch (psi) for 20–45 minutes depending on the size of the load and the contents.

Packs are usually wrapped in two layers of muslin or nonwoven wrappers. Materials need to be packed loosely to ensure good steam penetration. It is important to make sure that the autoclave chamber is not overpacked or packed too tightly. Place the items on the tray with space between packages so that steam can flow between items.

Once the sterilization cycle is complete, the autoclave will need to be vented and the items allowed to cool and dry. The instructions for running an autoclave will vary depending on the model. It is extremely important to follow all the manufacturer's instructions for operating and cleaning the autoclave.

The only way to ensure that sterilization has been achieved is to use proper technique and two sterilization indicators. One indicator must be placed inside each pack being sterilized. This should be used in conjunction with indicator-impregnated autoclave tape on the outside of each pack.

Preparing items for the autoclave

The ***indicator strip*** is used to ensure sterilization has taken place inside the pack. It ensures adequate penetration of the steam and indicates that the contents have been exposed to sterilization steam, that the pack reached the proper temperature and pressure for the proper time, and that the steam penetrated the entire pack (Figure 15.2).

Autoclave tape is useful for identifying packs and articles that have been exposed to steam but does not indicate whether the proper requirements of time, temperature, and pressure have been met. The autoclave tape looks like regular masking tape with white lines in it. Once sterilization has occurred, the white lines will turn black, which indicates exposure to steam. It is also important to mark the autoclave tape with your initials, the contents of the pack, and the date that it is being sterilized (Figures 15.3 and 15.4).

Wrapping a surgical pack

A surgical pack must be wrapped correctly to ensure the contents remain sterile. The following steps demonstrate this task.

Textbook for the Veterinary Assistant, Second Edition. Kara M. Burns and Lori Renda-Francis.
© 2022 John Wiley & Sons, Inc. Published 2022 by John Wiley & Sons, Inc.
Companion website: www.wiley.com/go/burns/textbookvetassistant2

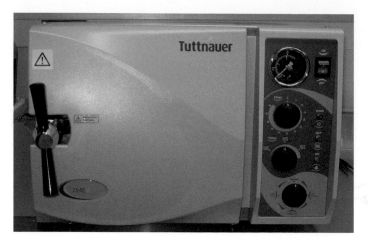

Figure 15.1   Autoclave. Source: Courtesy of Dr Lori Renda-Francis, LVT.

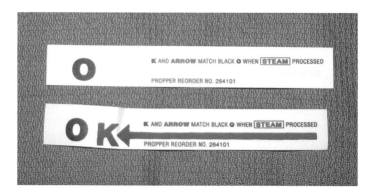

Figure 15.2   Indicator strip. Source: Courtesy of Dr Lori Renda-Francis, LVT.

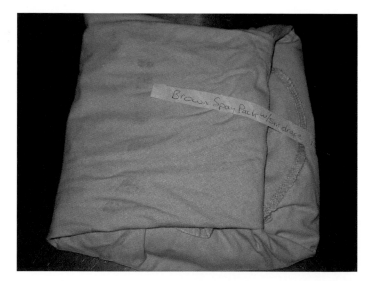

Figure 15.3   Surgical pack prior to autoclaving. Source: Courtesy of Dr Lori Renda-Francis, LVT.

1.   Place a pack wrap/towel diagonally on a flat surface.
2.   One method for assembling the instruments is to thread the handled instruments onto the Snook spay hook. Start with the largest instrument and work down to the smallest. Be sure all instruments are latched closed one notch before threading onto the spay hook.

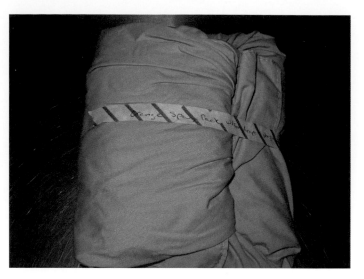

Figure 15.4   Surgical pack after autoclaving. Source: Courtesy of Dr Lori Renda-Francis, LVT.

3.   Place the instruments on the hook in the center of the wrap/ towel and spread the instruments out so they lie relatively flat. Place the scalpel blade handle and any tissue forceps next to the other instruments.
4.   Place the gauze, surgical drape, and indicator strip on top of the instruments.
5.   Fold the top corner of the wrap/towel down. Next, fold each side in, tucking the corners snug. (Think of wrapping a present.)
6.   Fold the bottom corner up. Leave a tab out for easy opening by the surgeon.
7.   Place another pack wrap diagonally on a flat surface.
8.   Place the wrapped instruments in the center of the pack wrap.
9.   A folded towel for the surgeon to dry his or her hands may be placed on top of the wrapped instruments.
10.   Fold the top corner of the pack wrap down.
11.   Next, fold each side in, tucking the corners snug. (Again, think of wrapping a present.)
12.   Fold the bottom corner up and tuck in like an envelope. Leave a tab out for easy opening.
13.   Apply autoclave tape around the center of the pack. Write the date, your initials, and contents on tape.

Sterile packs should be stored in a dust-free, dry, and well-ventilated area away from contaminated equipment. It is important to include the date because sterilized items are considered sterile for only 8 weeks if kept in a closed cabinet (less if they are left on an open shelf).

Cold sterilization

Cold sterilization refers to soaking instruments in a disinfecting solution. Several types of solutions are available. It is important to follow the instructions listed on the container. This method does not involve heat and will not produce the same effects as the autoclave. Sterility cannot be guaranteed with this method, so instruments in cold sterilization should be used only for minor procedures such as lacerations or dentals. The disinfectant solution needs to be changed periodically.

Instruments

As a veterinary assistant, you may be responsible for wrapping the packs. Therefore, you should know the different types of instruments used in veterinary medicine. Most hospitals have general packs used in most surgeries. Many hospitals also have specialized packs for procedures such as orthopedic (bone) surgery. Instruments fall into several general categories. Listed and shown below are the main instruments found in most general surgery packs.

Scissors (Figure 15.5)

Sharp operating scissors.

- Used for cutting inanimate objects like drapes or sutures.
- Blades can be straight or curved.
- Can be sharp or blunt-tipped.

Mayo dissecting scissors.

- Used for dissecting tissue
- Blades can be straight or curved.

Metzenbaum scissors.

- Used for delicate surgical dissection.
- Blades can be straight or curved.

Hemostats

These instruments are used to aid in controlling blood loss during a surgical procedure. They usually have varying serrations on the jaws and come in both straight and curved forms (Figure 15.6). Halstead mosquito forceps.

- Used to clamp small-diameter vessels.
- Small jaws with fine horizontal serrations.

Kelly forceps.

- Used for medium-sized vessels or small masses of tissue.
- Wide, horizontal serrations.

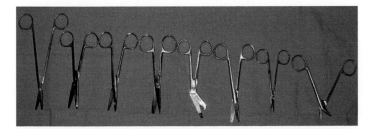

Figure 15.5 Surgical scissors. Source: Courtesy of Dr Lori Renda Francis, LVT.

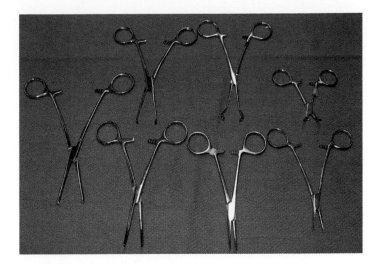

Figure 15.6 Hemostats. Source: Courtesy of Dr Lori Renda-Francis, LVT.

Rochester–Carmalt forceps.

- Used for very large vessels or tissue masses.
- Both horizontal and vertical serrations

Ferguson angiotribe.

- Not a true hemostat.
- Used to crush tissue and vessels that do not need to be viable.
- Has a raised jaw and a recessed jaw.

Needle holders

This instrument is used to hold the needle and suture material during a surgical procedure. It should also be used to place a scalpel blade onto a scalpel handle.
Olsen–Hegar.

- Has scissors built into jaws to allow the surgeon to cut the suture.

Mayo–Hegar.

- Lacks scissors in jaws.

Scalpel handle

These instruments hold the scalpel blade. They come in sizes 3 and 4. Blades #10–19 fit size 3 handles while blades #20–29 fit size 4 handles.

Thumb tissue forceps

These instruments are used to pick up and retract tissue for a short period of time. They resemble tweezers but should never be referred to as tweezers (Figure 15.7).
Debakey thumb tissue forceps.

- Used for the most delicate tissue.
- *Atraumatic*, grooved ends instead of teeth.

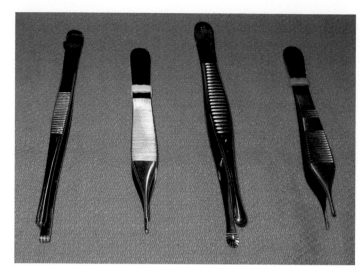

Figure 15.7 Thumb tissue forceps. Source: Courtesy of Dr Lori Renda-Francis, LVT.

Adson–Brown thumb tissue forceps.

- Used as a general surgery tissue forceps.
- Usually has two parallel rows of nine shallow teeth on both edges.

Adson 1 × 2 thumb tissue forceps.

- Used to grasp tissue firmly, can cause a fair amount of trauma if used too aggressively.
- Has one tooth on one tip and two teeth on the other.

Allis tissue forceps

This instrument is neither a tissue forceps nor a hemostat. It is used for grasping tissue in a traumatic way. These tissues are usually either going to be removed from the patient or are tough and can withstand some trauma. Allis tissue forceps have a ringed handle and tips that contain multiple interlocking teeth.

Towel clamps

These instruments are used to keep the sterile drapes or towels in place on the patient. They have both penetrating and nonpenetrating tips.
Backhaus towel clamps.

- Most common type, available in several sizes.
- Have penetrating tip.

Roeder towel clamps.

- Metal balls on the tips prevent them from penetrating tissue too deeply.

Snook spay hook

This hook-like instrument is used to located the **uterine horns** of a female patient and allow the surgeon to **exteriorize** them from the abdominal cavity. This instrument is used in a dog or cat ovariohysterectomy (spay).

Suture material and suture needles

It will be important for veterinary assistants to have a basic understanding of suture materials and the different types of suture needles.

Suture material

Suture material is used for many purposes such as stitching wounds or skin incisions, strengthening tissue or tying off specific blood vessels. Suture material comes in both an absorbable and a nonabsorbable type. Absorbable suture material is absorbed by the body over time and does not require removal. Nonabsorbable suture material remains strong and intact for long periods of time. Some common absorbable suture materials include surgical gut (also referred to as cat gut), Vicryl®, and PDS®. Some common nonabsorbable suture materials include Bronamid®, nylon, Prolene®, and stainless steel (Table 15.1).

The doctor will determine the type and size of suture to be used but the veterinary assistant will want to be familiar with all types used in the practice as you will be assisting in setting up for surgery.

The suture size is the measure of the diameter of the material, or how thick it is. It comes in a variety of sizes and is measured in gauges ranging from 7-0 (pronounced 7 aught) to a 3 gauge. So a 3-0 would be much smaller than a 3.

- 7-0 (smallest)
- 6-0
- 5-0
- 4-0
- 3-0
- 2-0
- 1-0
- 1
- 2
- 3 (largest)

Suture material can be packaged in individual foil wraps or in a spool for multi-use (Figures 15.8 and 15.9). The spool requires the surgeon to thread the needle and the individual packs may or may not contain swaged-on needles.

Suture needles

Surgical needles can be packaged in one of two ways. They can come preattached to the suture, which is called swaged on or swagged on (Figure 15.10). They can also come without the suture attached (Figure 15.11) which would mean that the surgeon would select the suture material and thread the needle.

Needles can also come with different type tips. They can be either a cutting needle or a taper needle. A cutting needle has sharp edges to allow it to pass through tough tissue (skin) with

Table 15.1 Common sutures used in veterinary medicine.

Generic name	Common trade name	Absorbent/nonabsorbent	Structure	Color
Chromic catgut	Gut	Absorbent	Monofilament	Brown
Polyglycolide	Vicryl®	Absorbent	Braided	Purple or undyed
Polydioxanone	PDS®	Absorbent	Monofilament	Purple or clear
Nylon	Ethilon®, Dermalon®	Nonabsorbent	Mono- or multifilament	Black, green, or blue
Silk	Many available	Nonabsorbent	Braided	Black
Polypropylene	Prolene®	Nonabsorbent	Monofilament	Blue

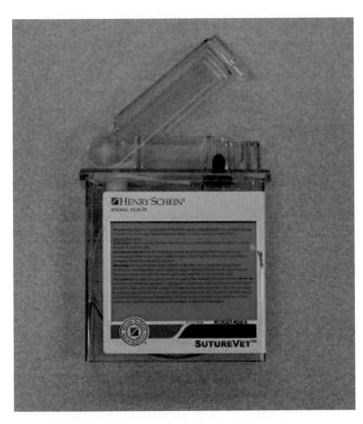

Figure 15.8 Suture cassette (spool). Source: Courtesy of Dr Lori Renda-Francis, LVT.

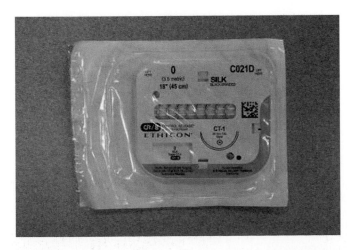

Figure 15.9 Individual suture pack with needle. Source: Courtesy of Dr Lori Renda-Francis, LVT.

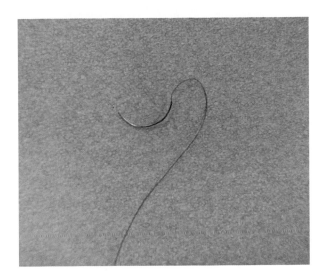

Figure 15.10 Swaged-on needle. Source: Courtesy of Dr Lori Renda-Francis, LVT.

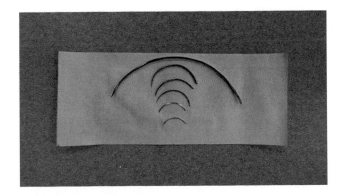

Figure 15.11 Suture needles. Source: Courtesy of Dr Lori Renda-Francis, LVT.

greater ease. A taper does not have cutting edges and passes through tissue without cutting. A needle rack is used to hold and contain free needles within the surgery pack.

Gowns and Drapes

As part of preparing surgical packs, you will be required to fold and pack surgical gowns and drapes for sterilization. They will need to be folded in a certain pattern to allow for ease of use and to maintain sterility. Following are the steps for folding surgical gowns and drapes. (Figures 15.12–15.19).

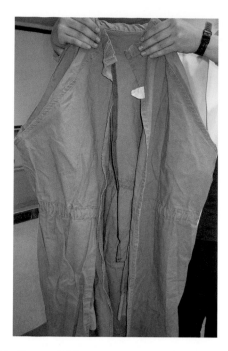

Figure 15.12   Steps to folding a gown. Source: Courtesy of Dr Lori Renda-Francis, LVT.

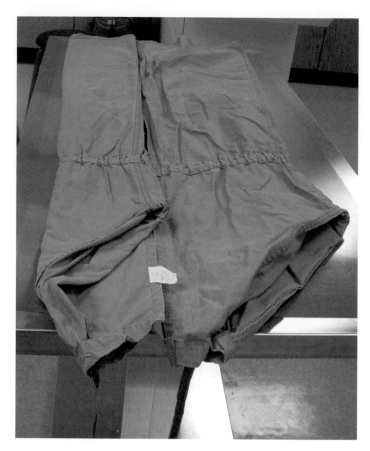

Figure 15.14   Steps to folding a gown. Source: Courtesy of Dr Lori Renda-Francis, LVT.

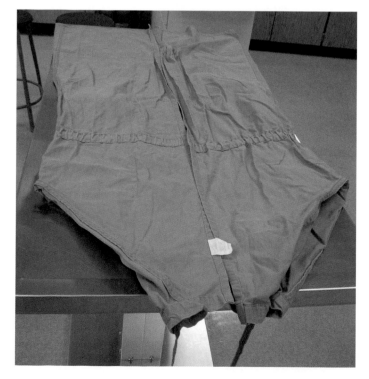

Figure 15.13   Steps to folding a gown. Source: Courtesy of Dr Lori Renda-Francis, LVT.

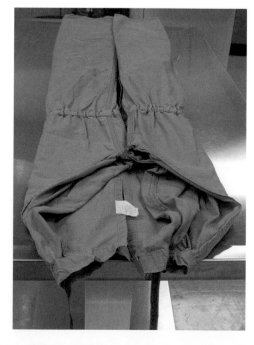

Figure 15.15   Steps to folding a gown. Source: Courtesy of Dr Lori Renda-Francis, LVT.

Folding a gown

1. Hold the gown so that the outside is facing away from you.
2. Fold the gown in half lengthwise twice. Be sure the inside of the gown is showing.

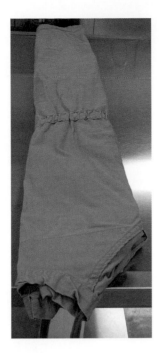

Figure 15.16   Steps to folding a gown. Source: Courtesy of Dr Lori Renda-Francis, LVT.

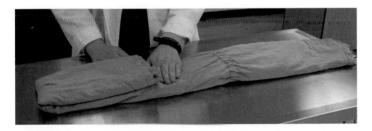

Figure 15.17   Steps to folding a gown. Source: Courtesy of Dr Lori Renda-Francis, LVT.

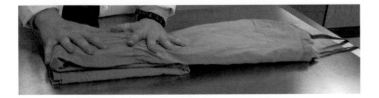

Figure 15.18   Steps to folding a gown. Source: Courtesy of Dr Lori Renda-Francis, LVT.

3. Lie the gown on a table and fold in half lengthwise again.
4. Next, fold it end to end, twice. The gown should be folded in such a way that the top, inside portion of the gown is up when the sterile pack is unwrapped. This is the area grasped by the surgeon.

Folding a surgical drape

1. Fold the drape in half lengthwise.
2. Fold each side of the drape lengthwise again, in an accordion-like fashion.

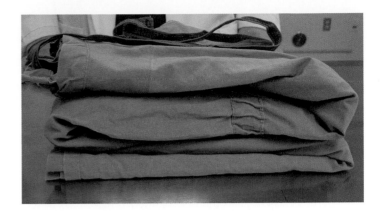

Figure 15.19   Steps to folding a gown. Source: Courtesy of Dr Lori Renda-Francis, LVT.

3. Fold the drape over, short end to short end.
4. Fold the drape short end to short end in an accordion-like fashion.

The sterile field

The sterile field is the area on and around the surgical table. Only sterile items and personnel who have properly scrubbed can come in contact with the sterile field. If anything nonsterile comes in contact with anything sterile, the sterility is voided. All non-sterile personnel must be extremely careful around the sterile field. Care must be taken to make sure your body or your hands do not touch or reach over any sterile item.

It is important for the entire surgical team to ensure that sterility is maintained. A "scrubbed-in" person is one who has scrubbed and donned a gown and gloves. Scrubbed-in people are considered part of the sterile surgical team and can touch only sterile items. A nonscrubbed or nonsterile person should touch only nonsterile items or areas and should never reach over or across a sterile item or field.

If at any point a break in sterility is suspected, it should be immediately brought to the veterinarian's attention, and steps need to be taken to reduce the risk of further contamination.

Preparing for surgery

All jewelery and nail polish should be removed prior to entering the surgery room and also ensure finger nails are clipped short and long hair pulled back out of the way. Before entering a surgery room, several items must be worn to ensure the risk of contamination is kept at a minimum. What is worn will depend on what role you will be playing during the surgical procedure. Caps and masks are worn by all people entering the surgical room. Shoes can be a major source of contamination so disposable shoe covers should also be worn. The cap and mask are not sterile, but they help prevent contamination by reducing the chance of contamination through saliva droplets and hair falling into the surgical site.

Surgical hand scrub

The veterinary surgeon and the sterile technician will perform a surgical scrub on their hands. The scrub will last between 5 and 7 minutes. Even though sterile surgical gloves will be worn, they cannot be relied upon solely to prevent contamination as it is possible that tiny holes or tears can occur. Once the surgical scrub is completed, they will use a sterile hand towel to dry their hands.

Gowning

The veterinary assistant would not routinely be asked to participate as a sterile assistant in surgery; however, it is important to be familiar with the different types of gowning procedures as you will be assisting with preparing and tying the sterile gowns.

Surgical gowns should be worn by all sterile surgical team members while in the surgical suite. Surgical gowns come in two main styles, reusable or disposable, and two types of ties, wraparound or tie behind. To ensure the gown stays sterile, the person wearing it must put it on in the manner outlined below. The front and sides of the gown are considered sterile areas. Care must be taken to avoid touching the sterile areas of the gown.

Sterile gowning steps

1. Lift the sterile gown out of its sterile wrapper or sterile pack. Avoid contamination.

2. Move into an area where the gown may be opened without contamination of self or gown.

3. Hold the gown away from your body and unfold it so that the inside is toward you.

4. Slip your hands into the arms of the gown while keeping them away from your body. Keep hands at shoulder level.

5. If a closed glove technique is performed, advance your hands up the sleeves of the gown until they reach the cuff. Do not put your hands through the cuff as this will not allow you to perform a closed glove technique as described in the next section. A nonsterile assistant will help pull the gown over your shoulders and fasten the neck of the gown.

6. Once the surgical gloves are on, the gown can be tied. The technique for tying the gown will depend on the style.

    a. With wraparound ties, hand the sterile right tab of the gown to the assistant, turn left 280° and then take back the tab. Finally, tie this to the other sterile tab to wrap the gown.

    b. With tie-behind gowns, the nonsterile assistant will tie the gown at the waistline, making sure to touch only the back of the gown.

Gloving

Once the surgical gown is on, you will need to apply surgical gloves. As with the gown, these gloves are sterile and care must be taken when putting them on. There are two types of gloving

techniques: closed gloving and open gloving. Closed gloving provides the best assurance against contamination because the bare skin on your arms and hands is never exposed during the process.

Closed gloving technique (Figures 15.20 and 15.21)

1. Keep your hands within the cuffs of the gown. With your left hand, you will pick up the right glove by the folded cuff.

2. While keeping your hand in the cuff of the gown, extend your right hand, palm facing up. The right glove is laid on the palm of the right hand, cuff to cuff with the gown sleeve. The fingers of the glove will point toward the elbow and the

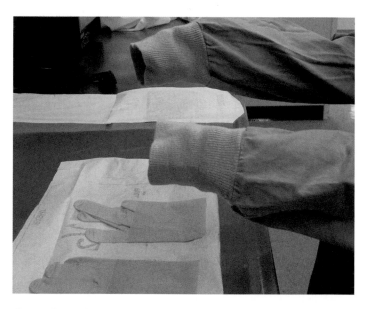

Figure 15.20 Closed gloving technique. Source: Courtesy of Dr Lori Renda-Francis, LVT.

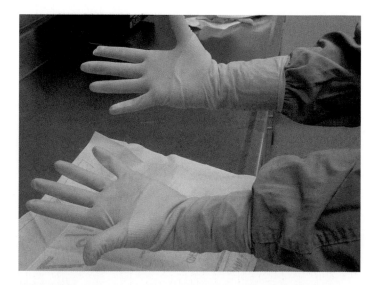

Figure 15.21 Closed gloving technique. Source: Courtesy of Dr Lori Renda-Francis, LVT.

thumb of the glove is positioned on top of the covered right thumb.

3. With your right hand still within the gown, grasp the inside of the cuff of the glove. With your left hand, fold the cuff of the glove over the back of the right hand.

4. With your left hand, pull the cuff of the right glove and sleeve of the right gown toward the elbow as your right hand slides into the glove. Do not adjust the glove until both gloves are on and sterility is ensured.

5. Using the gloved right hand, lift the left glove by its cuff and place on the palm of the left hand, again aligning it with the cuff of the gown. The gloved fingers should point toward the elbow and the left thumb of the glove over the covered left thumb.

6. With your left fingers still within the gown, grasp the inside of the glove and using the right hand, pull the left glove cuff over the back of the hand. Pull the glove cuff and gown sleeve toward your elbow as your left hand slides into the glove

7. Now that both gloves are on, pull glove cuffs over gown sleeves and adjust gloves for comfort.

Open gloving technique (Figures 15.22–15.25)

1. Open a sterile pack of gloves on a flat surface. Lift the right glove by grasping the inside of the cuff with the left hand.

2. Slide the right hand into the glove without touching the gown or the outside of the glove. As with the closed gloving technique, do not adjust glove or cuff until both gloves are on.

3. Next, lift the left glove by sliding fingers of gloved hand in between the upturned cuff and outside surface of glove.

4. While keeping the gloved fingers under the cuff, slide the glove onto your left hand and over the cuff of the gown.

5. With both gloves on, adjust the right glove by sliding the fingers of your left hand under the cuff that is still upturned and slide it over the cuff of the gown. Adjust both gloves for comfort.

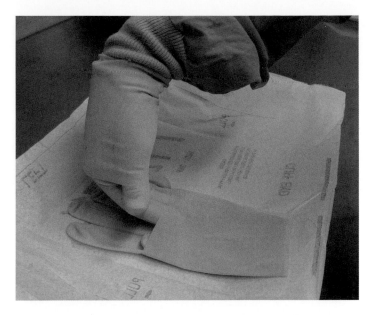

Figure 15.23 Open gloving technique. Source: Courtesy of Dr Lori Renda-Francis, LVT.

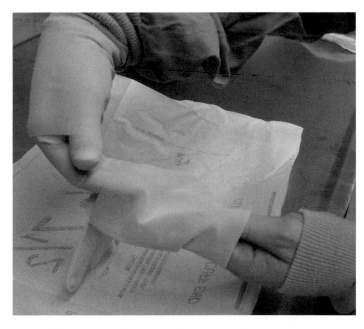

Figure 15.24 Open gloving technique. Source: Courtesy of Dr Lori Renda-Francis, LVT.

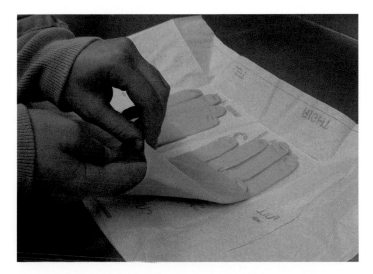

Figure 15.22 Open gloving technique. Source: Courtesy of Dr Lori Renda-Francis, LVT.

Opening and passing sterile items

The most important aspect regarding opening sterile items is the maintenance of sterility of both the items and the surgical team. Do not open sterile packs until the surgical team is prepared to receive them.

There are two common types of packs that you may be asked to open: peel-away pouches and those wrapped in drapes.

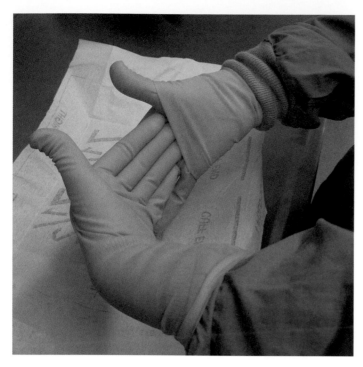

Figure 15.25   Open gloving technique. Source: Courtesy of Dr Lori Renda-Francis, LVT.

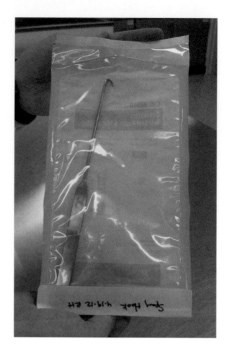

Figure 15.26   Sterile pouch. Source: Courtesy of Dr Lori Renda-Francis, LVT.

Opening peel-away pouches (Figure 15.26)

Many peel-away pouches will indicate which end to open. Holding the packet with both hands at the end where indicated, slowly peel back the two sides of the pouch. While opening the pouch, make sure to stabilize the item within so it does not slip out of the pouch or touch the nonsterile edges of the pouch. The item in the pouch can be handed directly to a surgical team member or placed on a flat, sterile, draped area. Suture material can be opened in the same fashion.

Opening drape wrapped packs

Depending on the size of the pack, some may be opened with one hand while others will need to be placed on a flat surgical stand or table. Small packs can be opened with one hand. By opening a pack with one hand, you will be able to pass the sterile item directly to a sterile surgical team member. To open the pack properly, hold the pack in one hand and slip your thumb under the taped fold. With the other hand, remove the tape. After removing the tape, lift the top fold and fold it back into the grasp of the other hand. Next, open the two side folds, again folding the flaps back in the grasp of the hand holding the pack. Finally, take the last corner tab and pull it back into the grasp of the handholding the pack. At this point, the sterile team member will take the enclosed sterile item.

With larger packs, you will need to place them on a clean, flat surface, such as a *Mayo stand* or surgical table. Place the pack on the flat surface with the folded, taped side facing up. Remove the tape. Open the distant folded edge first, making sure to avoid the

sterile contents within. Never reach over the sterile contents of the pack. After opening the distal edge, open the side flaps using only the exposed corners. Always open the tab closest to you last. Avoid reaching over the sterile field. If the pack is double-wrapped, a sterile member of the surgical team will be responsible for opening the interior wrap.

Preparing the patient

Surgical clipping

Once a patient has been anesthetized, the surgical site must be prepped. This consists of several steps. First, the hair must be removed from the surgical site. This is performed with a set of electric clippers and a #40 blade. This blade is sometimes referred to as a surgical clipper blade because it trims the hair short enough so that the surgical field will not become contaminated. Hair removal should be neat and symmetrical when possible. A client's impression of the surgical site, surgeon, and staff may be based solely on the clip. Clipping should be done against the grain of the hair. This will facilitate ease of removal and will not leave stubble that is too long and can lead to surgical complications and surgical site infections. How much hair is removed will often depend on what surgery is being performed. The general rule is two clipper widths in all directions from around the surgical site. When in doubt, ask the surgeon.

Surgical site preparation

Once the surgical site is clipped, a vacuum should be used to remove all the loose hair from the site. Once as much of the hair as possible is removed, the surgical area will be scrubbed. Because of the nature of an animal's skin, we cannot sterilize the area in the truest sense of the word. Our goal is to reduce the number of bacteria and other potential disease-causing agents as well as to remove dirt or oil from the skin at the surgical site.

The cleaning process is a multistep procedure. First, clean the skin with an antiseptic. The two most common ones used in veterinary medicine are povidone-iodine and chlorhexidine gluconate. Both of these products have few toxic effects on tissue, especially when diluted for surgical site cleansing. When scrubbing a surgical site, it is recommended to start at the center of the site, working your way out in ever enlarging circles. Make sure to never go over the same area twice to avoid cross-contamination. After an area is scrubbed with antiseptic, it should be rinsed. Sterile water or 70% isopropyl alcohol are commonly used. Again, this should be done starting from the middle of the surgical site and working your way out in a circular pattern. These steps are performed three times or until clean.

Once the surgical area is scrubbed, a final solution, usually povidone-iodine, is applied to the surgical site using a spray bottle. Do not wipe this solution off. The surgeon will remove this prior to making the incision.

After the patient is prepped, the animal will be moved to the surgical room. The patient will be placed on the surgical table in one of three main positions: sternal recumbency (on the belly), dorsal recumbency (on the back) or lateral recumbency (on the side). The patient's position will depend on the type of surgery being performed. The most common surgeries are within the abdomen, and thus most patients will be placed in dorsal recumbency. To help keep the patient in dorsal recumbency, a V-trough is commonly used. This piece of equipment is either placed on the table, or the table itself can be made into a V shape with an adjustment to its sides (Figures 15.27 and 15.28).

After the patient is placed in the proper position, its legs will need to be secured. Most often this is accomplished with ties to secure them to the surgical table. The ties are secured around the patient's carpus and tarsus, then to hooks on the surgical table.

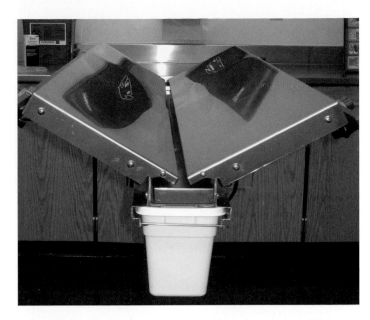

Figure 15.28 Table made into a V shape. Source: Courtesy of Dr Lori Renda-Francis, LVT.

The number of limbs secured by this method will depend on the animal's position on the table.

Postsurgical procedures

Following surgery and after the patient is off the surgical table, you may have several responsibilities. These may include monitoring the patient during recovery and cleaning the surgical room.

Postoperative monitoring

If you are asked to monitor the patient postoperatively, you should be familiar with the normal vital signs for the patient's species. Vitals to monitor in the postoperative period are respiration rate, heart rate, mucous membrane color, capillary refill time (CRT), and temperature. See Chapter 9 on physical examinations and animal nursing to refresh your memory on vital signs. Other changes to note are bleeding or swelling at the incision site. If any significant changes are noted in the patient, the technician and doctor should be notified immediately.

Surgical room clean-up

After the patient has been removed from the surgical room, it will need to be cleaned and prepared for the next surgery. All dirty instruments and equipment should be removed and taken to the prep area so that they can be cleaned. Any sharps (i.e., scalpel blades, needles) should be placed in the sharps container (Figure 15.29). All tissue or blood-saturated material (gauze, disposable drapes) must be removed from the *surgical kick bucket* and placed in a red biohazard bag (Figure 15.30).

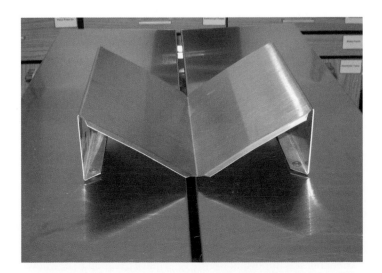

Figure 15.27 V-trough. Source: Courtesy of Dr Lori Renda-Francis, LVT.

The table, Mayo instrument stand, V-trough, or any other items that have come in contact with the patient or bodily fluids should be cleaned and disinfected. Solutions like dilute bleach or quaternary ammonium compounds such as Roccal® are most frequently used. Any items or materials used during surgery should be restocked. Finally, the floors should be swept and disinfected using one of the above-mentioned compounds.

Surgical positioning

As a veterinary assistant, you will be responsible for assisting in patient positioning in the surgery room and with transporting a surgical patient from the prep room to the surgery room.

In surgery, patients are positioned properly when the surgeon has optimal access to the surgical site that provides the best visualization and organ retraction during the procedure. Safe positioning should include knowledge, planning, and teamwork. Once an animal is transferred into the surgery suite, they should never be left alone.

The surgical technician should be knowledgeable about the patient's status, the procedure to be performed, and the preparation for the patient's procedure. You as the veterinary assistant will be assisting with this task.

There are several positions in which an animal will be placed, depending on the type of surgery that is going to be performed. We will cover some of the most common ones.

Dorsal recumbency is when the animal is placed on its back. It is used for most abdominal surgeries such as sterilization surgeries, exploratory laparotomies, cystotomies, mammary surgeries, and thyroidectomies. When the animal is in dorsal recumbency, the forelimbs are retracted and secured cranially and hindlimbs are secured caudally. A V-trough, also known as a thoracic positioner, may be necessary to stabilize pelvis or thorax or both. This is very helpful with large or deep-chested animals.

Lateral recumbency is when the animal is placed on its side with the forelegs pulled and secured cranially to stabilize and lift the ribcage. Hindlimbs are secured caudally. This position is often used for flank surgeries, feline neuters, renal surgery, amputations, and some other surgeries of the extremities. Many oral surgeries occur in this position, as well.

Sternal recumbency is when the patient is lying on its sternum or chest. Deep-chested animals may need additional surgical positioning devices to stabilize the thorax in this position. ***Anal sacculectomies***, spinal surgeries (especially lumbar disc), ophthalmic, aural and nasal surgeries, and cranial surgeries are commonly performed in this position.

Communication is the key to successful teamwork when positioning and transporting the patient to the surgical suite and each person on the team should be aware of their specific duties during the process to ensure that the patient is positioned and safely secured.

Surgical monitoring

The veterinary technician will be responsible for monitoring the patient but it is important for the veterinary assistant to be knowledgeable and aware of all aspects of the surgery room.

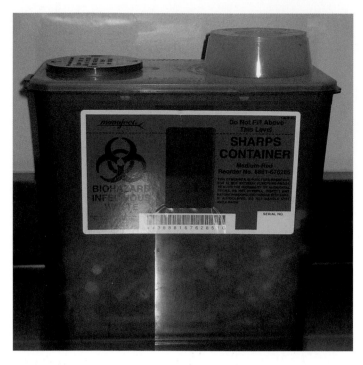

Figure 15.29   Sharps container. Source: Courtesy of Dr Lori Renda-Francis, LVT.

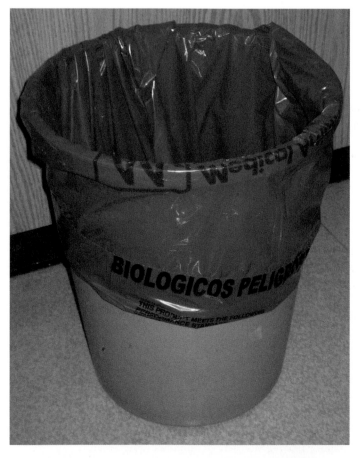

Figure 15.30   Biohazard bag. Source: Courtesy of Dr Lori Renda-Francis, LVT.

Because each animal may have a different reaction to anesthetic agents, and because the anesthetic drugs and the type of surgical procedure being performed may cause changes to a patient's status, it is important to use effective patient monitoring to trend a patient's vital signs and address cardiopulmonary issues at the first sign of a problem. A prompt response decreases the risk that a fatal error may occur. Monitoring tracks both the patient's response to anesthesia and their physiological condition. This allows for the maintenance of proper oxygenation throughout the procedure, preemptive pain management, and a swift and smooth anesthetic recovery.

According to the American College of Veterinary Anesthesia and Analgesia (ACVAA) and the American Animal Hospital Association (AAHA), patients should be monitored during sedation as well as general anesthesia. No piece of equipment can replace a skilled and observant anesthetist when it comes to monitoring. Circulation, ventilation, oxygenation, and analgesia are the parameters that should be monitored every 3–5 minutes throughout the anesthetic procedure. Anesthetic complications can be detected by monitoring these parameters.

You will notice that the veterinary technician will begin to monitor the patient prior to induction of anesthesia, through the surgery and through the recovery phase as well. Up to 60% of anesthetic deaths of dogs and cats occur postoperatively, and usually within the first 3 hours. Patients should continue to be monitored until they are alert, ambulatory, and their temperature is normal.

Monitoring a patient can include checking the temperature, pulse, auscultating the heart, blood pressure, and checking capillary refill time. It will also include the use of a variety of equipment. The veterinary technician will be routinely checking the depth of anesthesia. This can be done by monitoring the eye position, **palpebral reflex**, toe pinch, and jaw tone.

It is important for the veterinary assistant to be always vigilant and aware and to bring any concerns to the attention of the veterinary technician or veterinarian immediately.

Surgical log

The surgical log is a record of the anesthetic procedure that was performed. It contains the animal's **signalment**, the types of anesthetic agents used and their dosages, the amount administered as compared to the calculated dose, and the duration of the procedure. This log should be completed by the team member who is administering the anesthesia. The date should be recorded, as well as the initials of both the anesthetist and the overseeing veterinarian. The surgical log will remain a record of the animal's surgery as well as the experience of the technician and veterinarian.

Surgical room conduct

When entering the surgery room, everyone should be wearing a cap, mask, and shoe coverings. The surgeon and sterile veterinary technicians should also be wearing a gown and gloves.

Everyone in the surgery room should be aware of the following:

- Sterile personnel should only touch sterile items.
- Nonsterile personnel only touch nonsterile items.
- Sterile items should be grouped together and separated from nonsterile items to avoid contamination.
- If *any* doubt exists as to whether or not a specific item is sterile, it must be considered contaminated.
- If contamination occurs, it must be remedied immediately.
- Avoid sneezing and coughing. If a sneeze or cough cannot be avoided, turn your head away from the sterile zone.
- Do not move around the room or enter and leave the room unless necessary.
- Do not leave sterile fields unattended.
- Do not talk unless necessary. Talking increases bacterial contamination. It may also distract the surgeon. Saliva weakens the filtration of the surgical mask.
- Restrict body movements to those necessary. Arm and hand gestures increase air current which can increase risk of contamination.
- Foot covers should be worn in the surgical area.

www.wiley.com/go/burns/textbookvetassistant2

Please go to the companion website for assignments and a PowerPoint relating to the material in this chapter.

Chapter **16** Avian, Exotics, and Rodents

Avian

Birds are a very popular species as they provide companionship and are relatively easy pets to care for. Some species of birds can even be taught to interact with the owner and can learn some of the language which the owner speaks. Members of the psittacine or passerine families are usually the most common companion birds presenting to veterinary hospitals. Psittacines, or parrots, are the most popular companion birds. Psittacines are also referred to as hookbills due to the fact that their upper beak is curved. They also have a unique shape to their feet referred to as zygodactyl. Zygodactyl feet have the second and third toes facing forward and the first and fourth toes directed backward. Another popular companion bird is the passerine. These are small birds whose beak is pointed or slightly curved. They have feet that are known as anisodactyl, meaning three toes point forward and one toe points to the rear. Passerines are typically active. They enjoy moving around and/or flying around their cage.

Avian anatomy

Integument

The largest organ system of the body is the integument. The integument protects the underlying structures and organs. It is also a physical barrier between the body and the outside world. The bird's outside anatomy is made up of the skin, beak, claws, and feathers.

The skin of companion birds is delicate and is dry and slightly wrinkled. The area around the nostrils is known as the cere. Birds also do not have sweat glands. Some birds possess one major skin gland known as the uropygial gland which empties into a lone papilla located at the dorsal base of the tail. A lipoid sebaceous material secretes from this gland and is spread over feathers during preening, thus helping to waterproof the feathers. As stated, only some birds have this gland – it is absent in the ostrich, emu, woodpecker, and Amazon parrot.

The feathers found on birds have many functions. We know they are essential for flight. However, feathers also keep the skin safe from trauma and exposure. Furthermore, feathers also play a role in ***thermoregulation***, camouflage, and communication.

Birds have several types of feathers.

- Contour feathers – flight feathers or body feathers covering the body and wings.
- Remiges or primary flight feathers – located on the outer end of the wing.
- Secondary flight feathers – located on the wing between the body and the primaries
- Coverts or body feathers – provide surface coverage over the remainder of the body.
- Down feathers – provide insulation. Appear soft and fluffy. Powder down feathers break down and produce a white dusty powder.
- Molting – the periodic replacement of old feathers.
- Blood feathers – new, growing feathers with a vascular supply.
  - Blood feather shafts are dark and bleed profusely if broken.
  - May result in the death of the bird if not treated.

Textbook for the Veterinary Assistant, Second Edition. Kara M. Burns and Lori Renda-Francis.
© 2022 John Wiley & Sons, Inc. Published 2022 by John Wiley & Sons, Inc.
Companion website: www.wiley.com/go/burns/textbookvetassistant2

Musculoskeletal system

Avian skeletons are highly adapted. Many avian bones are pneumatized, meaning they contain air, thus resulting in a lighter skeleton. However, although the bones have thin walls which make them lighter, this also makes the bones more fragile. The beak is strengthened through the fusion of the bones in the skull. The neck of the bird is long and flexible. The keel (sternum) supports the pectoral muscles used in flight. Birds have a fused caudal vertebra called the synsacrum. This fusion is responsible for stabilizing the bird's back during flight.

Twenty percent of the bird's weight is found in the pectorals. The pectorals are the largest muscle in the body of an avian patient. The pectorals are often used by the health-care team to determine the bird's body condition.

Respiratory system

The respiratory system is unlike the respiratory system in other companion animals. The nares are located on either side of the beak and air enters through the nares. The **operculum** is located immediately behind the nares in the nasal cavity. After entering the nares, air passes over the operculum, through the sinus cavities, and enters the oral cavity through the choana. The choana is a V-shaped notch in the roof of the bird's mouth that directs air from the mouth and nasal cavities to the glottis. When the bird swallows, the choana closes. Visual observation will find the choana surrounded by sharp **papillae**.

Air will then travel through the glottis and down the trachea. The trachea in the bird is found on the left side of the cervical area. The avian trachea is mobile the entire length of the neck, consisting of complete cartilaginous rings that cannot expand. The syrinx, also known as the voice box, is found at the end of the trachea. Although birds do not talk as extensively as humans, they can produce vocalizations. Vocalizations in birds occur when air is forced over the syrinx and vibrating membranes during the expiratory phase of respiration. The complexity of a bird's vocalizations depends on the species and number of muscles in the syrinx.

As the air continues, it enters the small lungs, which are located near the dorsal spine. It is here that air exchange takes place. Birds' lungs do not inflate as they lack alveoli and lung lobes. Birds also lack a diaphragm. Inspiration of air occurs by the extension of the **intracostal joints** drawing in inspired air with a bellows-like action into the caudal air sacs. This bellows-like action takes place in the **coelom**. Active muscle contraction is needed for both inspiration and expiration in avians.

There are nine air sacs into which air flows. The air sacs are hollow spaces that have thin walls and are highly vascularized. The air sacs can be located as follows.

- Four paired air sacs:
    - cranial thoracic
    - caudal thoracic
    - cervical
    - abdominal.
- One air sac:
    - interclavicular – thoracic inlet between the clavicles.

Gas exchange does not occur in the air sacs in avians; rather, to move a breath completely through the respiratory system, the bird must complete two breath cycles. It is important to remember that normal breathing in birds should not be noticeable, and the beak should remain closed. After exercise, especially if the caged bird "escapes" and flies around the house before returning to its cage, there may be increased head and tail movement and increased abdominal effort. However, after a minute or two the bird's respiratory pattern should return to normal.

Digestive system

The avian species has a high metabolic rate requiring ingestion of large amounts of food. The beak anatomy will differ with the foraging strategies and diet make-up of the particular bird. In most birds, the beak is responsible for grasping food and pulverizing it. The tongue helps in this grasping and crushing process. The make-up of the mouth of a bird consists of the following.

- Hard, upper palate
- Soft, lower palate
- Unique tongue
- Taste buds scattered through the mouth
- Salivary glands

As a bird swallows, the food enters and travels though the esophagus. In many species the esophagus expands in the interclavicular space, thus creating the crop. The anatomy of the crop does vary among birds, but typically is a dilation of the esophagus, a single pouch or a double pouch. The crop is responsible for the softening of food and passes small portions of food into the true stomach, known as the proventriculus, where digestive acids and enzymes begin breaking down the food. Next, the food is passed into a thickly muscled organ that grinds the food into smaller particles, known as the gizzard or ventriculus. The small intestine is the major organ responsible for digestion and absorption of nutrients. Following the small intestine, as in other species, is the large intestine which terminates at the cloaca. The vent is the external opening of the cloaca, from which the droppings exit the body. Bird excrement, or droppings, consist of three components: liquid urine, cream consistency urates, and feces. The consistency of the droppings is variable dependent mainly upon the diet.

Circulatory system

The avian heart is approximately 1.5 times larger, relatively speaking, than the heart in mammals. The heart rate of birds is 250–350 beats per minute in large parrots and up to 1400 beats per minute in small avian species. Blood pressure also runs higher than companion animal counterparts. It is important to note that birds do not have lymph nodes and the lymphatic system is less extensive than in mammals. It is important to also note that the red blood cells differ from mammals, with bird red blood cells appearing oval in shape and containing a nucleus.

Office visit

Bird owners should always be advised to bring their bird to the hospital in a secured container. This is preferably in their cage, although oftentimes this is not possible and the bird is brought to the hospital in what the owner will refer to as a "travel cage or carrier." Small animal carriers are popular for bird owners to transport, as they are easy to clean and wooden perches are easy to add to the inside of a pet carrier. Insure the carrier has the water removed while transporting to avoid spillage, but have the owner leave newspapers in the carrier, as the droppings will be part of the overall examination at the hospital.

An avian physical examination includes three steps: a thorough history, a visual examination, a complete physical examination. As with any examination, one of the most important steps is to obtain a detailed history from the owner. Nutrition and husbandry-related problems are very common findings and can lead to various medical conditions. Client education by the health-care team is crucial to working with and overcoming many of the issues related to nutrition and husbandry.

Physical examination of birds during an office visit also includes watching the bird in the exam room. A great deal of information can be found from observation of the bird's behaviors and appearance. Transportation to the hospital is a very stressful event for the bird so watch carefully to insure the bird recovers from this stressful trip. Healthy birds should have a regular respiratory rate with no increased or forced effort. Watch as the bird stands. Is it trying to stand on its perch or is it wobbly, trying to sleep, or falling off the perch? Remember to evaluate the droppings in the transport cage as well. Stressed birds will produce mostly urine. Remember the history that was taken especially concerning the diet. Birds that eat strictly seed diets typically have drier droppings. Look for blood and parasites. Undigested seeds also may indicate disease. The urine color should be clear, with the urates appearing white to possibly tan.

Restraint

As with all animals, proper restraint techniques are important for the safety of the handler and the person performing examinations or treatments, but most importantly for the safety and wellbeing of the patient. Restraint is a large stressor for avian patients, so knowing the avian patient and proper restraint and capture techniques will help to decrease pain and stress.

All escape routes should be closed and the room should be sealed. Hiding places to which the bird may flee should be identified and closed off. To capture and restrain an avian patient, it is recommended to use a towel. Towels of different sizes relative to the size of the bird are indicated. Using a towel to capture a bird helps to reduce fear of hands in the future. Gloves are *not* recommended, as a fear of hands may develop with gloves and the wearer loses much of their tactile sensation which is extremely important when handling birds.

A slow approach with the towel in hand is best. Do not try to capture a bird that is sitting on the owner, as this may result in

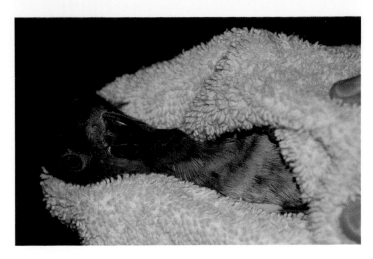

Figure 16.1   Meyer's parrot in towel restraint. Courtesy Kara M Burns, LVT, VTS (Nutrition).

behavioral issues of the bird toward the owner and may lead to the bird biting or attacking the owner. Remember to use a calm and soothing tone when approaching a bird. Confidence should be displayed, especially when trying to capture and restrain a large bird – they can detect fear and hesitation. The hand (in the towel) should grasp the head of the bird toward the cervical (lower) end of the head but do not choke around the neck. Hold the sides of the head firmly, but ensure the bird is able to breathe (Figure 16.1). Oftentimes, letting the bird bite the excess towel offers a distraction. For small birds, use the remainder of the hand to control the body and make sure the towel is wrapped around the bird to control the wings and feet. Larger birds should remain controlled with the opposite hand holding the towel that is wrapped around the body. The person restraining the bird should be monitoring the bird's respirations and stress level the entire time it is restrained. Observe the avian patient closely for signs of stress, **hypoxia**, and hyperthermia. Hands should be moved accordingly to allow the examiner to exam the bird at a faster pace.

Restraint is a very stressful experience for a bird. Allow the examiner to move as quickly as possible to insure the bird is restrained as little as possible. It is typical for a bird to show signs of stress when the restraint is released and the bird is placed back in its carrier. Open beak breathing, holding wings away from body, and fluffing of feathers may be exhibited but the bird should recover rather quickly, so be aware if the bird exhibits these behaviors for a while after returning to its cage.

Nutrition

Problems associated with nutrition are very common in birds kept as pets. Psittacine and passerine species have unique nutritional requirements and if owners are not familiar with the proper care and feeding of the species owned, the bird is at risk for disease or malnutrition. Each avian species has differing nutritional demands and it is important to review the needs of the specific breed of bird with the owner.

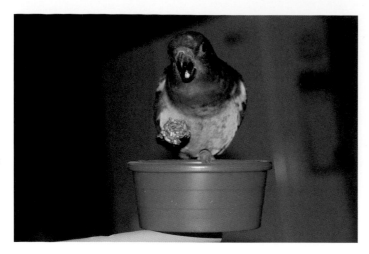

Figure 16.2 Meyer's parrot clutching pellet/seed ball. Courtesy of Kara M Burns, LVT, VTS (Nutrition).

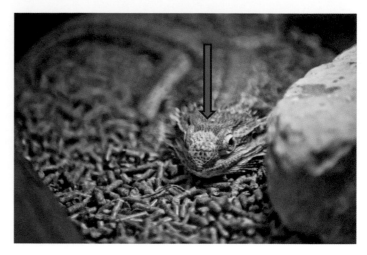

Figure 16.3 Bearded dragon shedding skin – arrow points to skin on nose ready to shed. Source: Courtesy of Kara M. Burns, LVT, VTS (Nutrition).

Smaller birds have a higher metabolic rate and higher energy requirements than larger birds. Subsequently, small birds are best suited to have continuous access to food. Seed diets are popular, but many are deficient in certain nutrients and seed is not the natural diet of birds kept as pets. Seed diets are mainly composed of sunflower seeds which are low in calcium and vitamin A, and high in fat (Figure 16.2). This type of diet leads to obesity and specific deficiencies in birds. Birds in captivity may also select specific foods from a variety offered by the owner. This also leads to nutritional deficiencies. Birds will select items to eat on the basis of water content, texture, color, and taste as opposed to nutrient content, thus resulting in the potential for severe nutrient imbalance.

Pelleted diets offer the best all-round solution for companion birds as they are formulated diets that include the nutrients recommended for specific species of companion birds. These diets are also formulated along the lifestage/lifestyle philosophy and are available not only for specific species but also according to age, lifestyle, reproductive status, etc. Commercially formulated pelleted diets include vitamins, so vitamin supplementation is contraindicated. If the owner is feeding a seed diet, the recommendation to transition to pelleted foods should be discussed. Veterinary health-care team members play a huge role in educating and offering support to bird owners transitioning from a seed diet to a pelleted diet. Although this is challenging, the benefits of proper nutrition, as in companion mammals, result in a longer, healthier life of the bird.

Fresh water should be available at all times. The owner should be educated to place the water dish above perches. This will decrease the amount of fecal contamination, as birds, like other companion animals, should have clean, fresh water available to them.

Reptiles, Amphibians, and Fish

Reptiles

In recent years the popularity and ownership of reptiles have increased tremendously. There are a number of common reptile species kept in captivity today and it is imperative that veterinary health-care team members have knowledge of these species and the health-care and husbandry issues that will help to keep them healthy.

It is important to recognize that reptiles cannot generate their own body heat, and consequently must obtain heat from their environment. Reptiles move in and out of the shade or heat to help regulate their body temperature. Each species of reptile has a temperature range required for their metabolism to function properly, known as the preferred optimum temperature zone (POTZ). Reptile skin is covered by a protective layer of keratinous scales. The outermost layer is shed regularly, but whether it is shed all at once or in pieces is dependent upon the type of reptile (i.e., snakes will shed their skin all at once while lizards shed their skin in pieces) (Figure 16.3).

Reptiles do not have a diaphragm separating the thoracic and abdominal cavities. They have one cavity – the coelom. The majority of reptiles have a network of vessels known as the renal portal system which distribute medications to the entire body if these medications are injected caudal to the kidneys. However, this can be extremely detrimental to the kidneys if the medication is ***nephrotoxic***. The excrement of reptiles, similar to birds, is composed of three components: urine, urates, and feces. The excrement exits the body through the cloaca.

As with other species, one of the most common reasons for a reptile to present to a veterinary hospital is due to illness from poor nutrition and poor husbandry. Again, there is a huge role for veterinary health-care team members to educate owners on proper nutrition and husbandry for the health and longevity of reptiles.

It is recommended to house reptiles in a cage appropriate for the species, which is easy to clean and disinfect. The cleaning should be routine, and any excrement or debris should be taken out daily. All reptiles have the ability to shed *Salmonella* spp. so care should be taken when cleaning and handling reptiles and their environments. It is imperative that this is discussed with the owner and documented in the medical record. Logs, plants, rocks, etc. are often placed in the cage and the type and size will vary by species. The bedding should also be easy to remove and clean. Shavings should be avoided in reptiles, as this can cause a respiratory irritation or worse. Lighting is extremely important when working with reptiles. Reptiles cannot metabolize nutrients or synthesize vitamin D properly without ultraviolet (UV) lighting. A full-spectrum bulb placed approximately 2 feet away from the reptile is ideal.

Due to the *ectothermic* nature of reptiles, a heated area for the reptile to "bask" is necessary. The reptile will move among the heated and nonheated areas to regulate its own body temperature. Be careful to educate owners regarding the heat intensity as certain heating elements sold for reptiles may cause thermal burns.

Physical examination of reptiles is similar to that of companion small mammals. It is good practice to simply observe the reptile in its environment before removing and restraining it. It is best to begin the examination at the head and move toward the tail. The eyes, ears, and oral cavity should be examined followed by the coelomic cavity. The limbs, appendages, and tail should be palpated. Note any swelling or deformities and abnormalities as you move down the body. The heart rate and respiratory rate should be evaluated and captured on the medical record.

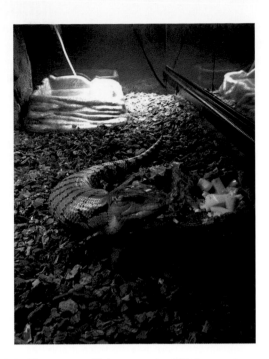

Figure 16.4 Blue tongue skink cage and nutrition example.

Restraint

Most snakes can be picked up in the transport carrier, especially when dealing with nonaggressive snakes. For aggressive snakes, a towel may be used by tossing the towel over the snake and finding the head of the snake. Once the head is located and restrained, it is safe to remove from the carrier. It is best to gently grasp the snake behind the head with one hand and support the body with the other hand.

Aquatic turtles, also known as chelonians, are considered easy to capture. However, restraining chelonians involves controlling the head. To gain control of the head, the health-care team member should put their thumb on one side of the cranial neck portion and the index finger (or fingers if a larger animal) on the other side of the neck at the base of the skull.

Lizards typically can be held with two hands and removed from the transport carrier. However, some lizards are aggressive, or the species' natural defenses prevent one from simply picking up the lizard. In this instance, long-sleeved shirts, gloves, and a towel may be necessary. Frightened lizards may try to bite or scratch with their long claws. It is recommended to keep one hand on the neck, immediately behind the base of the skull, to prevent being bitten. Do not try to capture a lizard by the tail. Many species have a natural response to "drop" their tail to escape, and this may happen if they view the restrainer as a predator. Restraint of lizards can be obtained by placing one hand again around the neck and pectoral region and the other hand supporting the body near the pelvic region. Apply only enough pressure to keep the lizard restrained, as too much pressure may damage the spine of lizards.

Nutrition

As with other species, inadequate diet and nutrition can cause a multitude of disease conditions in reptiles. Diets are typically species specific, so it is important to familiarize oneself with the specific reptile species and educate the owner as to the proper diet needed to provide for a healthy long life. As with all species, clean fresh water should be available at all times and the water should be changed at least once a day.

Snakes are carnivores and feed on whole prey. Eating the entire prey allows for added nutrients such as calcium. Snakes will defecate the parts of the prey they do not use. Supplementation is typically not necessary when feeding whole prey such as rats, mice, etc.

The feeding of lizards is dependent upon the species. Herbivores should be fed a variety of dark leafy greens and vegetables (Figure 16.4). Insectivores will eat mealworms, crickets, etc. Carnivorous lizard species should be fed prey consisting of the bones, contents of the GI tract, muscle, and fur. Lizards that fall into the omnivore family should be fed dark leafy greens and insects. It is important to remind reptile owners to not feed the same foods every day – reptiles prefer variety.

Aquatic turtles are omnivorous and will eat fish, algae, leafy greens, etc. There are commercial foods available for aquatic turtles which should be fed in moderation. Educate turtle owners to insure these commercial foods have the essential nutrients. Any food items with animal proteins should *not* be fed to aquatic turtles.

Amphibians

The class Amphibia is divided into three orders: Anura (frogs and toads), Caudata (salamanders, newts, and sirens), and Gymnophiona (caecilians). There are over 4000 extant species, but very few (one-tenth) are ever held in captivity.

Amphibians' bodies are consistent with those of other vertebrates. But for veterinary team members, as with any exotic animal species, knowledge regarding the nuances of species variation for some anatomical and physiological traits can be helpful when developing a diagnostic or treatment plan for an amphibian patient. For example, amphibians do not have distinct thoracic and abdominal cavities. Instead, they have a single coelomic cavity. This information is important when considering surgery.

Four limbs are present, but there may be variable hindlimb lengths. The length depends on species locomotory modes; longer hindlegs occur in animals that jump. The forelimbs possess a fused radius and ulna (radioulna), whereas the hindlimbs have a fused tibia and fibula (tibiofibula). The forefeet possess four phalanges on each foot, whereas the hindfeet have five phalanges. The **hyoid apparatus** in some species is adapted to eject the tongue for prey capture. Vertebrae are separated into three fused regions: presacral, sacral, and postsacral. Amphibians do not have diaphragms.

Anatomical modifications of the skin vary among species, but the basic integument has a thin keratin layer and a relatively thin basal epidermal layer. There is a significant subcutaneous layer that can accumulate fluid. In some species, this is normal (as a fluid reservoir); however, it may also indicate a pathological condition. This again reminds us that we must know our amphibian species. **Ecdysis** occurs regularly, and keratophagy (consuming the shed skin) may occur. The skin may contain venom glands for predator avoidance.

In anurans, three modes of respiration occur: **buccopharyngeal**, **pulmonic**, and **cutaneous**; the mode used is dependent upon species variability and environment. Anurans have a short trachea, thus impacting clinical procedures such as tracheal intubation and washes. Two equally sized lungs are present. Amphibians have a simple, short alimentary system that empties into a cloaca. Amphibians have **mesonephric** kidneys and cannot concentrate urine above the solute concentration of the plasma. The kidney is a dual filter for coelomic and vascular fluid, and this has implications when administering drugs via the coelomic cavity.

Fish

Fish represent the largest class of vertebrates, with more than 20 000 different species. This group also represents the largest number of species kept in captivity. While there may be tens or even hundreds of different species from another class of vertebrates kept in captivity, there are likely more than 1000 different species of fish that have been maintained in captivity. There are three major groups of fish kept in captivity: freshwater, brackish water, and saltwater. The fundamental difference among the three groups is the relative density of the water in which they live. Some fish can move between fresh water to brackish water or salt water to brackish water, but relatively few fish can live in the two extremes (fresh water and salt water).

Freshwater tropical fish represent the largest numbers of animals typically found in home aquaria. Generally, this group of fishes is readily available for a small to moderate investment and can be easily maintained by the novice aquarist or hobbyist.

There are approximately 23 categories of marine tropical fish. These 23 groups can be arbitrarily divided into four major groups by their feeding attributes and compatibility with other species.

The first category of marine tropical fish is the "rapid eater" and includes the angelfish (e.g., *Pomacanthus* spp.), damselfish (e.g., *Amblyglyphidodon* spp.), groupers (e.g., *Cephalopholis* spp., *Variola* spp.), etc. These fish do well if kept at low densities in the aquarium or if they are provided a large area where overcrowding is not an issue. Hostile interaction is a major concern for these animals, as they can be very food aggressive. These animals may be kept together quite readily if provided an abundance of food and a diverse diet.

The "slow eaters" represent the largest subgroup of marine tropical fish. This group includes the anemone clown fish (e.g., *Amphiprion ocellaris*), parrotfish (e.g., *Sparisoma* spp.), puffers (e.g., *Carinotetraodon* spp., *Tetraodon* spp., *Colomesus* spp.), etc. Compatibility is a concern with this group of animals. They do best if maintained in large displays with a large amount of hiding area. Although these fish are grouped based on their feeding strategy, there remains a great deal of variability in the diets of these animals.

Another group with extreme feeding habits includes those animals that have difficulty competing for food. This group includes the more unusual species, such as the seahorses (*Hippocampus* spp.), jawfishes (*Opistognathus* spp., *Stalix* spp., *Lonchopisthus* spp.), pipefish (*Stigmatopora* spp., *Lissocampus* spp., *Corythoichthys* spp.), etc. These fish are typically slow swimmers and are easily outcompeted by faster swimming fish. Members of this group should be housed together with similar species and monitored closely to ensure that they obtain sufficient calories.

The last group to be categorized as marine tropicals includes the snappers (e.g., *Lutjanus* spp., *Pristipomoides* spp., *Nemadactylus* spp., *Etelis* spp.) and grunts (e.g., *Haemulon* spp.). These are larger, territorial schooling fish that are most often kept at public facilities. They can best be described as "gluttons" because of how they feed and the almost insatiable hunger they exhibit. They are virtually fearless in their feeding habits and will attempt to remove food from the jaws of even large predators.

Rabbits

Rabbits are popular pets because they are small, relatively easy to care for, fastidious, quiet mannered, and can be litterbox trained (Figure 16.5). Pet rabbits have unique, lively, and affectionate personalities that make them ideal pets for mature children and adults. Handling pet rabbits when they are young will likely make them more comfortable with humans later in life. In contrast, wild rabbits, no matter their age, do not become comfortable with human interaction.

Rabbits have very thin and delicate skin, covered with fine fur composed of both a soft undercoat and stiff guard hairs. Veterinary technicians must take care when clipping fur because the skin is prone to tearing. Rabbits' feet are covered with thick coarse fur that protects the plantar and palmar surfaces of the

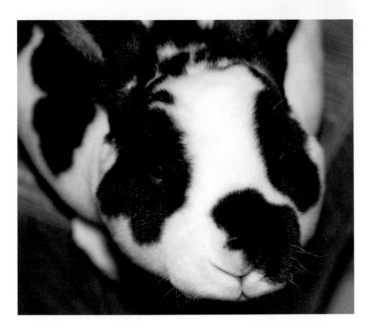

Figure 16.5   Domestic rabbit. Courtesy of Kara M Burns, LVT, VTS (Nutrition).

feet. Because they lack footpads, rabbits should be provided soft padded areas within their enclosures. Rabbits' claws are nonretractable, thus making declawing an inappropriate procedure. Certain breeds of female rabbits have a dewlap, which is analogous to a second chin. Female rabbits may pluck fur from the dewlap during the breeding season to build a nest. Male and female rabbits may have three types of scent glands, including a single chin gland, paired inguinal glands, and paired anal glands. The glands are used to mark the rabbit's territory.

The ears represent a large amount of the animal's surface area. Because rabbits are low in the food web, these large ears serve an important function in assisting the animal with identifying potential predators. In addition, rabbits' ears are highly vascularized and serve an important role in thermoregulation via *vasoconstriction* and *vasodilation*. Rabbit ears are very sensitive and delicate and should never be used for restraint.

Rabbits have a wide field of vision, ideal for a prey species. With the lateral positioning of their eyes and their large corneas, rabbits have an overlapping field of vision of 190°. Although rabbits are visually acute within this region, they cannot visualize items below the horizon, including the area below their nose. Instead, rabbits use their highly sensitive *vibrissae* and lips as tactile structures to distinguish food items. Rabbits possess good night vision and some color vision. They have functional third eyelids that partially close with sleep or while under anesthesia. Tear drainage from the eyes occurs via the *nasolacrimal gland*.

Rabbits have a light skeleton surrounded by a very well-developed muscular system, which makes the vertebrae and long bones susceptible to fractures. To minimize the likelihood of injury, the hindlegs should always be supported when transporting the rabbit. The number of vertebrae varies between breeds, from 12 to 13 thoracic and 6 to 7 lumbar vertebrae. The *epaxial* and large muscles of the hindlimbs can be used for intramuscular injections.

Two pairs of upper incisor teeth differentiate *lagomorphs* from rodents. The smaller, second upper incisors (peg teeth) are found behind the first. These peg teeth lack a cutting edge. Rabbit teeth are *hypsodont*. Malocclusion and overgrowth commonly occur with the incisor teeth as these can grow 10–12 cm a year during the rabbit's life. Rabbit teeth are developed for a high-fiber, herbivorous diet. Rabbits are herbivorous hindgut fermenters and have a GI system like horses. The rabbit's GI tract consists of a noncompartmentalized stomach and a large cecum. The simple stomach has thin walls and indistinctly separated glandular and nonglandular areas. It is important to note with owners that rabbits are unable to vomit due to a well-developed *cardiac sphincter*.

There are no US-approved vaccines for domestic rabbits. It is recommended that all house rabbits receive an annual physical examination, and as they become geriatric (>4 years), a twice a year examination is recommended. Additionally, a serum chemistry panel, complete blood counts (CBCs), and fecal exams for parasites are also recommended annually. Ovariohysterectomy or orchiectomy should also be recommended for all nonbreeding rabbits to decrease aggression, decrease the incidence of scent marking with urine and feces, and avoid unwanted pregnancy, pseudopregnancy, and neoplasia.

When adding new rabbits into an existing population, it is always recommended to quarantine the new additions for a minimum of 90 days. Separating new arrivals can decrease the likelihood of introducing infectious diseases and parasites to a standing population of rabbits. Before the rabbits are released from quarantine, they should have a CBC and chemistry profile done, and have 3–5 negative (2 weeks apart) fecal examinations consecutively. The client should be made aware that even a 90-day quarantine may be insufficient to detect some infectious diseases.

Rabbits' owners should be educated that enclosures should be cleaned daily. Organic material should be removed before disinfectant is applied. Fresh substrate should be offered either daily or as it is soiled. The cage may be disinfected with mild soap and water or a dilute bleach solution (1:32). The disinfectant should have a minimum of 3–5 minutes of contact time to increase the effectiveness of the compound. The solutions should be thoroughly rinsed away, and the surface of the cage dried.

Restraint

Rabbit physical restraint needs to be carefully performed to avoid injury to the animal. Because rabbits have a well-developed muscular system and thin cortical bone, they are subject to vertebral and long bone fractures if restrained incorrectly. Because most skeletal injuries associated with incorrect restraint occur in the lumbar vertebrae, it is important to firmly restrain the hindlegs. Rabbits should be handled in a manner similar to cats; place one hand under the forelimbs and use the other hand to hold the rear legs against the body. Always place the rabbit onto a nonslip surface to ensure that it has good footing. To restrain the animal, lightly scruff it and support its dorsum with the same arm. The opposite arm is used to support the body and rear legs.

Nutrition

Nutritional management of a rabbit should provide sufficient fiber to support normal GI motility as well as to ensure sufficient amounts and types of digestible nutrients are available to the cecal microflora for fermentation. Rabbits also need enrichment and thus, the diet should stimulate normal foraging behavior throughout the day.

Rabbits derive amino acids directly from the foods they ingest, as well as from cecotrophs. Essential amino acids in the rabbit include arginine, glycine, histidine, isoleucine, leucine, lysine, methionine, phenylalanine, threonine, tryptophan, and valine. Grasses tend to contain limited amounts of methionine and isoleucine but are abundant in arginine, glutamine, and lysine. Synthetic amino acids are added to commercial mixes for rabbits as these cereals are often low in methionine and lysine. Conversely, legumes are high in lysine and may be used to balance low lysine levels in cereal-based diets. Rabbits can digest forage-based protein because of the increase in protein digestibility that occurs as a result of cecotrophy. An appropriate protein level for pet rabbits is 12–16% dry matter basis (DMB). For lactating does, the level may increase to 18–19% protein DMB.

Although simple sugars and starches can be used for energy, excessive levels of these should not be fed. Lagomorphs have a rapid gut transit time resulting in starch and simple sugars not being completely digested in the small intestine. These are then directed into the cecum, where they may be used for fermentation by the cecal microorganisms. Carbohydrate overload in the cecum predisposes to *enterotoxemia*, especially in young animals. Low-energy grains such as oats are recommended for the rabbits' diet as opposed to corn or wheat. Care should be taken to not process the grains too finely.

Fiber is an essential nutrient for the maintenance of GI health. It also helps to promote normal dental attrition and encourages normal foraging behavior, thus decreasing the potential for behavioral issues. The digestion of fiber in rabbits overall is poor; however, indigestible fiber is essential for stimulating gut motility and helping to control gut transit time. Manufacturing processes play a role in the digestibility of commercial rabbit foods. For example, the finer the grinding, the longer the gut transit and cecal retention times which lead to greater potential for *cecal dysbiosis*.

In the dietary management of rabbits, balance must be established between providing enough indigestible fiber to maintain normal motility, cell regeneration, secretion, absorption, and excretion while simultaneously providing enough digestible fiber for sufficient bacterial fermentation in the gut. The total dietary fiber levels recommended for pet rabbits is 20–25% DMB. Healthcare team members should educate owners to provide an ad libitum source of indigestible fiber (e.g., grass and/or hay). Also, owners should insure the amounts of other dietary components are limited. This will ensure that the rabbit actually eats the primary fiber source. Commercial foods used as a portion of the diet should preferably have a crude fiber content of >18% DMB, with indigestible fiber at >12.5% DMB.

Fat provides another source of energy and increases palatability. Fat also decreases dustiness and crumbling of commercially manufactured pellets. As with other species, rabbits are prone to obesity. They are also at risk for *hepatic lipidosis*. Consequently high-fat diets must be avoided. The recommended level of fat for rabbits is 2.5–4% DMB.

In the nutritional management of rabbits, vitamins A, D, and E are important and should be part of the dietary make-up. Gut bacteria synthesize B vitamins in sufficient quantities so adding B vitamins to commercial foods may be unnecessary. Vitamin K synthesis in the gut is not as efficient. Therefore, vitamin K is often added to the commercial formulation by the rabbit food manufacturer. Vitamins A and E are readily destroyed by oxidation, so it is imperative that food preparation and storage methods prevent losses from excess light or heat. The recommendation is to store rabbit feed at 15 °C (60 °F) and feed within 90 days of milling. If the food is composed of more than 30% alfalfa meal there should be sufficient vitamin A in the form of the precursor beta-carotene. However, if the alfalfa is over a year post harvest, vitamin A deficiency can occur.

Guinea pigs

Guinea pigs have wide bodies with short limbs (Figure 16.6). A distinctive anatomical characteristic is the number of digits on the front and rear feet (four digits front feet and three digits rear). Tails are usually very short or absent. The guinea pig has a short, flat nose, laterally placed eyes, and hairless external pinnae. Adult guinea pigs usually weigh between 700 and 1200 g, with the males being slightly larger than females. The average life span of the companion guinea pig is approximately 5–7 years.

The dentition of the guinea pig is described as aradicular hypsodont (e.g., all teeth have a relatively long crown and are "open rooted"). The maxilla is slightly wider than the mandible, and the occlusal angle of the premolars and molars is marked compared to other rodent species. The dental formula of the guinea pig is 2(I 1/1, C 0/0, PM 1/1, M 3/3) = 20. The maxillary incisors are much shorter than those set in the mandible. The molars and premolars are not easily visualized without special instrumentation because of the small size of the oral cavity and tendency for the involution of the buccal surface.

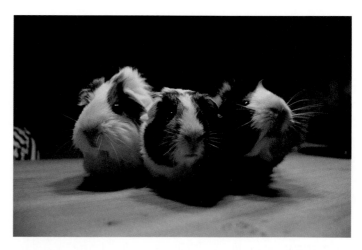

Figure 16.6 Guinea pigs. Source: Photo by Karlijn Prot on Unsplash.

Females are sexually mature at 6 weeks of age, whereas males on average reach puberty approximately 4 weeks later. Gestation is long, when compared to other rodents, at 68 days. As a result of this long gestation period, young are *precocial* when born. Juvenile pigs usually eat solid foods by 4–5 days of age. Litter sizes range from one to six, with an average of 3–4 young. A female guinea pig should deliver her first young before she is 6 months of age. If birth has not occurred before 6 months of age, the pubic symphysis becomes mineralized, with future pregnancies resulting in an inability of the sow to naturally deliver the babies. Female guinea pigs that become pregnant after 6 months of age invariably require cesarean section deliveries.

Guinea pigs are best housed in well-ventilated, wire-sided cages with solid bottoms. Wire-bottom cages may also be used but care must be taken to ensure that the mesh is small enough that a limb cannot become entrapped. An area of solid flooring should be provided, as uninterrupted time on wire mesh may predispose the guinea pig to pododermatitis. Adequate space is needed in the enclosure for the guinea pig to move about unencumbered with enough space for a hide box. Hide boxes or a secluded space is required for prey species (e.g., rodents) to reduce stress that may lead to disease problems. Bedding that contains aromatic oils (e.g., cedar and pine shavings) should not be used, as they can act as contact and respiratory irritants. Appropriate bedding materials include recycled newspaper products, shredded paper, and aspen shavings.

The enclosure should be cleaned thoroughly on a regular basis, at least twice per week, because unsanitary conditions predispose the guinea pig to *pododermatitis*, respiratory, and other health problems. If housed indoors, guinea pig enclosures do not require a cover, as these animals do not typically jump or climb. However, the sides of the enclosure should be high enough to prevent escape (approximately 25 cm). Heavy food containers are recommended to make dumping of the receptacle more difficult. All food containers should be easy to disinfect and cleaned regularly, as guinea pigs have a habit of soiling their food bowls. Most guinea pigs readily accept drinking water from a sipper bottle, which will decrease spillage and keep feces, urine, and bedding from contaminating the water.

Guinea pigs are very susceptible to hyperthermia and should never be housed in temperatures greater than 80 °F. High humidity can also exacerbate a guinea pig's sensitivity to elevated temperatures by increasing the heat index. All animals are very sensitive to environmental and/or nutritional changes. Therefore, if changes have to be made, gradual exposure of the animal to the changes is recommended.

Nutrition

An appropriate guinea pig diet includes a formulated, pelleted diet for that species, high-quality hay (e.g., timothy, orchard grass, oat) ad libitum, and ample fresh vegetables. As the animal's food intake is more dependent on volume consumed rather than calories consumed, a pet fed a predominantly pelleted diet (higher nutritional concentration) tends to become obese. Fruits and grains should make up a very small portion (<10%) of the total diet and be offered only as treats.

Because guinea pigs lack the enzyme L-gulonolactone oxidase, they are unable to synthesize ascorbic acid from glucose. Therefore, they require supplemental vitamin C in their diets. Although commercial guinea pig pellets are manufactured with vitamin C, the supplement often degrades rapidly, especially if the pellets are subjected to high heat and humidity. Vitamin C placed in drinking water also degrades rapidly and should be changed daily. To ensure that a guinea pig is receiving a proper amount of vitamin C, it is necessary to supplement a diet of pellets and hay with plenty of fresh foods. Many green, leafy vegetables, such as kale, mustard greens, dandelion greens, parsley, etc., are excellent sources of ascorbic acid. The vitamin C requirement of an adult, nonbreeding guinea pig is 10 mg/kg/day.

Many health problems of guinea pigs are related to improper husbandry. During a routine veterinary visit, the owners should be asked to provide a detailed description of the animal's housing environment, including substrate, frequency of cleaning, ambient temperature, and exercise time. The diet history is also important. Owners should be asked not only what the guinea pig is offered, but also in what proportions and of what foods the animal eats.

Restraint

Most guinea pigs are docile and do not require aggressive restraint. Often a hand on the animal's dorsum is adequate to restrain a guinea pig patient on the examination table. When transporting a guinea pig, support the body with one hand under the thorax and abdomen while placing the other hand on the back to prevent the patient from falling or jumping.

Annual examination

Guinea pigs are not routinely vaccinated for infectious diseases. Owners should be encouraged to have annual examinations that include an oral examination and a complete blood count. Guinea pigs are adept at hiding illness, and routine evaluations by a qualified veterinarian may help in detecting abnormalities early.

Mice and rats

Mice and rats are not as common as pets as other rodents. The prevalence and type of mouse and rat diseases seen in clinical practice are quite different from those seen in a research setting. The diagnosis and treatment of pet mice and rats involve evaluation and care of an individual animal from a household, not the health management of rodents from a research colony. Most problems in mice and rats are *dermatopathies*, respiratory infections, and *neoplasia*.

Male rats are sexually mature by 6–10 weeks, female rats by 8–12 weeks. The breeding life of both male and female rats is 9–12 months. Estrous cycle length in female rats is 4–5 days, and estrus lasts 10–20 hours. Female rats ovulate ~10–20 eggs. Gestation lasts 21–23 days; pseudopregnancy from sterile matings lasts 12 days. Rats have an average litter size of 8–18 pups. Weaning takes place at ~21 days. Mice have an average litter size of 5–12 pups. Weaning takes place at ~21 days. Male rodents show a constant libido after sexual maturity; in contrast, females are receptive to copulation only during estrus. Males cannot fertilize females until 6–8 weeks after reaching puberty.

The average life span of mice is 18–24 months and of rats 18–36 months. Restricting dietary calories without compromising overall nutrition results in increased life span. Obesity in pet rats and mice is common, and calorie-restricted pets live significantly longer lives.

Owners must combine frequent bedding changes with good husbandry such as regular cage cleaning, low animal density, and low environmental temperature and humidity. This will reduce toxic or odor-causing gases such as ammonia from building up, because urease-positive bacteria in the feces act to break down urea in the urine.

Size and manipulability of bedding material are the main determinants of mice and rats' choices. Mice and rats avoid bedding consisting of small particles, whereas they prefer bedding consisting of large, fibrous particles. When exposed to different types of nesting materials such as paper strips, cornhusks, sawdust, and wood materials (shavings, peelings, and chips), rats choose long strips of soft paper. They also select opaque or semiopaque nest boxes rather than transparent nest boxes. Mice show no preference between paper and wood-derived materials but show a clear preference for materials that they can manipulate such as paper tissues, string, and wood materials (shavings, peelings, and chips). Many mice will combine two preferred nesting materials to make complex nests. Mice typically dislike wire-bottomed cages.

Environmental enrichment is important for both mice and rats. Rats will use more enrichment devices than mice, but they usually stop using the devices after 3–4 days. Rotation of enrichment toys and introduction of novel devices are recommended as they pique their curiosity. Food treats are also valuable enrichment items. These can range from simple, inexpensive treats such as a daily piece of a breakfast cereal to formulated nutritious or calorie-free treats. Pet rodents accustomed to handling will eat food treats out of the owner's hand. This daily routine can allow owners to detect subtle changes in the pet's behavior, but too many treats are not healthy. Sick rodents effectively hide signs of disease. Sick rats do not show the same interest in their daily treat, and this can alert the owner early to disease when it is still treatable and/or reversible.

Nutrition

Rats and mice are omnivores and will eat food of both plant and animal origin. Formulated pelleted diets for laboratory rodents are convenient and nutritionally balanced diets for early life and reproduction. However, laboratory rodent diets are relatively high in fat and low in fiber, and when provided ad libitum, they cause obesity. Consequently, the amount of pelleted diet owners provide daily should be limited. Diets formulated specifically for pet rodents are now commercially available. Owners should supplement their pet's diet with feeds high in fiber such as vegetables, limited amounts of fruit, and occasional treats.

Gerbils

Gerbils are also known as jirds or sand rats. The pet and laboratory gerbil is *Meriones unguiculates*, commonly known as the Mongolian gerbil. There are 14 species in the genus *Meriones*.

Externally, gerbils are quite rat-like. The head and body length is 95–180 mm, and tail length is 100–193 mm. The average weight is 50–55 g for females and 60 g for males. The covering of fur on the tail is short near the base and progressively longer toward the tip so that it is slightly bushy. Coloration of upper parts varies from pale, clear yellowish through sandy and gray. The sides of the body are generally lighter than the back. Gerbils have a high degree of resistance to heat stress and dehydration.

Gerbils tend to pair bond, and when older females lose their mate, getting them to accept another is often impossible. Early-maturing females are more likely to breed successfully on first pairing, and the lifetime *fecundity* of early-maturing females is more than twice that of their late-maturing littermates. Two-thirds of the early-maturing females that do not reproduce after a first pairing will become pregnant after a second pairing, but only 10% of late-maturing females do so.

The gestation period of nonlactating gerbils is 24–26 days, but lactating females always have a prolonged gestation of 27 days. Litter size ranges from three to seven animals. Young gerbils suckle for ~21 days and begin to eat solid foods at 16 days. In general, day 25 is considered suitable for weaning. The normal life span of a gerbil is 2–3 years.

Gerbils thrive on commercially available pelleted rodent diets with 18–20% protein but may have deficiency problems when fed primarily home-made diets, sunflower seeds, or table scraps, which lack specific nutrients. Sunflower seeds are high in fat and low in calcium. Pelleted chow (5 g/day) has been recommended to avoid obesity. Gerbils will develop high blood cholesterol concentrations on diets containing >4% fat. This is manifest as *lipemia* and is more pronounced in males.

Gerbils excrete little urine, and fecal pellets are hard and dry. Their cages require less frequent cleaning than other pet and laboratory rodents. Gerbils adapt to a wide range of ambient temperatures. Because they have a propensity to develop nasal dermatitis at relative humidity >50%, a low humidity is advisable.

Gerbils require sandbathing to keep their coats from becoming oily. They often stand erect on their hindlimbs, so it is important that cages have a solid bottom and that the floor-to-lid height is tall enough to allow for this behavior.

Sick animals are often isolated from others and may demonstrate weight loss, hunched posture, lethargy, rough fur, labored breathing, and a loss of exploratory behavior. Early signs of illness involve changes in the color, consistency, odor, and amount of urine and feces. The perineal area should be checked for fecal or urine stains or discharges from the vulva in females. Fecal samples may be taken for parasite detection and bacterial culture. The fur and skin should be examined for alopecia, fight wounds or other trauma, ectoparasites, and elasticity for evidence of dehydration. The oral cavity should be checked for overgrown teeth. Ears and eyes should be examined for discharges or inflammation. Feet should be examined for sores and overgrown or broken nails. The abdomen should be palpated for masses. Normal body temperature is 98–102 °F (37–39 °C). Respiratory rate or signs of labored breathing should be noted. The thorax can be auscultated with a pediatric stethoscope. Gerbil tails are fragile, and only the base of the tail should be grasped during handling to avoid injury.

Hamsters

The most common pet and research hamster is the golden or Syrian hamster (*Mesocricetus auratus*). Syrian hamsters have a head and body length of 170–180 mm and tail length of 12 mm. They range in weight from 110 to 140 g, and females are larger than males. Wild Syrian hamsters have a light, reddish brown dorsal coat, and the underparts are white. The skin of Syrian hamsters is very loose.

Other species now common as pets are the dwarf hamsters such as the Djungarian (*Phodopus sungorus*) and Roborovsky (Proborovskii) hamsters. They are small (<100 g body weight), have a docile disposition, do not attempt to bite or run away, thrive in captivity, and make good pets.

Female Syrian hamsters are heavier than males and generally are aggressive toward other hamsters. Estrus lasts ~1 day, and the gestation period is 16–19 days. The litter size ranges from two to 16, with an average of nine. Cannibalism of young accounts for nearly all preweaning mortality. Cold ambient temperatures (<10 °C/50 °F), lean diets, and low body weight during pregnancy increase cannibalism. Disturbing the mother by handling the young or nest, and not providing adequate nesting material, warmth, food, or water, often results in cannibalism. Syrian hamsters are prolific breeders, and there may be 3–5 litters/year. The young are weaned at 20 days and capable of reproducing at 7–8 weeks. The life span of Syrian hamsters is 2–3 years.

Syrian hamsters are omnivorous, eating many kinds of green vegetation, seeds, fruit, and meat. Exposure to cold stimulates hamsters to gather food, and they will often hibernate at temperatures <5 °C (41 °F). Syrian hamsters do not fatten before hibernation and will starve unless they waken periodically to eat. Hibernating animals remain sensitive to external stimuli and are usually aroused if handled. Syrian hamsters have prominent depositions of brown fat beneath and between the shoulder blades, in the *axilla*, and in the neck and perirenal areas.

Syrian hamsters are active chewers and skillful at escaping from their cages. Glass water tubes are not recommended for Syrian hamsters, because they will readily bite through glass. Stainless steel sipper tubes close to the floor are recommended. Because Syrian hamsters have broad muzzles that often prevent them eating from feed hoppers, feed pellets are placed on the floor of their cage. Hamsters are naturally *coprophagic*. Deep bedding that is appropriate for burrowing is recommended.

Diarrhea may occur in Syrian hamsters of any age and is known as "wet tail," although this euphemism is frequently used to describe the disease in young hamsters. Proliferative ileitis is the most significant intestinal disease of 3–10-week-old Syrian hamsters and results in high mortality. It is caused by the intracellular bacterium *Lawsonia intracellularis*. Treatment involves correcting life-threatening electrolyte imbalance and dehydration, administering antibiotics, and force feeding.

Ferrets

The ferret, *Mustela putorius furo*, has been domesticated for more than 2000 years. Ferrets have proven to be an important model in biomedical research, and much of what is known today about the ferret is based on this use. Recently, the ferret's popularity as a household pet has risen dramatically because of its amicable nature, small size, and relative ease of housing and care. As the number of pet ferrets increases, so does the need for proper veterinary care.

Ferrets have a long, slender body with short muscular legs, a long thin tail, small eyes, and short ears. They are very lively and active creatures, playing hard about 25% of the day and utilizing the remaining 75% for sleep. Ferrets are very curious and often investigate the smallest of spaces with ease, given their tubular-shaped, flexible bodies. They may be vocal at times, eliciting a chirp with excitement during play, a hiss of warning when threatened, or a scream when a painful stimulus is experienced. Ferrets normally walk with their torso elevated off the ground in a slightly hunched posture. This posture is exaggerated during play, when they distinctly arch their backs, bringing their front and rear feet closer together, and move around with a characteristic bounce.

Ferrets are highly social creatures and require a time commitment to maintain their welfare. To be good house pets, ferrets need to be socialized and handled from a young age; establishing familiarity with people may help to control aggressive behavior. A sturdy, escape-proof cage is essential to protect your ferret as they are very adept at squeezing through tiny spaces.

Ferret owners should arrange to have their pet descented and spayed or neutered. Descenting, or removal of the anal glands, helps control the naturally strong, musky odor that many people find objectionable. Regular bathing is essential, even when the scent glands are removed. Unneutered male ferrets (hobs) have a very strong, musky odor and are aggressive. Intact, unspayed females (jills) never go out of heat if they are not bred, and this can lead to life-threatening bone marrow disease.

Ferrets measure 44–46 cm from nose to tail tip. Males are larger than females with the average male weight of 1–2 kg and the average female weight of 0.5–1 kg. The weight may be less in the neutered male or greater in the spayed female. There is a seasonal fluctuation in body weight of 40% loss in the summer and gain in the winter in intact animals. The musky odor of ferrets originates from the presence of many sebaceous glands in the skin. The number of these glands increases in the breeding season in the intact animal, resulting in a stronger body odor, yellow discoloration, and oiliness of the fur.

Clean, social, and affectionate, ferrets can make excellent house pets, but require knowledgeable owners because they have special needs. They are naturally curious and can establish strong bonds with people. Ferrets normally live for between 5 and 9 years.

When educating potential owners regarding selecting a ferret, ensure they look for a bright, alert, and active individual. The ferret should have a shiny, lush hair coat and be healthy weight and well fed. Remind potential owners that if any ferrets in the select group appear sickly, do not consider adopting even the healthy-looking animals as a pet, as they may develop signs of illness later. Educate the owner that the ferret should be energetic and inquisitive.

It is important that potential owners understand that a ferret with a dull and rough hair coat, or an animal that is too thin, potbellied, or sluggish, may very well be sick. Be sure the owner knows to check below the tail for dampness as this may be indicative of GI issues, especially diarrhea. The owner should check the potential ferret for parasites such as fleas. It is imperative that the future ferret owner ensures an environment that is clean and well maintained. The food and water should be fresh and plentiful. It is important to ascertain if the ferret has had regular human contact and avoid selecting a ferret that bites hard or frequently during handling.

Owners should be educated regarding diet to keep the ferret healthy. The veterinary team should communicate that a good-quality ferret food or kitten food is a well-balanced dietary choice. Encourage future ferret owners to consult with the veterinary team, as they are best qualified to evaluate the health of the ferret. Additionally, the veterinary team can advise potential owners about nutrition, proper immunization, parasite control, sterilization, socialization, training, grooming, and other care that may be necessary to ensure the welfare of the ferret.

Remember to educate pet owners about the ferret's environment and the need for proper housing. Veterinary teams must remind potential owners that ferrets love to chew and should be aware of the ferret's whereabouts at all times. With this education, we are trying to educate the owner about potential hazards in the environment. Electric cords and furniture are very tempting, dangerous, and expensive chew toys. A cage is necessary for housebreaking the ferret. Remind them that many ferrets can be litterbox trained. Also, to avoid danger and heartbreak, the potential owner should be educated that ferrets are amazing escape artists and will squeeze through small openings or even open cage latches; therefore, it is important to test the cage to keep the ferret securely inside. Ferrets are naturally curious and are likely to crawl into ducts or underneath appliances. These can be dangerous places and make it difficult or even impossible to access and retrieve the pet. If allowing the ferret to roam in the kitchen, remind them to block off access to areas under the stove, refrigerator, and other appliances.

Hedgehogs

Hedgehogs are nocturnal and hide in burrows during daylight hours. At night they search out their preferred food of insects, earthworms, slugs, and snails. Males and females are territorial and prefer to live individually. They are active diggers and swim and jog around their natural habitat.

Healthy hedgehogs are very active; 2 × 3 ft are minimum floor dimensions for a cage. Hedgehogs are able to climb and can escape through small holes, so the cage must be secure and lidded. A hiding place is essential. The cage substrate should be soft and absorbent. Recycled newspaper bedding is a good choice; aspen shavings, alfalfa pellets, and hay are other options. Natural plant litters used for cats make the best litter substrate. Clay, clumping-type litter, or sand may stick to the animal and should not be used. Many hedgehogs defecate in their hide boxes and exercise wheels, so daily spot cleaning is often necessary. Exercise wheels with solid metal or plastic running surfaces are highly recommended. Hedgehog legs can become entrapped in wire wheels. Hedgehogs should be let out daily for exercise. Cardboard tubes, straw, safe climbing structures, swimming tubs, and other toys provide interest. Dirty hedgehogs may be bathed with a mild pet shampoo and use of a soft-bristle vegetable brush.

The ideal diet is a commercially prepared hedgehog food. If hedgehog food is not used, premium food for less active cats or dog food are alternatives. Food should be rationed to prevent obesity. In addition to the main diet, ~1–2 tsp (5–10 mL) of varied moist foods and/or invertebrate prey (e.g., canned cat or dog food, cooked meat or egg, low-fat cottage cheese, mealworms, earthworms, waxworms, gut-loaded crickets) and ~1 tsp (5 mL) of vegetable/fruit mix (e.g., beans, cooked carrots, squash, peas, tomatoes, leafy greens, banana, grape, apple, pear, berries) should also be provided daily.

Sugar gliders

Sugar gliders are highly social and best housed in pairs or small groups. The female sugar glider has a pouch in which the young are raised. Sugar gliders are not routine subjects for biomedical research, and there are a few US states that prohibit ownership of sugar gliders by private individuals.

Sugar gliders have a gliding membrane, the patagium, between the front and hindlimbs. This structure is responsible for the ability of the animal to glide through the air for distances up to 50 m. Eyes are large, widely spaced, and somewhat protruding, giving them a wide field of vision, especially at night. The second and third digits are fused to assist with gliding. The tail serves as a stabilization aid during gliding and is somewhat prehensile. The sugar glider life span is quite long, with 10–12 years not unusual in captivity. Their ears move independently and are highly sensitive to sound. They also have a great sense of smell to locate food, sense predators, and recognize both their territory and their colony-mates.

Sugar gliders are omnivorous and feed on sugar-rich plant and insect exudates (sap, gum, nectar, manna, pollen) and invertebrates as a source of protein. They are hindgut fermenters and possess a well-developed cecum that utilizes bacterial fermentation to break down complex polysaccharides contained in gum.

Chinchillas

Chinchillas are popular as pets and used in biomedical research in limited numbers. In the 1940s and 1950s, chinchillas were used to develop a vaccine for cholera. They have also been used by the US National Aeronautics and Space Administration (NASA) for sleep research studies; much of the knowledge gained from those studies has been applied to assisting astronauts on their missions.

Chinchillas are slender-bodied, medium-size rodents with short forelimbs and long muscular hindlimbs that give the animal a rabbit-like appearance. The head, eyes, and ears are relatively large, and the **bullae** are greatly expanded. Chinchillas have long gestation periods and deliver fully furred young with open eyes.

Chinchillas like to live in burrows or rock crevices and are well adapted for running. They dust bathe, are vegetarian, and are active throughout the year. The female chinchilla has an estrous cycle of 38 days. Females are **seasonally polyestrous**, and the breeding season is November to May in the northern hemisphere. The gestation period averages 111 days. Generally, the female will have two litters a year with 1–6 young (average two) per litter. Young become sexually mature at 8 months of age. Chinchillas have a long life span, reported to be up to 20 years.

Chinchillas are very tolerant of cold but sensitive to heat. The ambient temperature range to which chinchillas are adapted is 65–80 °F (18.3–26.7 °C). Exposure to higher ambient temperatures, especially in the presence of high humidity, can result in heatstroke.

Chinchillas are easily housed in either wire mesh-bottom or solid-bottom cages, although solid-bottom cages are recommended for pregnant females about to have young. Wire mesh spacing in cages should be narrow, because tibial fractures commonly occur in young chinchillas that catch a hindleg in wide floor mesh grating. Chinchillas are shy animals and need a place to hide when in captivity. Because they have a habit of dust bathing, a box containing a mixture of silver sand and Fuller's earth (9:1), 2–4 inches deep should be placed in the cage daily. Dust baths should be provided for ~30 min/day.

Chinchillas have a high requirement for dietary fiber. Their diet should mainly consist of high-quality grass hay. Pelleted chinchilla diets are commercially available and should be used to supplement the diet. Guinea pig or rabbit pelleted diets have also been used successfully. Like rabbits and guinea pigs, chinchillas produce two types of fecal pellets: one nitrogen-rich intended for cecotrophy, and one nitrogen-poor delivered as fecal pellets.

References

Ackerman, N., Aspinall, V. 2016. *Aspinall's Complete Textbook of Veterinary Nursing*, 3rd edition. Elsevier, Edinburgh.

Burns, K.M. 2014. Nutrition for companion birds. *RVT Journal*, Summer, 6–9.

Mitchell, M., Tully, T.N. 2016. *Current Therapy in Exotic Pet Practice*. Elsevier, St Louis, MO.

Quesenberry, K.E., Carpenter, J.W. 2012. *Ferrets, Rabbits, and Rodents: Clinical Medicine and Surgery*, 3rd edition. Saunders, St Louis, MO.

Wortinger, A., Burns, K.M. 2015. *Nutrition and Disease Management for Veterinary Technicians and Nurses*, 2nd edition. Wiley-Blackwell, Ames, IA.

Resources

www.cliniciansbrief.com/columns/91/avian-physical-examination – article reviewing proper PE for birds

www.cliniciansbrief.com/article/avian-venipuncture – article reviewing proper venipuncture techniques for birds

www.atdove.org/video/avian-restraint-and-exam – avian examination with restraint techniques

www.cliniciansbrief.com/article/image-gallery-avian-restraint – images of proper restraint for birds

www.youtube.com/watch?v=fF8-dW42ipM – parrot restraint video

https://lafeber.com/vet/exotic-animal-history/ – exotic animal history

https://lafeber.com/vet/video/?fwp_content_type=video&fwp_species=reptiles-amphibians&fwp_procedures=restraint-handling – restraint and handling of reptiles and amphibians

https://lafeber.com/vet/amphibian-history-form/ – history taking form for amphibians

www.fishvets.org/default.asp?id=1 – American Association of Fish Veterinarians

http://veterinarymedicine.dvm360.com/performing-basic-examination-fish – physical exam of fish

https://lafeber.com/vet/rabbit-restraint/ – article and video showing proper restraint of a rabbit

https://lafeber.com/vet/behavior-basics-clinical-approach-guinea-pig/ – article on examination of the guinea pig

www.research.psu.edu/arp/training/videos/guinea-pig-handling.html – video of guinea pig restraint

www.jove.com/video/2771/manual-restraint-common-compound-administration-routes-mice – Manual Restraint and Common Compound Administration Routes in Mice and Rats

www.research.psu.edu/arp/training/videos/handling-and-restraint-of-mice.html – handling and restraint of mice

www.aaha.org/pet_owner/pet_health_library/other/general_health/caring_for_your_gerbil.aspx – general gerbil care from the American Animal Hospital Association

www.aaha.org/pet_owner/pet_health_library/other/general_health/ferret_care.aspx – general care of the ferret

https://vet.purdue.edu/vth/files/documents/Sugar%20Gliders.pdf – article on general care for sugar gliders

https://lafeber.com/vet/chinchillas-101/ – basic care for chinchillas

https://lafeber.com/vet/chinchillas/ – client education handout for chinchillas

with website

www.wiley.com/go/burns/textbookvetassistant2

Please go to the companion website for assignments and a PowerPoint relating to the material in this chapter.

Chapter 17 Equine

All species of horse belong to the class Mammalia and have a great deal in common with other mammals. The domesticated horse of today differs in certain anatomical features such as the specialized digestive tract that allows consumption of grass and grains and an elongated single-digit limb that enables rapid escape from predators. The veterinary health-care team must be familiar with the uniqueness of the horse to provide proper care and management.

Skeletal system

The equine skeleton can be divided into two main sections: the axial skeleton, which consists of the skull, spine, ribcage, and pelvis; and the appendicular skeleton, which consists of the bones of the limbs (Figure 17.1).

The skull of the horse is made up of a number of bones joined together by fibrous joints allowing for little movement between them. The main function of the skull is to protect the brain, inner ear, parts of the eye, and the nasal passages. The majority of the skull is made up of the following:

- mandible (the lower jaw)
- maxilla, incisive, and palatine bones (the upper jaw, hard palate, and base of the nasal cavity)
- nasal bone
- frontal bone
- supraorbital process
- temporal bone
- occipital bone
- hyoid bones.

The nasal septum divides the nasal cavity into two compartments, and a bony, membranous septum splits the maxillary sinus into rostral and caudal compartments. The maxillary sinus links with the nasal cavity through an opening in the **middle nasal meatus**.

The dentition of the horse begins with deciduous teeth, replaced by permanent teeth. The dental formulas are as follows:

$$\text{Decidous teeth} - \left(I\frac{3}{3}PM\frac{3}{3} \right) \times 2 = 24$$

$$\text{Permanent teeth} - \left(I\frac{3}{3}C\frac{1}{1}PM\frac{3}{3}V\frac{4}{3}M\frac{3}{3} \right) \times 2 = 40 \text{ V } 42$$

Horses' teeth are all of the same height, and they do not have a surface covering of enamel; this is known as hypsodontic teeth. Hypsodontic teeth create an abrasive surface, which aids in the grinding of plant material, and include vast reserve crowns which allow the teeth to grow continually for many years, ensuring a long working life. The **occlusal surfaces** are worn down by approximately 2–3 mm per year as the horse chews. The extent of tooth wear and tooth appearance aids in estimating the age of the horse. Canine teeth may be absent in the mare.

The vertebral column is similar to that of other mammals in that it is made up of groups of vertebra, and serves to house the spinal cord, support the skull and thorax, and provide attachment for the pelvis and insertion of many muscles. See Figure 17.1 for the complete equine skeleton. The vertebral formula is represented as the following: C-7, T-18, L-6, S-5, Ca 15-20.

The horse has 18 pairs of ribs.

Textbook for the Veterinary Assistant, Second Edition. Kara M. Burns and Lori Renda-Francis.
© 2022 John Wiley & Sons, Inc. Published 2022 by John Wiley & Sons, Inc.
Companion website: www.wiley.com/go/burns/textbookvetassistant2

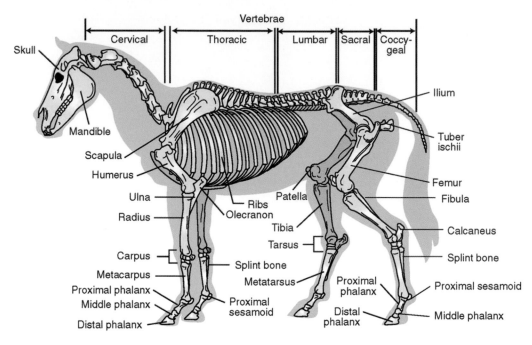

Figure 17.1 Equine skeleton. Source: Colville, T.P, Bassert J.M. 2016. *Clinical Anatomy and Physiology for Veterinary Technicians*, 3rd edition. Mosby, St Louis, MO.

The appendicular skeleton is made up of the limbs which allow for abundant leverage to maximize speed. The forelimb is attached to the trunk by the scapula; the scapula is attached by muscles. The forelimb is made up of the following bones, proximal to distal:

- scapula
- humerus
- ulna and radius
- proximal row of carpal bones (medial to lateral): radial carpal bone, intermediate carpal bone, ulnar carpal bone, accessory carpal bone
- distal row of carpal bones (medial to lateral): first carpal bone (may be absent), second carpal bone, third carpal bone, fourth carpal bone
- metacarpal bones (medial to lateral): second metacarpal bone, third metacarpal bone (the cannon bone), fourth metacarpal bone. Second and fourth metacarpal bones also known as medial and lateral splint bones
- medial and lateral proximal sesamoid bones
- proximal phalanx (P1, long pastern)
- middle phalanx (P2, short pastern)
- distal sesamoid bone (navicular bone)
- distal phalanx (P3, coffin bone).

The hindlimb attaches to the body by the pelvic girdle, which is composed of three fused bones: ilium, ischium, and pubis. The equine hindlimb is made up of the following bones, proximal to distal:

- femur
- patella
- tibia and fibula

- calcaneus
- talus
- central tarsal bone
- first and second tarsal bones, which are fused
- third tarsal bone
- fourth tarsal bone
- second metatarsal bone – or medial splint bone
- third metatarsal bone – or cannon bone
- fourth metatarsal bone – or lateral splint bone
- medial and lateral proximal sesamoid bones – on plantar surface
- proximal phalanx (P1, long pastern)
- middle phalanx (P2, short pastern)
- distal sesamoid bone (navicular bone)
- distal phalanx (P3, coffin bone).

The horse foot has a bony base composed of the distal half of the middle phalanx, complete distal phalanx, and distal sesamoid bone. Within the foot are the digital cushion and the navicular bursa, which are soft tissue structures. A highly vascular modified dermis known as the corium covers this. The corium is made up of the perioplic corium, coronary corium, laminar corium, solar corium, and corium of the frog. The hoof is the insensitive ***cornified*** layer of the epidermis that covers the distal end of the digit. The insensitive structures of the hoof include the periople, walls, bars, laminae, sole, and frog. These are produced by the ***germinative*** layer of the epidermis, which lies close to the corium of the same name. It is well supplied with capillaries and nerves.

Digestive tract

The digestive tract of the horse is similar to that of cats and dogs, which was covered in Chapter 3. The digestive system of the horse has evolved to deal with a poor-quality diet eaten over a long period of time. Thus horse digestion is a slow but consistent process. Horses historically roamed large areas of land, grazing, while at the same time being aware of their surroundings and potential predators. This resulted in the need to be able to flee at a moment's notice.

The digestive system of the horse is divided into the foregut and the hindgut. The foregut encompasses the mouth, esophagus, stomach, and small intestine, and its function is similar to that of other monogastric mammalian species. The hindgut is made up of the large intestine (cecum and colon) and rectum. The cecum and colon function as an extensive microbial fermentation vat that allows for bacterial digestion of complex carbohydrates that cannot be digested by the rest of the gut. The cecum is located at the junction of the small intestine and large intestine. Material that is not digested in the stomach and small intestines passes into the cecum. The cecum has billions of bacteria and protozoa responsible for digesting fiber, cellulose, and the remaining soluble carbohydrates that were not broken down and absorbed in the stomach and small intestine. Microbes in the cecum and colon synthesize B vitamins. The microbes also metabolize nitrogen and produce protein. Little, if any, absorption of amino acids occurs in the large intestine.

It is important for health-care team members to remember that feed passes through the foregut of the horse quickly and passes through the hindgut slowly. This may become problematic due to the fact that the majority of nutrient absorption takes place in the foregut. The horse's digestive tract was designed for grazing, so small amounts of forage pass through the gut continuously, and digestion is fairly efficient. With domestication of the horse came owner convenience. Most owners feed their horses once or twice a day. Consequently, large amounts of food are passing through the GI tract at one time. Veterinary health-care teams must be aware that this may cause less efficient digestion and absorption in the horse leading to *colic*.

Nutrition

The feeding of horses is complex. Horses should be fed a precise amount and balance of nutrients. Today's companion horses ingest a variety of feeds ranging in physical form from forage with a high moisture content to cereals with high amounts of starch to hay with physically long fibrous stems. Horses are nonruminant *herbivores* and naturally spend 60–75% of their day grazing. Typically, they ingest approximately 2% of their body weight (dry matter basis) per day while grazing.

The nutritional structure of the horse differs from that of the cat or dog. There are multiple compartments making up the digestive tract of the horse, and each compartment has its own function in terms of utilizing ingested feed. The oral cavity is responsible for physically processing foods into smaller particles (~1.6 mm), which allows for passage through the esophagus and increases the surface area for the small intestinal enzymatic action. The oral cavity breaks down structural carbohydrates for bacterial fermentation in the large intestine. The horse averages 60 000 chews per day and it is only during chewing that salivation is activated. However, due to the increased chewing in the equine species, a horse will produce an average of 5–10 liters of saliva per day. This acts as a lubricant for food passage in the esophagus.

The diets formulated for horses contain on average 5% fat and 7–12% protein, with carbohydrate being the major source of energy (around 80%). This is a result of the evolution of horses to eating grass and other forages. Grass and hays serve as a strong foundation for the feeding of horses. Protein is required mainly in the building and replacement of tissues and although some may consider protein to be an expensive source of energy, dietary protein and fat contribute to meeting the physiological energy demands of the horse. Protein converts into intermediary acids and can be converted to glucose. Fat can aid in meeting energy demands following its hydrolysis to glycerol and fatty acids. The glycerol, glucose, and fatty acids can be utilized by the cell for energy.

Carbohydrate digestion and fermentation yield mostly glucose and acetic, propionic, and butyric *volatile fatty acids*. The *portal venous system* collects these nutrients, and a proportion of them are removed from the blood as they pass through the liver. Both propionate and glucose contribute to glycogen (liver starch) reserves, and acetate and butyrate bolster the fat pool and comprise primary energy sources for many tissues.

Key nutritional factors for horses

The key nutrients in regard to the horse are water, energy, protein, minerals, and vitamins. Water is the most important nutrient for any mammalian species. There should be fresh, abundant water available at all times. Horses drink on average 25 liters per day. In conditions of extreme heat or stress, they may drink 100 liters per day. It is essential that health-care team members remind owners that the more grain their horse eats, the more water intake the horse will need.

Energy is measured in terms of digestible energy (DE) and fed in kilocalories. The amount of DE horses need is dependent upon various factors: physiological state, activity level, environment, and the size of the individual horse. The majority of energy utilized by the horse is from carbohydrates ingested through the horse's natural feed. Table 17.1 shows the amount of kcal/kg in various carbohydrate feeds.

Table 17.1 Energy in carbohydrates.

Feed	kcal/kg
Oats	3000
Alfalfa (early bloom)	2100
Bermuda grass hay	1800
Corn cobs	1250

Fats provide the horse with high-density energy. In equines, fat should not exceed 20% of the total diet or 30% of concentrate. Health-care team members should understand that fat in excess of these percentages will likely result in decreased palatability and loose stools.

Protein amounts are typically expressed as "crude protein" (CP) and are expressed as % dry matter (DM). Again, the amount of protein needed by an individual horse is dependent upon physiological state, type of diet, age, and quality of diet. The closer the proportions of each of the various essential amino acids in the dietary protein conform to the requirements of the tissues, the higher the quality of the protein.

Calcium and phosphorus are considered together because of their interdependent role as the main elements of the crystal apatite, which provides the building blocks for the skeletal system. The requirement for calcium and phosphorus is dependent upon the physiological state of the horse. The average adult horse weighing approximately 500 kg will need around 20 g of calcium and 14 g of phosphorus per day. It is important to balance the ratio of calcium to phosphorus; a mature horse needs a ratio of 1.1:1 to 6:1. The recommended ratio for a growing horse is 1.1:1 to 3:1.

Sodium and chloride are very important electrolytes. Chloride concentration in the extracellular fluid is directly related to that of sodium. Rarely do companion animals have an excess or deficiency of sodium or chloride; however, these are both conditions of which to be aware. Daily sodium requirements are recommended at approximately 0.18–0.36% DM. If the requirements for sodium are met, a deficiency of chloride will seldom occur. Good sources of sodium and chloride can be found in grains with premixture. Salt blocks are another way for owners to provide sodium.

Potassium is the main intracellular cation. Potassium deficiencies in equines are rare, and excess potassium is not usually a problem either. However, excess potassium can lead to hyperkalemic periodic paralysis, which causes episodic weakness in horses accompanied by elevated serum potassium concentration. This syndrome appears to be more common in American quarter horses and their hybrids. Forages are approximately 1–4% potassium. Cereals are relatively poor sources of potassium.

Selenium is a trace element needed as an antioxidant. The requirement is 1–2 mg/day for a 500 kg horse or 0.1–2 ppm. Deficiencies in selenium produce pale, weak muscles in foals and a yellowing of the *depot fat*, known as white muscle disease. It is imperative that pregnant mares receive adequate amounts of selenium in their diet. Selenium is highly toxic to animals, with the minimum toxic dose at 2–5 mg/kg feed. Skin, coat, and hoof abnormalities are the result of excess selenium.

Grazing horses derive vitamin A from *carotenoid* pigments present in herbage. The principal one is beta-carotene, with 1 mg of beta-carotene equating to 400 IU of vitamin A. Horses that graze for 4–6 weeks build up a 3–6-month supply of vitamin A in the liver.

Requirements for vitamin A vary during certain life stages: mature horses require 30 IU/kg body weight; horses in the gestation/lactation stage require 60 IU/kg body weight; and growing horses require ~50 IU/kg body weight.

Vitamin E (alpha-tocopherol) functions as a cellular antioxidant in conjunction with vitamin A and selenium and is required for normal immune function. Fresh green forage and the germ of cereal grains are rich sources of vitamin E. Adult horses require 80–100 IU/kg DM. Although deficiencies are rare, two neurological disorders of horses can be caused by vitamin E deficiencies: equine degenerative myeloencephalopathy and equine motor neuron disease. These diseases are seen in horses that do not have access to pastures, are consuming poor-quality hay, or have low concentrations of circulating alpha-tocopherol.

Types of feed

There are three types of feed with which health-care team members should be familiar: roughages, concentrates, and complete feeds. Roughages include grasses and forage *legumes* cut for hay. Most common species of grass are suitable, but the preferred are the more popular and productive grasses such as rye grasses, fescues, timothy, and cocksfoot. Permanent pasture species are satisfactory as well and include meadow grasses, brome, bent grass, and foxtails. Legumes include red, white, alsike, crimson clovers, trefoils, lucerne, and sainfoin. Roughages are relatively low in energy and have more than 18% crude fiber. Roughages are considered to be the foundation to an equine feeding program. Quality hay can provide energy for the maintenance requirements of the horse. Legumes and nonlegume grasses that are well managed and fertilized (proteinaceous roughages) provide greater than 10% CP as opposed to carbonaceous grasses (those that are not well maintained or fertilized), which provide less than 10% CP (Figure 17.2).

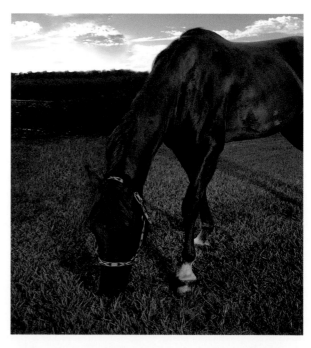

Figure 17.2 Grazing. Source: Courtesy of Kara M. Burns, LVT, VTS (Nutrition).

Veterinary technicians and assistants should understand and educate clients on the quality of roughage using the following guidelines:

- free of mold
- soft and pliable to the touch
- leafy with fine stems (2/3E, 34 protein)
- pleasant, fragrant aroma
- bright green, not brown or yellow.

Another key point to communicate to owners is the fact that excess handling of roughages can result in loss of one-quarter of the leaves; loss of one-fourth to one-third of the energy and protein; and loss of 90% of beta-carotene.

Concentrates are typically a cereal grain that may or may not have supplemented protein, minerals, and vitamins. Concentrates are high in energy (typically 50% greater than forage) and are less than 18% crude fiber. Concentrates are used as a supplement if forage is insufficient in nutrients, especially energy and protein. Concentrates are needed more often in certain life stages, such as gestation (especially later in the gestation period), lactation, and growth, as well as in work horses. A rule of thumb is to not exceed a 50:50 concentrate-to-roughage weight ratio. As always, anything new in the diet should be introduced and transitioned in slowly. It is important for health-care team members and owners alike to be aware of the fact that excess concentrate may lead to *laminitis*, colic, *rhabdomyolysis*, developmental orthopedic disease, and obesity.

Complete feeds are typically a mixture of roughage and concentrate, usually 80% roughage to 20% concentrate mixture. Complete feeds are manufactured by completely grinding the food and formulating it into a pellet, making a convenient, all-in-one feed. There is often an increased cost for the convenience. Because the complete feed is pelleted or wafered, attention must be given to the potential risks associated with inadequate particle size, including colic, choking risk, wood chewing, and coprophagy (eating stool).

Behavior and handling

The horse has the "fight or flight" instinct. The eyes lie on each side of the head above the mouth which allows the horse to graze while watching for predators. The field of vision of a horse is nearly 360° but the binocular vision is approximately 60–70° in front of the horse. Binocular vision is required for a horse to be able to judge distance. Outside the range of 60–70°, the horse must move its head and its body to see a threat. Horses have also adapted to sleeping while standing. This ensures a quick response to or escape from a potential threat. The veterinary team must be aware of these characteristics when attempting to handle a horse. Horses will adapt their body language to warn off potential predators or unwanted beings. A horse may turn its hindquarters to ward off a threat or may even charge with its head down. Blatant aggression in horses is not a common occurrence.

Horses are social beings and typically move around in herds (Figure 17.3). Social contact with other horses is important to the

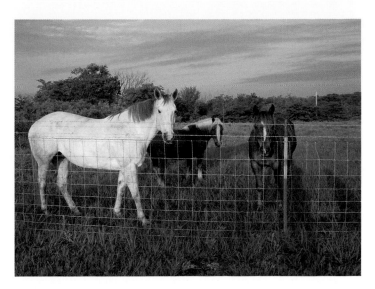

Figure 17.3 Small herd of companion animal horses. Source: Courtesy of Kara M. Burns, LVT, VTS (Nutrition).

health of a horse. If a horse is isolated, stress may manifest through unwanted "vices" or behaviors.

Horses communicate through their senses. They are keenly aware of their environment and any changes that may occur. Olfactory (smell) senses play a large role in the social context of horses, and smell helps to identify individuals and their degree of dominance as well as the location of potential rivals.

The veterinary health-care team should not approach from the blind spot directly behind the horse. As stated, the horse, as it detects new things, will raise its head and attempt to observe the new things in its vision. The most important rule for approaching a horse is to avoid startling it. People approaching can make their presence known to the horse by talking to it.

The ear *pinna* is very mobile and is used to locate the source of a sound. This can also be advantageous for health-care team members approaching a horse. The response and position of the ear are very important methods of communication and oftentimes will let the individual know the attitude of the horse. If the ears are back, the horse may be upset or aggressive.

Health-care team members must know and recognize normal behavior in the horse. Eye position, nostrils, and ear position are critical to understanding what the horse is feeling. Alertness, willingness, unwillingness, and even menace can be expressed through ear position. Neighing and snorting have a large range of expression. Horses can also express feelings through their mouth (e.g., baring of teeth), forefeet (e.g., stamping, pawing, etc.), hind feet, and tail carriage.

Mutual grooming provides a means of maintaining the social network and hierarchy of the herd. Grooming helps to strengthen the bonds of friendship between horses of similar age and social rank. The most preferred grooming sites are concentrated near the autonomic nervous system's longest nerve – vagus (X). Stimulation of this nerve has been shown to decrease the heart rate and relax the horse.

The key to handling horses is anticipation of the body language and facial expressions (as described above). Most horses will behave and react positively if approached with firmness and kindness. Horses instinctively know if a person lacks confidence. It is recommended to stand close to the horse, near the head and away from the hind legs and on the "near" (left) side. It is best to not stand in front of the horse. If the horse becomes agitated, it may attempt to kick with its front foot. Preparation is key. Health-care team members should know what they need to do and have the proper equipment with which to complete the procedure.

The health-care team member should first touch the horse on the withers with arm oustretched at shoulder height (Figure 17.4). The team member should talk softly as he or she moves slowly toward the horse, taking care not to rush. To halter the horse, one's hand should be placed on the lower neck and a rope looped around the neck. Typically, horses will accept that they have been caught and will be more accepting of having a halter placed on them. The halter is a simple restraint device for horses, and a lead rope should be fastened to the halter – a horse should never be led by the halter only. The lead rope should be held close to the horse's head with the remaining rope loosely held in the other hand. The excess rope should never be wrapped around the hand in case the horse suddenly moves or pulls away.

Another common method of restraint is a lead shank with a nose chain, lip chain, and nose twitch. Horses that are fractious respond well to a lead shank with a nose chain. Lip chains are used in controlling young racehorses and stallions. With this restraint, the chain portion of the lead shank is placed under the upper lip of the horse and constant, steady pressure is applied.

When restraint is necessary for veterinary procedures, a nose twitch helps by providing immobilization. A humane twitch is composed of metal and others have wooden handles with either a chain or a rope at the end. Humane twitches are best when working with weanlings, as the twitch is small and the pressure

it exerts is mild. Twitches should be held firmly and lead ropes used to stabilize the horse's head. Nose twitches are used to restrain the horse for procedures such as placing a nasogastric tube, performing a rectal examination, suturing a wound, and so forth.

If a horse must be tied, the equipment must be strong and sound. A chain over or under the nose should never be used. The halter, rope, and what these are tied to must be able to withstand heavy pressure. If they are not sturdy, there is a risk of breakage and freeing the horse. The horse should be tied at shoulder level or higher to stop it from pawing at the restraint and getting a foot over the rope. Horses should be tied with a relatively short rope. The area surrounding the horse should be examined for potential objects that may spook the horse once it is tied. The health-care team should prevent the horse from having too much rope and potentially getting into trouble. A quick-release knot is typically used for tying the horse. Horses that are tied up should never be left unattended.

Horses' feet should be cleaned and inspected daily and thus the horse should be trained to pick up its feet. The handler should, as always, talk to the horse as he or she approaches. To lift a forefoot, the handler should stand facing the hind end and run his or her hand closest to the body of the horse down over the elbow, back of the knee, and tendons until the fetlock is reached. The handler can tug at the fetlock and give the command "Up." As the horse lifts its foot, the handler should catch the toe of the hoof and support it with the other hand. The horse should be encouraged to stand square to prevent it from leaning on the person while its foot is elevated. The foot should be held securely until the cleaning and inspection are finished.

To lift the hind foot, the handler should face the rear and run his or her hand down the flank or rump area, and then to the back leg, to the point of the hock, and then to the anterior portion of the cannon bone until the medial part of the fetlock. The same process of tugging at the fetlock can be repeated on the hind feet. It is best to begin training foals early. It has been shown that when a horse realizes this behavior is required, they will learn to lift their feet when they are asked.

Nursing care and husbandry of horses

Physical examination of the horse is similar to that of small companion animals. This examination will allow the veterinary health-care team, the owner, and the horse to establish a relationship and determine the health of the patient. The rectal temperature, respiratory rate, and heart rate should be taken and recorded. Vital assessments are ideally taken before and after light exercise. The thorax and abdomen should be auscultated. The weight of the horse should be determined, and the musculoskeletal system and integument evaluated. An ophthalmic and dental examination should also be a part of the physical examination.

Bedding for horses can be composed of a variety of materials. Care should be taken to keep the bedding clean and free of dust. A quick checklist for equine bedding should include the following:

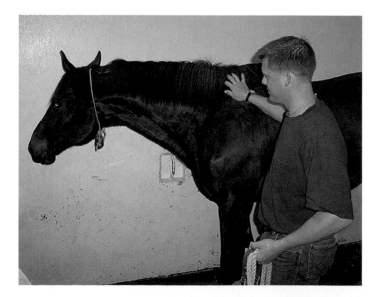

Figure 17.4 Approach to the horse from the left, or near, side. Note the right hand leads to touch the horse at the withers. The left hand holds the halter and lead rope low and to the handler's side. Source: McCurnin, D.M., Bassert, J.M. 2009. *McCurnin's Clinical Textbook for Veterinary Technicians*, 7th edition. Saunders Elsevier, St Louis, MO.

- warm
- absorbent
- soft
- easy to manage
- nontoxic
- dust-free
- compostable.

Pine shavings are adequate and used often but have a tendency to be very dusty. In horses with respiratory problems or open wounds, pine shavings or any bedding that produces dust should not be utilized. For these horses, shredded paper bedding or a bedding that is low in dust and not likely to stick to or clog an open wound is recommended. Owners who use wood shavings should obtain them from a trustworthy source. If black walnut shavings are incorporated into the wood shavings, the risk of laminitis may be increased. Mares with newborn foals are often bedded on straw. Care should be taken to insure that a deep layer of bedding is available for mares and foals. Soiled bedding should be removed and clean bedding added at least once a day. Adult horses that are recumbent should be kept on a deep layer of bedding in an attempt to reduce or prevent the formation of decubital ulcers.

Fly control is best achieved through the education of the owner to keep the barn as clean as possible and remove manure regularly. Topical fly sprays are available, but owners should be made aware of the harm of repellants that use organophosphates as the pesticide. This is especially true for owners of sick or debilitated horses and foals. Fly masks are available for the face and ears of sensitive horses.

Grooming should be a part of the daily regimen of the horse, unless a disease condition prohibits this activity. This is a great human–animal bond activity and provides for maintenance of skin and coat. Grooming begins with the removal of any dried sweat or mud with a rubber curry comb moved in a circular motion on the horse. A stiff bristled brush can then be used to remove dirt and loose hair. Metal curry combs should not be used on the head or distal limb of the horse. The grooming session should be finished with a soft brush or a damp cloth to remove remaining dust from the horse's coat. The tail and mane should be groomed with a stiff brush or metal mane comb.

Horse hooves should be picked clean daily with the use of a hoof pick. As discussed earlier, the horse can be taught to lift the leg to enable the groomer to pick the hoof. The hoof should be cleaned through the removal of dirt and debris from the lateral and central sulci (Figure 17.5). Cleaning should begin at the heel and work toward the toe. If horses' feet are not cleaned frequently or if they are standing in damp bedding or muddy soil, their chance of developing the degenerative condition known as thrush is increased.

Owner education by the veterinary health-care team is crucial to maintaining good health, proper nutrition, and proper husbandry in equine patients. The veterinary team must be familiar with the distinctiveness of the equine species in order to provide proper nursing care and management.

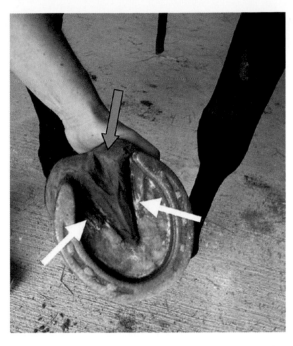

Figure 17.5 Central sulcus (green arrow) and lateral sulci (white arrows) of the frog. Source: Sirois, M. 2010. *Principles and Practice of Veterinary Technology*, 3rd edition. Mosby, St Louis, MO.

References

Ashton, L. 2016. Equine behavior and handling. In: *Aspinall's Complete Textbook of Veterinary Nursing*, 3rd edition. Ackerman, N., Aspinall, V. (eds). Elsevier Butterworth Heinemann, Edinburgh.

Colville, T., Bassert, J.M. 2016. *Clinical Anatomy and Physiology for Veterinary Technicians*, 3rd edition. Elsevier, St Louis, MO.

Burns, K.M. 2011. Equine nutrition. *Canadian Veterinary Technician*, Fall, 3:4.

Gordon, M.B., Young, J.K., Davison, K.E., Raub, R.H. 2009. Equine nutrition. In: *Equine Manual for Veterinary Technicians*. Reeder, D. et al. (eds). Wiley-Blackwell, Ames, IA.

Ellis, A.K., McCommon, G.W. 2018. Preventive health programs. In: *McCurnin's Clincal Textbook for Veterinary Technicians*, 9th edition. Bassert, J.M., Beal, A.D., Samples, O.A. (eds). Elsevier Saunders, St Louis, MO.

Phillips, C. 2016. Equine anatomy and physiology. In: *Aspinall's Complete Textbook of Veterinary Nursing*, 3rd edition. Ackerman, N., Aspinall, V. (eds). Elsevier Butterworth Heinemann, Edinburgh.

Pippard, C. 2016. Equine nutrition. In: *Aspinall's Complete Textbook of Veterinary Nursing*, 3rd edition. Ackerman, N., Aspinall, V. (eds). Elsevier Butterworth Heinemann, Edinburgh.

Scorer, T. 2016. Stable design and management. In: *Aspinall's Complete Textbook of Veterinary Nursing*, 3rd edition. Ackerman, N., Aspinall, V. (eds). Elsevier Butterworth Heinemann, Edinburgh.

Sirois, M. (ed.) 2017. Nursing care of horses. In: *Principles and Practice of Veterinary Technology*, 4th edition. Elsevier, St Louis, MO.

Todd-Jenkins, K., Dugan, B. 2018. Restraint and handling of animals. In: *McCurnin's Clincal Textbook for Veterinary Technicians*, 9th edition. Bassert, J.M., Beal, A.D., Samples, O.A. (eds). Elsevier Saunders, St Louis, MO.

Wortinger, A.E., Burns, K.M. 2015. Equine. In: *Nutrition and Disease Management for Veterinary Technicians and Nurses*, 2nd Edition. Wortinger, A., Burns, K.M. (eds). John Wiley & Sons, Inc., Ames, IA.

Zimmel, D. 2009. General horse management. In: *Equine Manual for Veterinary Technicians*. Reeder, D. et al. (eds). Wiley-Blackwell, Ames, IA.

www.wiley.com/go/burns/textbookvetassistant2

Please go to the companion website for assignments and a PowerPoint relating to the material in this chapter.

Chapter **18** Preparing for Internships and Employment

There are many parts to the internship/job search process including interviews, resumés, and cover letters. Interviews are necessary but often nerve-wracking. Many people have "butterflies" when speaking to people in an unfamiliar setting. This may be compounded if you are generally an introverted person. You will often be interviewing with the office manager or head technician instead of the owner of the practice. This is especially true in larger practices.

Interview

There are several steps you can take to overcome any nervousness. First, be prepared. Be sure you know what job you are applying for. Try to research the hospital(s) to which you are applying. If the hospital has a website, be sure to visit it. Show the interviewer you have done your homework about the hospital. It is also a good idea to bring an extra copy of your resumé with you to the interview.

Practicing your interview may help calm your anxiety as well as preparing you to cover the main points you would like to get across to the interviewer. Don't cram the night before your interview. Have friends or family members practice with you. Tell them why you would be the best person for the position.

Many people ignore the basics prior to an interview. These include grooming, eating well prior to the interview, and getting enough sleep the night before. Lack of any one of these areas will affect your interview. You may come across as less than enthusiastic about the position. In many cases, it may make any anxiety you have worse. Looking and feeling good will help boost your confidence.

You are applying for a position in a professional setting and therefore you should dress accordingly. Yes, in most hospitals, the employees wear scrubs but you should dress professionally for an interview. It is better to be overdressed than to appear slovenly to the interviewer.

Finally, don't fear the interviewer. As mentioned earlier, the person interviewing you will most likely be the practice manager or head technician. The interviewer does not want to see you fail – this is a common misconception. Viewing the person interviewing you as the enemy will increase your anxiety. Relax and keep your wits about you. If mistakes happen during an interview, be prepared to make light of them. Employers aren't looking for the perfect employee but one who is flexible and resilient. How you handle yourself in an interview will show your future employer how you will handle yourself on the job, especially in a stressful situation.

Resumé writing

One of the most important aspects of obtaining an internship or job is a precise, well-organized and well-written resumé. There are several websites that offer basic resumé writing templates and styles (see Resources section). Select one that best suits you and the position you are applying for. Some templates may be better suited for professional or medical situations. You may find in some sources a template for a curriculum vitae or CV. Though similar to a resumé, a CV differs in several ways. It tends to act as a record of scholarly activities and is more suited for use by a veterinarian or licensed veterinary technician. A resumé will suffice when applying for a VA position or internship.

No matter which template you choose, resumés should contain the following information.

Textbook for the Veterinary Assistant, Second Edition. Kara M. Burns and Lori Renda-Francis.
© 2022 John Wiley & Sons, Inc. Published 2022 by John Wiley & Sons, Inc.
Companion website: www.wiley.com/go/burns/textbookvetassistant2

Education

List any degrees you have obtained or are currently working on. Be sure to list the school, location, and years attended.

Experience/work history

List any previous positions held. List the name of the company and any skills you feel will be pertinent to the position you are attempting to obtain.

Achievement/awards

List any academic or professional achievements or awards that pertain to the field of work you are applying to.

Skills

Note any skills you have that may be beneficial to your potential employer. This section may be combined in the experience/work history section.

References

Here you will list people your potential employer can contact to obtain further information regarding you as a person. A minimum of three people should be listed. Choose people you feel will give you a favorable review. Often references are listed as available upon request.

You may find many templates that contain an objective statement at the beginning of the resumé. Many professionals find this to be a dated practice and forgo it altogether. Instead, they state their objective in a cover letter as will be discussed later in the section. Ideally, keep your resumé to a single page of information. If the resumé is too long, a potential employer may pass it by. Many employers look for a few key words when scanning a resume. You need to sell yourself in the most succinct way.

Dos and don'ts of resumé writing

- DO make your resumé as clear and concise as possible. Make every word count.
- DO try to look at examples of resumés other people have written, especially people in a professional field.
- DO take time to make a high-quality, uncluttered resumé. Style matters. A resumé should appear professional.
- DO check for errors and spelling mistakes. Have someone else read the resumé. That person may note weaknesses, typographical errors, or inconsistencies in style. Proofread every new version you make.
- DON'T give excessive details about professional experience by reiterating every task you performed at every job.
- DON'T list irrelevant information about yourself.

- DON'T include the reason for leaving your last position.
- DON'T include minor accomplishments. This may give the appearance of padding.
- DON'T list all previous employment. List any from the past 5–7 years and those that may be directly applicable to the position you are applying for.
- DON'T print the resumé on colored or busy paper or use fancy typefaces.

Cover letter

While a resumé is a summary of your credentials, a tailored cover letter should be a brief description of why you are applying to a specific hospital and what your ultimate goals are. Use the cover letter to market yourself. Your aim with the letter is to demonstrate why your education skills and work experience qualify you for the position. When possible, find out who you will be interviewing with and address the letter to the interviewer. If this is impossible, address the letter to the practice owner. By calling the hospital, you can find out who usually performs the interviews.

Mary A. Smith
2065 Huron Rd.
Warren, MI 48089
(h) (555) 411-1212
smithma@email.com
1/1/2012

Jane Anderson, D.V.M.
Main Animal Hospital
15479 Main Ave.
Detroit, MI 48221

Dear Dr. Anderson,

I am writing to inquire about obtaining a position as an intern/veterinary assistant with your hospital. I learned of your hospital through the college's internship registry.

I am currently a student in County Community College's veterinary assistant program.

I have attached my resume to provide a brief account of my experience. I hope you will consider me for a position. I look forward to the opportunity to meet with you and discuss my qualifications in person. I can be reached at the e-mail address or phone number listed on my resume. The best time to contact me is after three o'clock weekdays. Thank you for your time.

Sincerely,

Mary A. Smith

Figure 18.1 Example cover letter.

There are some basic points to remember when writing a cover letter. Use standard business-letter format printed in one typeface. Avoid decorative typefaces and stick to standard font sizes, usually 10–12. Use terms and phrases that may be meaningful to your prospective internship site or possible place of employment. Minimize the use of abbreviations and contractions. Try to be concise. Always check for grammatical errors, and be sure to sign the letter.

Most cover letters will contain two or three paragraphs covering your main points. First, identify the position for which you are applying. When possible, state how you learned of the position. Next, summarize why you are the best candidate for the position. Try to target the internship/job description and explain how your skills relate to the position's requirements. Finally, always thank the person for considering your resumé and offer to provide further information. Be sure to include your email address, phone number, and the best time you can be reached. An example of a cover letter is presented in Figure 18.1.

References

Career Services, University of Pennsylvania. Making the Most of Your Internship. www.vpul.upenn.edu/careerservices/jobsandinternships/makingmostofinternship.php

Counseling and Wellness Services, Center for Advising and Career Development, Washington State University, Pullman, WA. Resume and Cover Letter Packet. https://s3.wp.wsu.edu/uploads/sites/167/2015/08/Resume-Packet.pdf

Resources

office.microsoft.com
www.resumetemplates.org
www.instantresumetemplates.com
www.vetmed.wsu.edu/academic/counseling/CareertResume1.pdf

www.wiley.com/go/burns/textbookvetassistant2

Please go to the companion website for assignments and a PowerPoint relating to the material in this chapter.

Chapter **19** Inventory

When you think of your love of animals and of pursuing a career as a veterinary assistant to help them, you probably don't think of inventory. The fact is, inventory is very important to all veterinary practices. Having an accurate account of all drugs, supplies, and equipment on hand is one of the crucial factors in running a cost-efficient business. It determines customer satisfaction and is a tool in maintaining financial control. It is important to be able to meet customer demand both immediate and long term by being properly stocked for emergencies.

Animal patients and their owners will be your customers. To serve all their needs efficiently, an individual will usually be assigned to be the practice inventory manager. It could be the veterinarian, the practice manager, licensed veterinary technician, or veterinary assistant. This person will be responsible for all product ordering, maintaining functioning levels of inventory, planning, and budgeting. The budget must allow for maintaining current stock as well as the occasional hard-to-find item. It is very important to have a protocol in place that ensures supply levels are maintained so that stock isn't diminished so low that you are unable to provide for the demands of your patients. If you are the person who manages your clinic's inventory then pat yourself on the back. You obviously are a responsible, detail-oriented individual with an important job. Inventory management is a useful skill that can increase your value as an employee. Inventory experience will also enhance your resumé, making you more competitive when you look for future employment.

What will be inventoried in your clinic or hospital?

The answer is . . . almost everything: drugs, medical supplies, pet food, office supplies, and so on. It is good practice to keep track of everything. An inventory provides information about which drugs and supplies are available for use. It also keeps track of drugs and supplies on order and is a useful tool in the development of reorder points and purchasing. Responsibilities of inventory usually encompass maintaining the drug inventory, including a separate inventory for controlled substances, maintaining a supply and equipment inventory, a pet food inventory, a file of manufactures and distributors, and a database of sales representatives serving as your contacts for products you use and sell. Other responsibilities of inventory involve unpacking deliveries, writing expiry dates on all items, removing expired items from stock, data entry to record all drugs and supplies, returning any expired drugs, accounting for damaged goods, and returning all defective products.

A well-run pharmacy

Working with your clinic's sales representatives can help you establish a well-run pharmacy (Figure 19.1). The availability of drugs and supplies is the goal, and maintaining an effective turnover rate is of crucial importance to achieving this. Turnover rates

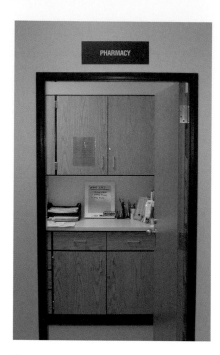

Figure 19.1 Pharmacy. Source: Courtesy of Dr Lori Renda-Francis, LVT.

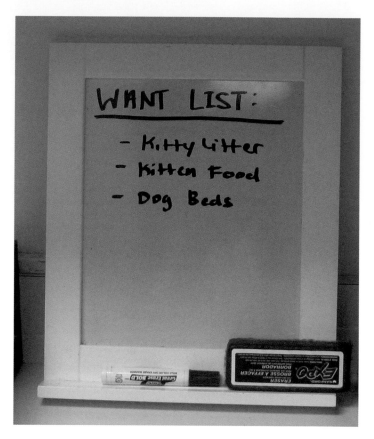

Figure 19.2 Want list. Source: Courtesy of Dr Lori Renda-Francis, LVT.

indicate how quickly a drug is used and can be difficult to predict. It is very important to have a good working relationship with your clinic's sales representatives. In addition to placing orders on existing medications, the sales representative will inform you about special deals and educate staff regarding new or emerging drugs with pertinent product information.

A veterinary assistant can become even more valuable to the veterinary team by being informed about all products the sales representatives handle. You may help determine order quantity, or how much of a certain drug or product is needed. Many drugs come in several sizes. For example, various brands of tablets and capsules can come in 100, 500, or 1000-count containers. It is important to keep track of which drugs are commonly dispensed and at what frequency. Then an informed decision can be made regarding effective order quantity. Once the inventory manager knows this information, it is important to determine a reorder point. Reorder point planning with a sales representative uses information regarding product demand to help decide when to automatically reorder products to avoid shortages or wasteful overages.

The want list

Another way to ensure a well-run pharmacy is to utilize a "want list." This is a list for anyone working in the clinic to record anything that is running low. Quite often, the want list is on a white board in a location for everyone to see (Figure 19.2). As an assistant, one of your jobs will be to help monitor current inventory. Yet another measure in running an efficient pharmacy is a plan to help insure client demand is met during an emergency situation. Your clinic should maintain a good professional relationship with other nearby veterinary clinics as well as human hospitals. These connections can provide a much-needed safety net when

emergencies arise. The practice of borrowing (or lending) seldom used drugs and supplies is a good idea because it saves time (record keeping is seldom needed in such cases) and money.

The veterinary assistant's role

A veterinary assistant should be familiar with various aspects of inventory. As previously mentioned, you will be monitoring current inventory. You will also help provide information regarding inventory turnover rate. This involves keeping track of quantities of drugs and supplies used over a period of time along with the cost of each item. You will participate in inventory counts which take place in most veterinary hospitals at least once a year. The majority of hospitals take a physical count more often than that. Your goal should be to have an active inventory with a high turnover rate. A high turnover rate will ensure a lower monetary investment in supplies.

Shortages are a problem no clinic wants. To try and avoid this, many practices intentionally maintain a higher inventory than actually needed. One advantage to ordering in greater numbers is financial; usually price incentives increase the more you order so ordering more can seem like a good deal. However, there are a few problems with maintaining a higher inventory. One is the budget. Even though you may get a price break, it means that a lot of the clinic's budget may be bound up with inventory only to be spread thin in other areas of the practice. Also, a higher inventory can lead to a greater potential problem of drugs and products expiring before they can be used due to a lower than expected turnover rate. The inventory manager should always make adjustments in maintaining stock for high-demand and low-demand periods. Careful planning is crucial in order to avoid wasteful and expensive mistakes.

Drug inventory

You should spend time learning the various types of drugs that a veterinary facility usually has in its inventory. Some of the most potent drugs are called controlled substances. According to the DEA, "A controlled substance is placed in its respective schedule based on whether it has a currently accepted medical use in treatment in the United States and its relative abuse potential and likelihood of causing dependence." These drugs or chemical substances are strictly regulated under the federal US drug policy, the Comprehensive Drug Abuse Prevention and Control Act passed in 1970. The US government has established five groups (known as schedules) of controlled substances. Many different potent prescription and illegal drugs fall into these five schedules. The following are the criteria for each controlled substance schedule.

Schedule I

- The drug or other substance has a high potential for abuse.
- The drug or other substance has no currently accepted medical use in treatment in the United States.
- There is a lack of accepted safety for use of the drug or other substance under medical supervision.
- Some examples of substances listed in schedule I: heroin, lysergic acid diethylamide (LSD), marijuana, peyote, methaqualone.

Schedule II

- The drug or other substance has a high potential for abuse.
- The drug or other substance has a currently accepted medical use in treatment in the United States or a currently accepted medical use with severe restrictions.
- Abuse of the drug or other substances may lead to severe psychological or physical dependence.

Examples of schedule II *narcotics* include morphine and opium. Other schedule II narcotic substances and their common name brand products include hydromorphone (Dilaudid®), methadone (Dolophine®), meperidine (Demerol®), oxycodone (OxyContin®), and fentanyl (Sublimaze® or Duragesic®).

Examples of schedule II *stimulants* include amphetamine (Dexedrine®, Adderall®), methamphetamine (Desoxyn®), and methylphenidate (Ritalin®).

Other schedule II substances include cocaine and pentobarbital.

Schedule III

- The drug or other substance has a potential for abuse less than the drugs or other substances in schedules I and II.
- The drug or other substance has a currently accepted medical use in treatment in the United States.
- Abuse of the drug or other substance may lead to moderate or low physical dependence or high psychological dependence.

Examples of schedule III *narcotics* include Vicodin® and Tylenol® with codeine. Also included are buprenorphine products (Suboxone® and Subutex®) used to treat opioid addiction.

Examples of schedule III *nonnarcotics* include ketamine and anabolic steroids such as oxandrolone (Oxandrin®).

Schedule IV

- The drug or other substance has a low potential for abuse relative to the drugs or other substances in schedule III.
- The drug or other substance has a currently accepted medical use in treatment in the United States.
- Abuse of the drug or other substance may lead to limited physical dependence or psychological dependence relative to the drugs or other substances in schedule III. An example of a schedule IV narcotic is propoxyphene (Darvon® and Darvocet-N® 100).

Other schedule IV substances include alprazolam (Xanax®), clonazepam (Klonopin®), diazepam (Valium®), lorazepam (Ativan®), midazolam (Versed®), temazepam (Restoril®), and triazolam (Halcion®).

Schedule V

- The drug or other substance has a low potential for abuse relative to the drugs or other substances in schedule IV.
- The drug or other substance has a currently accepted medical use in treatment in the United States.
- Abuse of the drug or other substance may lead to limited physical dependence or psychological dependence relative to the drugs or other substances in schedule IV.

Schedule IV medications consist primarily of preparations containing limited quantities of certain narcotics. These are generally used for antitussive, antidiarrheal, and analgesic purposes. Examples include cough preparations containing not more than 200 mg of codeine per 100 ml or per 100 g (Robitussin® and Phenergan® with codeine).

It is important to know that all veterinarians must legally obtain a DEA license in order to purchase or dispense a controlled substance. A controlled substance inventory is required by law and by federal agencies. Due to their abuse and addiction, potential controlled substances require a detailed protocol for secure storage. Schedule I, II, III, IV, and V controlled substances

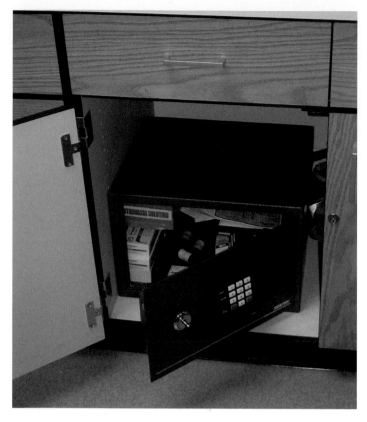

Figure 19.3 Safe, opened. Source: Courtesy of Dr Lori Renda-Francis, LVT.

must be stored in a locked, steel cabinet or a locked substantially constructed cabinet (Figure 19.3).

By law, all controlled substances must carry a specific label designating their schedule.

All noncontrolled drugs should be accurately maintained in a separate drug inventory. For this inventory, the pharmacy is quite often divided into various categories such as antibiotics, sedatives, vaccines, ear medications, eye medications, etc.

A separate vaccine log should also be in place to track all vaccine services offered at your clinic.

Heartworm and parasite prevention treatments should be maintained in yet another inventory.

As a valuable veterinary assistant, it is imperative that you understand the drug inventory protocols in place at your clinic. They encompass several categories and are directly responsible for client safety and satisfaction.

Human versus computer: both needed!

Maintaining your clinic's inventory can at times seem overwhelming. What is the best way to do the job? Ideally, inventory is managed by both manual and computer work. Inventory management software is a highly effective tool in most clinics today. Going green with paperless computer-based systems for tracking product levels, orders, returns, back orders, and so forth is an efficient way to manage your clinic's needs. There are several veterinary computer-based inventory systems available. Computer-based inventory management software will help you effectively and easily track product and supply counts, which will save time and money.

However, there are a few disadvantages to take into account. Initial expense is one; veterinary inventory software programs are expensive so the initial budgeting for them can be an issue. Also, computer-based programs, although very detailed and precise, are complicated and can require extra training. This requires an employee to become proficient which can be quite time-consuming. Unfortunately, such software cannot verbally alert you when you're almost out of something. As a veterinary assistant, your input on day-to-day stock levels is very important. Never underestimate your part in maintaining a functioning inventory!

In addition to utilizing an inventory software program, it is very important to do a clinic-wide manual inventory count. This means literally counting everything in your clinic. It is helpful to organize items to be counted into several categories, such as vaccinations, pet food, oral medications, supplies, and so on. Be sure to update your previous totals as soon as you're finished.

As you can see, both methods of inventory tracking work together and are critical to successful inventory planning.

Organizing inventory

There's no such thing as a "little job." Veterinary assistants quite often will play a major role in organizing inventory storage. When thinking about inventory and keeping supplies on hand, your clinic's storage facility space must be factored in. Physical limitations such as space (large boxes of products can take up large spaces) can greatly influence order quantity. Also, several items will require proper temperature control when stored. Some can be stored at room temperature while others must be refrigerated.

As a veterinary assistant, you may be the designated employee responsible for the storage of vaccines and other items that require refrigeration. It is important to know that when storing vaccines and other temperature-sensitive products, you must read and follow the manufacturer's directions for each product, specifically regarding temperature and light exposure. Again, the importance of every aspect of inventory control is crucial because a casual approach to product knowledge can mean major problems for your clinic. Improper storage of vaccines can result in vaccine failures, which can result in possible adverse reactions post vaccination as well as product spoilage. All of this directly impacts the veterinary practice with needless waste, useless expenses, lost clientele, and, most importantly, disappointing results for the animals you want to help.

Aside from vaccines, all the other drugs, supplies, and equipment must be organized and stored. Ideally, you should plan to place items on shelves in groups that make sense. If this is done effectively, it makes locating a particular medication or supply much easier. For example, on one shelf you might arrange all eye medications, ear medications, ear wash, and so on. On another shelf, arrange all anesthetics. Still another shelf might have all antibiotics and cough tabs. ***Analgesics*** should have their own area on the shelf as well. Intuitive arrangement of products saves time and is a component in easing the flow of a busy workplace.

Veterinary assistants are vital health-care team members in veterinary practices. Veterinarians will depend on you for assistance in many aspects of their work. Your knowledge and understanding of your clinic's inventory are very important to your job. Your input in maintaining a well-organized and successful inventory will help ensure a well-organized and successful veterinary practice of which you will be proud.

References

American Association of Equine Practitioners. Vaccine Storage and Handling. www.aaep.org/vaccine storagehandling.htm

Beal, A.D., Viviano, K.R. 2018. Pharmacology and pharmacy. In: *McCurnin's Clinical Textbook for Veterinary Technicians*, 9th edition. Bassert, J.A., Beal, A.D., Samples, O.M. (eds). Elsevier, St Louis, MO.

Prendergast H. 2020. Inventory management. In: *Front Office Management for the Veterinary Team*, 3rd edition. Elsevier, St Louis, MO.

US Department of Justice Drug Enforcement Administration Office of Diversion Control. Controlled Substance Schedules. www.deadiversion. usdoj.gov/schedules/index.html

www.wiley.com/go/burns/textbookvetassistant2

Please go to the companion website for assignments and a PowerPoint relating to the material in this chapter.

Chapter 20 Euthanasia and Pet Loss

Euthanasia is one of the most difficult procedures to be performed by the veterinary health-care team. The term has its origin from two Greek words: *eu*, meaning good or right, and *thanatos*, meaning death. There are numerous factors that must be considered by the pet owner, veterinarian, and health-care team prior to the decision to euthanize an animal. As the name implies, euthanasia is meant to be an "easier" death. However, euthanasia is widely recognized as one of the most stressful procedures that veterinarians and health-care team members must perform. Each health-care team member also must remember the stress to the pet owner and the stages of grief that all involved will confront.

The human–animal bond is a very strong emotional bond that ties animals and human beings together in a manner beneficial to both (Figure 20.1). The bond is formed through respect, trust, devotion, and love. In today's society, many owners treat pets as their children and/or their closest friends. The veterinary health-care team helps to strengthen the human–animal bond and with each visit educates owners further on how to properly care for their pet. As the bond forms between the owner and pet, over a lifetime of visits to the veterinary hospital, the bond also strengthens between the pet, owner, and health-care team. Consequently, it becomes very difficult for empathetic team members to face euthanasia of a beloved lifelong patient.

Veterinary teams become attached to patients and their families, especially if they have seen the patient from puppy/kittenhood. Oftentimes, these patients are not just "patients" but extended family members with whom a bond has been established. Euthanasia can lead to compassion fatigue and burnout in veterinary health-care team members. However, the focus on performing a euthanasia has been shifted to ensure the pet's last moments are comfortable and peaceful. Today, pet owners expect that veterinary professionals will provide a death worthy of the pet's life. Our profession has recognized that pet deaths needed to be more meaningful – the kind of experience that leaves the entire veterinary team feeling they provided the best medicine possible and supported the client throughout the life and death of the patient. The focus of the veterinary team has shifted to the human–animal bond which, especially at the time of euthanasia, is a rare gem of connectedness and intimacy. The shift in attention has allowed for teams to slow down, to listen to stories, to take deep breaths in quiet reflection in an otherwise chaotic schedule. Euthanasia, while sad and heartbreaking, can lead to rich personal satisfaction when performed well. When love is at the heart of our work, the veterinary profession finds peace, even when life is lost.

Although euthanasia is aimed at providing reduced stress and pain for the patient, the thought of losing their best friend or family member often overwhelms owners. The pet owner will look to the health-care team, especially the veterinarian, for guidance as to the appropriate time to end a pet's suffering. The remainder of the team will be relied upon for emotional support. The owner's grief must be handled with empathy, compassion, and sensitivity. All members of the health-care team must understand the process of euthanasia in their hospital as well as the signs of grief in themselves, their colleagues, and the pet owner.

Deciding to euthanize a beloved pet is one of the hardest decisions pet owners will ever face. There are a host of reasons that play a role in making the decision, including financial reasons, fear of eventual outcomes of a disease, and the decision to let a pet

Textbook for the Veterinary Assistant, Second Edition. Kara M. Burns and Lori Renda-Francis.
© 2022 John Wiley & Sons, Inc. Published 2022 by John Wiley & Sons, Inc.
Companion website: www.wiley.com/go/burns/textbookvetassistant2

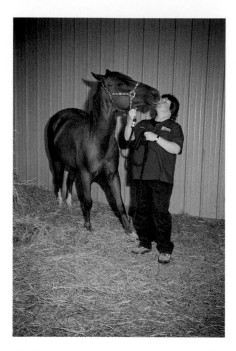

Figure 20.1 The human–animal bond between a technician and her horse. Source: Courtesy of Kara M. Burns, LVT, VTS (Nutrition).

die naturally. The majority of owners who choose euthanasia do so out of the belief that their pet is suffering. The owner will look to the veterinary health-care team for counsel during the decision-making process. The team should listen to the client's concerns and assist the client professionally and with compassion and respect.

The owner will want to be fully educated on the euthanasia process – how euthanasia is performed, whether the animal will feel any pain, how long euthanasia may take, and what happens to the body after euthanasia. This discussion is best handled by the credentialed veterinary technician or the veterinarian. The veterinary team member should discuss all options with the owner but not make the decision for the owner. Open-ended questions play a large role in communicating with the client, getting to the root of the question, and helping the client with this very difficult decision. The pet owner will go through the stages of grief before, during, and following the euthanasia of their pet. It is important for health-care team members to reassure the pet owner that these stages are normal and expected and that the owner is encouraged to talk about their feelings if desired.

Once the owner makes an informed decision, the hospital team must support the decision and the owner, even if the decision is not what you would have decided. All health-care team members interacting with clients, pets, and extended families must exhibit a caring, calm, and empathetic manner.
Once the decision has been made to euthanize an animal, the pet owner has a number of further decisions to make.

- Where should the euthanasia take place?
- Are the client and/or other members of the family planning to be present?
- What is the plan for the body following the euthanasia?

- Is there a certain way the owner would like the patient memorialized?
- Is a *necropsy* warranted and, if so, approved by the pet owner?
- What are the plans for payment?

Communication and empathy are the keys to limiting the stress and fear associated with euthanasia. The veterinary health-care team should communicate with the client in an attempt to educate them on the procedure and to avoid the unexpected as much as possible.

Prior to the actual euthanasia, the health-care team should discuss what will happen during the procedure in detail. Each step should be discussed, with care given to what the client will see, as well as some of the unpleasant occurrences that may arise. Owners may not realize that their pet may urinate, defecate, twitch, or vocalize as it becomes unconscious. This can be quite disturbing to a pet owner, but the health-care team can assist by explaining ahead of time what may occur during the procedure. This will help to inform the client of what to expect and to alleviate the perception that these bodily functions are indicative of pain and suffering. The key point is to plan for the unexpected and to prepare the client through open channels of communication.

The euthanasia should be planned as much as possible at a time and place convenient for the owner. If it is to be performed at the veterinary hospital, try to avoid high traffic or busy times. Allow for the owner to spend time before and after with the pet. The use of a client consultation room will be less stark than a sterile examination room. Limit the amount of distractions and noise as much as possible. Prepare everything for the veterinarian and the pet owner in advance to insure a smooth procedure.

Once the preparations are complete, all health-care team members must know their role and responsibilities and perform their duties with the greatest skill, concern, and professionalism. As mentioned earlier, all members should plan for the unexpected. Be sure to let the client know it is encouraged to talk to the pet, or if the owner is not present, let them know that someone was with the pet, talking to it and soothing it throughout the procedure.

Clients, whether present during euthanasia or not, appreciate reassurance from the team that their pet is in fact deceased. The veterinarian will auscultate the animal's *thorax* and/or shine a pen light into the animal's eyes before pronouncing that a patient is deceased. Owners who are not present for the procedure oftentimes request to see the body of the deceased pet following euthanasia. Permit time for this as it allows closure and alleviates fears on the owner's part that the pet is not deceased. Ensure the pet is presentable before bringing the owner to see the body. Clean the pet as much as possible, remove any catheters, and close the animal's mouth and eyes. Lay the pet on a clean blanket or towel. Treat the pet and owner with respect and dignity throughout the entire process. Do not place the deceased pet in a body bag with the owner present or where the owner can see what is being done. Knowing this will happen and seeing this happen to a beloved pet are two different sensory perceptions. If the owner plans to bring the patient home for burial, communicate the details of how the body is wrapped and whether there are any signs of surgery or trauma. Owners who state they will not look at the body often change their mind before burying the body, so it is important that they know what to expect.

Ensure the team offers the appropriate environment for the owner to begin grieving. Let the owner know that emotions are expected and that crying is necessary and part of the grieving process. Have tissues at the ready for the pet owner and family. Do not try to say the "right thing" as this is very difficult, and each person is different in how they feel and what they believe in regard to their pet's passing – truly, there is no right thing to say. Rather, ease the owner's mind by assuring that the animal's death was painless, and focus on some of the positive memories of the pet and owner. Gentle gestures and words let the client know that the team understands the pain, the team cares, and that the owner is not alone. If the owner comes to the euthanasia unaccompanied by another person, it is best to arrange beforehand for another person to drive the grieving owner home. This allows for a safer trip home and ensures that the owner is not alone. A follow-up phone call to see how the owner is doing and to answer any questions that may have arisen is a wonderful service that the team can provide to a grieving owner. A sympathy card sent to the owner signed by the health care team of the hospital is a thoughtful gesture that shows the care and compassion of the veterinary health-care team.

Many veterinary hospitals like to assist clients in remembering and memorializing their pet. If the pet has succumbed to a certain disease condition, a donation in that pet's memory to a foundation researching a cure for that disease is often a thoughtful way to remember the pet. Other ways include taking a paw print of the pet, either with paint or in clay, and giving this to the owner. Adding this to a poem or a picture of the pet is a wonderful way to express the care and sympathy of the hospital team to the pet owner (Figure 20.2).

If the owner elects to have the pet's body cremated, there are generally two options: mass cremation or private cremation. Private cremation allows for the ashes to be returned to the owner. Health-care teams must remember that it is very difficult for owners to return to the hospital and pick up the ashes of their deceased pet. It is best that the phone call to the owner be brief and direct: "Fluffy's ashes have been returned to the veterinary hospital and are available for you to pick up at your convenience." It is imperative that the health-care team know where the ashes are located in the hospital and that the patient and owner's name are readily visible on the cremation container. All team members should be expecting the owner and remember that when the owner comes to "pick up Fluffy," it is for Fluffy's ashes, not for a current patient. It is painful enough for an owner to return to the hospital to pick up the ashes; to have to explain that "Fluffy" refers to remains rather than a live pet makes it even more difficult.

Euthanasia is also extremely stressful on the health-care team in the hospital. In fact, frequent euthanasia procedures are the primary cause of staff burnout in small animal practice. Veterinarians and veterinary technicians/nurses take an oath which includes promoting animal welfare and preventing animal suffering. However, this oath can become a burden when team members focus on helping patients and clients, but neglect to take care of themselves. As mentioned, euthanizing a patient is one of many stressful experiences in the veterinary hospital that contribute to compassion fatigue. Compassion fatigue is a condition which individuals in helping professions experience. These individuals give of themselves – sometimes totally – and do not give anything to themselves which results in depleting internal resources. This is not healthy behavior – for our families, our patients, our clients, our hospital – but most important this is not healthy for us as individuals. Therefore, veterinary professionals need ways to cope with such stress.

All euthanasia procedures – smooth as well as difficult – are stressful for the health-care team. Team members involved in euthanasia should be allowed to decide if they are prepared to participate at any given procedure, especially from an emotional standpoint. Additionally, each veterinarian's perceptions on euthanasia may differ, so it is important to know his/her stance prior to accepting a position with that hospital or working with that veterinarian. Communication again is the key to decreasing the amount of stress related to euthanasia in a veterinary hospital. If there are differing views among team members, these should be discussed honestly and openly. Also, the stress of euthanasia in a veterinary hospital is eased through discussions with coworkers and colleagues. The health-care team members need outlets to discuss their emotions surrounding euthanasia in an open and safe environment, so meetings or sessions to help the team cope with and deal with their emotions is a very healthy approach for all involved. This will also help the team to understand what others in the hospital are feeling and how they are dealing with this stressful procedure.

All team members should be encouraged to find other outlets to deal with the stress of work and euthanasia. Some ideas that have helped veterinary team members are helping clients deal with their grief, educating colleagues on dealing with euthanasia, discussing feelings and emotions with coworkers who experience the same stress, engaging in hobbies outside work, and, very importantly, taking time off.

In general, people are not comfortable talking about death but the veterinary health-care team must discuss death, participate in it, and support pet owners and colleagues through it on a weekly and in many cases daily basis. Very few health-care team members have degrees or training in psychology, especially as it relates to death and grieving. Empathy and compassion are two strong tools to help owners and colleagues through this very difficult experience.

The veterinary is responsible for promoting healthy decision making regarding the euthanasia procedure with companion animals. This healthy decision making is important for the team's wellness, for ensuring a humane and respectful outcome for the pet, and for strengthening the human–animal bond. In order to discuss with pet owners when euthanasia is an alternative to continued suffering, the veterinary team need to develop and maintain empathic, professional relationships with their clients. Understanding the human–animal bond between the pet and the owner is one of the most important roles in determining the outcome for each animal, owner, and veterinary team member.

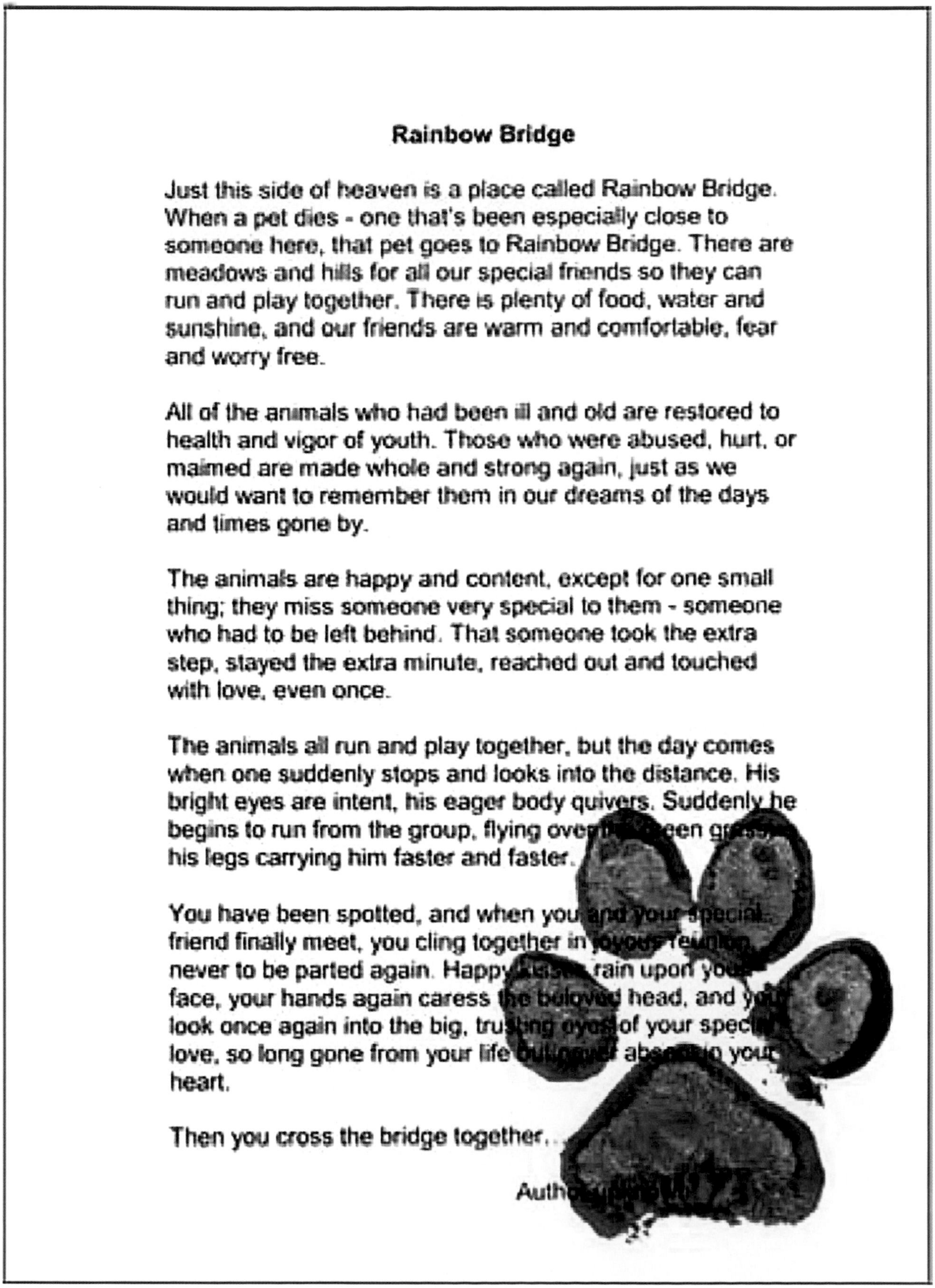

Rainbow Bridge

Just this side of heaven is a place called Rainbow Bridge. When a pet dies - one that's been especially close to someone here, that pet goes to Rainbow Bridge. There are meadows and hills for all our special friends so they can run and play together. There is plenty of food, water and sunshine, and our friends are warm and comfortable, fear and worry free.

All of the animals who had been ill and old are restored to health and vigor of youth. Those who were abused, hurt, or maimed are made whole and strong again, just as we would want to remember them in our dreams of the days and times gone by.

The animals are happy and content, except for one small thing; they miss someone very special to them - someone who had to be left behind. That someone took the extra step, stayed the extra minute, reached out and touched with love, even once.

The animals all run and play together, but the day comes when one suddenly stops and looks into the distance. His bright eyes are intent, his eager body quivers. Suddenly he begins to run from the group, flying over the green grass, his legs carrying him faster and faster.

You have been spotted, and when you and your special friend finally meet, you cling together in joyous reunion, never to be parted again. Happy kisses rain upon your face, your hands again caress the beloved head, and you look once again into the big, trusting eyes of your special love, so long gone from your life but never absent in your heart.

Then you cross the bridge together...

Author unknown

Figure 20.2   The Rainbow Bridge poem with a pet's paw print. Source: Prendergast, H. 2011. *Front Office Management for the Veterinary Team*. Elsevier, St Louis, MO.

The continued strengthening of the human–animal bond, not only between the pet and owner but also between the patient and health-care team member, has complicated the ethical conundrum surrounding euthanasia. Euthanasia is an emotional, psychological, and economic issue with which all team members wrestle. Many in the profession experience stress as they grapple with the challenge of ending an animal's life too soon, or waiting too long. Additionally, the team must manage the client's expectations while assisting with their emotional needs. The veterinary team adapt best when they develop strategies for putting end-of-life decisions and experiences into perspective. This aids in preventing or dealing with burnout. It is important for all team members to have a working knowledge of ethical values, principles, and decision-making strategies.

The five stages of grief

Grief evolves through a series of stages, which may or may not appear sequentially and have no set timetable. Each individual will go through the stages at his or her own pace. Health-care team members must understand that the time until the acceptance of a pet's death is highly variable, and it may take 18 months or longer for an individual's grief to resolve. Also, the grief process is highly emotional and impacts a person's mind, body, and spirit. To say there are five stages of grief implies a process with an end goal of letting go, reinvesting, emotional growth, and emotional reattachment.

The five stages of grief are as follows:

1. denial
2. anger
3. bargaining
4. depression
5. acceptance.

Denial

This is a normal defense mechanism and is a conscious or unconscious refusal to accept facts, information, or the reality of the situation. The owner simply cannot or will not believe the severity of the diagnosis or prognosis.

Anger

The second stage occurs when the individual recognizes the denial and is beginning to accept the reality of the situation. This acceptance, however, reveals itself through anger. Anger can manifest in different ways and may make it difficult for the individual's support system due to feelings (oftentimes misplaced) of anger and sometimes rage. Individuals may be angry with themselves or with others and especially those who are close to them. Veterinary health-care team members must remember to remain detached and nonjudgmental when dealing with a person experiencing anger from grief.

Bargaining

This stage centers on the hope that the individual can somehow postpone or reverse the reality of death. Oftentimes negotiation for an extended life is made with a higher power, and miracles are asked for by the pet owner. This stage of grief is often a difficult one for health-care team members, as the client will most likely have a lot of questions and "solutions" (typically found on the internet or suggested by a close relative). Patience and compassion are crucial during the bargaining stage.

Depression

This stage finds the pet owner beginning to understand that death is inevitable. The owner may become silent, withdrawn, and spend much of the time crying and grieving. This stage allows the pet owner to disconnect from the beloved pet. This is an important stage, and the health-care team should not try to "cheer up" an individual who is in this stage. The owner's grief must be processed. It is natural to feel sadness, regret, fear, and uncertainty during this stage. Feeling and/or expressing these emotions shows that the owner has begun to accept the situation, and they must be allowed to feel and express these emotions.

Acceptance

In this last stage, individuals begin to come to terms with the loss of a beloved pet. The pet is not and will not be forgotten but rather will always have a special place in the heart of the owner, and new attachments can be made without hesitation.

Clients should be allowed to grieve and supported through the grief process. They should also be reminded that the process is normal and that all individuals go through a similar process. The stage length will vary from owner to owner, but the process is the same. The veterinary health-care team gives support to the client through the compassionate acts of listening and assuring owners that their emotions and feelings are normal. The majority of clients will eventually reach a point when they are ready for a new pet and realize this new pet is not a replacement for the deceased pet but rather a testament to the love shared with the deceased pet.

References

Anderson, M. 1994. *Coping with Sorrow on the Loss of Your Pet*, 2nd edition. Peregrine Press, Los Angeles, CA.

Kübler-Ross, E. 1969. *On Death and Dying*. Macmillan, New York.

Kübler-Ross, E. and Kessler, D. 2005. *On Grief and Grieving: Finding the Meaning of Grief Through the Five Stages of Less*. Simon & Schuster, New York.

Pattengale, P. 2005. *Tasks for the Veterinary Assistant*. Lippincott Williams & Wilkins, Philadelphia, PA.

Prendergast, H. 2011. Interacting with a grieving client. In: *Front Office Management for the Veterinary Team*. Elsevier, St Louis, MO, pp. 242–250.

Taboada, J. 2006. Client bereavement and the human–animal bond. In: *Clinical Textbook for Veterinary Technicians*, 6th edition. McCurnin, D.M., Bassert, J.M. (eds). Elsevier Saunders, St Louis, MO, pp. 1177–1189.

Taboada, J. 2006. Euthanasia. In: *Clinical Textbook for Veterinary Technicians*, 6th edition. McCurnin, D.M., Bassert, J.M. (eds). Elsevier Saunders, St Louis, MO, pp. 1167–1176.

Tefend-Campbell, M. 2011. Nursing care of dogs and cats. In: *Principles and Practice of Veterinary Technology*, 3rd edition. Sirois, M. (ed.). Elsevier, St Louis, MO, pp. 606–645.

www.wiley.com/go/burns/textbookvetassistant2

Please go to the companion website for assignments and a PowerPoint relating to the material in this chapter.

Chapter **21** Client Management

The most important person in a veterinary hospital is the client. Clients will return again and again for routine veterinary care and when their pet is ill if, and only if, they are satisfied with the services provided. Veterinary medicine truly revolves around people. Veterinary professionals who dislike working with people and their animals' problems should not be in this field. Clients are the lifeblood of the practice. A practice will collapse unless old clients are retained and new clients are continually entering the practice. Loyalty is won with teamwork, hard work, and dedicated service to each client. Before the basic concepts of client management are discussed, it may be helpful to learn how to evaluate and relate to your client.

Evaluating your clients

Careful evaluation of your clients will give you the tools needed to handle them properly. It is important to realize not all clients are pleasant to work with. In any service business, some people are always in a poor frame of mind. The saying goes that 5% of clients cause 95% of our problems. This 5% causes many people to become negative and eventually leave their practice or, worse, continue to practice, dwelling on unpleasant client experiences.

The foundation to effectively interacting with your clients is to learn how to identify with them. No two clients are the same, but many tend to fall into one or more of these categories.

The "A" clients are your dream clients, but they account for only approximately 10% of the clients you will meet. They are the clients who practice preventive medicine, seek professional advice on everything, and are generally concerned about their animal. These clients will be your most rewarding. They will appreciate all your efforts and provide you with the momentum to continually serve your clients and their patients.

The "B" client is the most common, making up about 50% of your clients. This is the client who is good to work with but has some financial limitations. This client practices some preventive medicine and usually seeks professional advice for most conditions. "B" clients are concerned about their pet and follow most recommendations. These clients will pay if given some time allowances. When good communications are maintained, this client will become very loyal. If client communication breaks down, "B" clients will sometimes become demanding and start shopping around.

The "C" client is usually the second most common client, making up approximately 25% of your client base. This client practices little preventive medicine and only occasionally seeks professional advice. They are more concerned with cost than with the animal's health. They follow some recommendations but limit their spending. The "C" client can sometimes be converted to an "A" or "B" through client education.

The "D" client accounts for approximately 12% of your client base. These are the most frustrating type of client and generally are those who have no business owning a pet. These are the clients who desire no preventive care. They seek veterinary attention only when their pet is near death or when their neighbor's advice fails. They are not too concerned about the animal and follow few recommendations. They have difficulty paying their bills, have no intention of paying their bills, or may agree to pay but never follow through. It is very rare that a "D" client can be converted to a "C" client. The "D" client should always be given the best service possible, but limitations offered by the client should be carefully followed.

The "S" client is the special client. This client is much like "A" and "B" but generally has difficulty paying for services. These clients are usually retired or on a fixed income and can sometimes offer to try and work off their bill by working at the clinic, volunteering to walk dogs, clean cages, or do laundry or other tasks. They are the Good Samaritans and can be very appreciative of anything you can do to help their pet.

When working with your clients, it might be helpful to keep these categories in mind and know that, although some people may never change, there are many people who will, if handled appropriately. Your job is to effectively communicate with them on their level and provide the best information available about their pets. Every patient and client should be handled to the best of your ability and at the level of care their owners desire.

The challenge comes when you have an angry client. It may be helpful to keep the above categories in mind when dealing with this client. Generally, when someone walks through the doors of the veterinary practice looking for fault or being difficult to please, there is an underlying cause. There may have been an issue from a prior visit, a traffic incident on the way there, the pet may not handle the car ride easily and be very stressed, or many other reasons. If a client is confrontational, it is best to try and appreciate where the client is coming from. Repeat the client's complaint so he or she knows that you understand, and then relay it to the appropriate management staff member. In most cases, it is best to put an angry client issue into the hands of the practice manager, owner, veterinarian, or veterinary technician on duty, depending on the issue of concern. Generally, when a client is upset, just putting him or her in communication with someone in charge will begin to diffuse the situation so it can be handled appropriately. The best thing for you to do until a problem is delegated to the proper person is to remain calm and keep a professional, pleasant demeanor.

Client management; essential skills for the veterinary assistant

Communication is the key to success. The veterinary assistant may be put in situations that require extensive communication with a client. It is crucial to have good communication skills. When talking to a client, always introduce or identify yourself. Giving someone your name provides a connection to the client. Eye contact is critical to assure the client that you are listening. It is tempting to multitask when your mind is on many different patients, but you should never allow clients to feel that the time you spend with them is an inconvenience. Focus on your clients, their needs, and the needs of their pet. Always relay accurate information. Be honest. If a client asks a question and you don't know the answer, say you are uncertain but will find out. Never be too proud to admit you don't know something. Your patients are too important to give out wrong information.

Exceptional telephone etiquette is a very important consideration when managing your clients (see Chapter 5). When a client phones into a veterinary hospital, it is important to communicate in a pleasant, professional manner. Always answer using the name of the veterinary hospital and, again, always identify yourself. Never place a client on hold without asking first if he or she *can* hold. A client calling in for an emergency is not going to be able to wait and should never be put directly on hold without being asked first. It is always a good idea to let callers know how many calls there are ahead of them. After listening to the reason for a client's call, it is a good idea to repeat the reason for calling. This not only clarifies for you the reason for the call, it also gives clients comfort that you understand their needs. Never hang up on clients before you know all their needs have been met and that they understand everything you have told them.

Personal presentation is another important consideration when effectively managing clients. Always maintain a neat, clean, and professional appearance. This should involve a clean and pressed uniform, clean shoes, and neat hair. If your hair is long, it should be pulled back, and you should always wear a name tag that is visible to the client.

Always maintain a good attitude when communicating with your clients. Your attitude toward yourself will reflect to your clients. If you are excited, happy, and positive about yourself and what you are doing, this will dominate your client relations. Enthusiasm is one of the most infectious conditions we have. Enthusiasm is caught, not taught!

Proper patient handling is extremely important in reassuring your clients that you will responsibly care for their animals. The way you handle them will make a big difference in the confidence a client will have in you. Treat every patient as if it were your own pet. Call patients by name and make sure you refer to them by the appropriate gender. There needs to be a level of compassion, confidence, and commitment when you handle your patients. No matter what type of client you encounter, the level of care and compassion should be the same for all your patients. You may be called upon to admit patients into the exam rooms for appointments or outpatient procedures and admit and discharge patients for hospitalization, surgery, or special procedures. Handling the animal is only part of it. You need to be effective in communication efforts by taking accurate histories, ensuring proper documentation in the form of signed financial estimates and procedure authorization forms, explaining protocols accurately, and ensuring correct client contact information is obtained.

Employee roles

As you can see, patient management and client management go hand in hand. The role of each employee in the hospital plays a crucial part in the overall experience a patient and client will have while in your care. From the time a client walks in the door to the time of discharge, there is a general protocol for which staff member handles each part of the client's visit, and this protocol may be helpful in the successful management of your clients and patients.

The receptionist is generally the first to have contact with clients as they enter the practice. He or she should be pleasant and welcoming to both the client and the patient. The receptionist should move the client and patient as quickly as possible into an exam room. Emergencies should be given priority upon entering the clinic. Not all emergencies are actual emergencies, but according to the client they may be and should be assessed and handled as such. The receptionist or veterinary assistant should always notify the veterinary technician or veterinarian of a possible emergency so that the patient can be properly triaged.

The veterinary assistant may be the staff member entering the exam room initially. The assistant should always wear a name tag and introduce him or herself. A brief history and chief complaint or reason the client and patient are there should be noted. The veterinary assistant may also obtain a patient's weight, temperature, pulse, and respiration. From that point on, the assistant will focus on assisting the veterinary technician and veterinarian in any way necessary to ensure excellent patient care.

The veterinary technician may also enter the exam room initially. The technician should also wear a name tag and introduce him or herself. A brief history and chief complaint should be noted if they have not already been taken by the veterinary assistant. The technician may also obtain a patient's weight, temperature, pulse, respiration, and even blood pressure on initial exam if this has not been done by the veterinary assistant. A brief, physical examination may also be done. If any preexam diagnostic tests are indicated prior to the client seeing the veterinarian, the veterinary technician will ensure they are completed.

Every member of the healthcare team should wear a name tag and introduce themselves to the client. If working with a pet owner and a veterinary technician and/or veterinary assistant, the veterinarian should be introduced by the veterinary assistant or veterinary technician. The veterinarian will do a complete physical exam and address any concerns the client is having about the pet. The veterinarian will order the diagnostic tests deemed necessary based upon the patient's history, the client's chief complaint, and the physical examination findings. The technician will carry out all the necessary diagnostic tests, which may include drawing blood or collecting other patient samples for any laboratory testing indicated, taking any necessary radiographs or any other diagnostic tests desired. The veterinary assistant will assist the technician with restraint and setting up the diagnostic procedures. The veterinarian will then return to go over the results of the diagnostic testing and give a diagnosis and treatment recommendations.

The veterinary technician will then be responsible for preparing the client and patient for discharge. This may include client education regarding the veterinarian's diagnosis, prescribed medications or at-home therapy, or protocols recommended.

The veterinary assistant may be responsible for preparing the prescribed medications, obtaining necessary signed authorizations, or preparing the patient for discharge. Owners judge the care that an animal has received by the condition and appearance of the animal at the time of dismissal. Any foul odors, bloodstains, or so forth need to be addressed prior to discharging any patient.

As you can see, client management is the lifeblood of a practice. The descriptions of the roles of the veterinary staff are very general but are commonly followed in practice with the same goal in mind: to provide excellent patient care while ensuring client satisfaction. This common goal can be reached only when ultimate teamwork is achieved. Teamwork is the common denominator of a successful practice, and success is determined by a busy appointment schedule, clients who return again and again to entrust their pets to the care of the hospital, and word-of-mouth recommendations to friends and family from those clients. Patient management and client management go hand in hand and are the purpose of our profession.

References

Bassert, J.M. 2018. Veterinary medical records. In: *McCurnin's Clinical Textbook for Veterinary Technicians*, 9th edition. Bassert, J.M., Beal, A.D., Samples, O.M. (eds). Elsevier Saunders, St Louis, MO, pp. 77–104.

Prendergast, H. 2020. Veterinary healthcare team members. In: *Front Office Management for the Veterinary Team*, 3rd edition. Elsevier, St Louis, MO, pp. 2–11.

Sirois, M. (ed.). 2017. Practice management. In: *Principles and Practice of Veterinary Technology*, 4th edition. Elsevier, St Louis, MO, pp. 26–55.

www.wiley.com/go/burns/textbookvetassistant2

Please go to the companion website for assignments and a PowerPoint relating to the material in this chapter.

Chapter 22 Medical Records

The most important document in the veterinary hospital and in veterinary medicine is the client–patient–veterinarian/veterinary health-care team medical record. The medical record is a permanent written description of the medical services recommended and administered in the client–patient–health-care team relationship. Medical records serve as a legal document of that relationship. Medical records can be paper or computerized, but both serve the same purpose.

The medical record's purpose is to provide accurate and detailed patient information for the veterinary health-care team and patient owner, to alert the health-care team to specific disease conditions and/or special needs in the patient, and to serve as documentation should the patient be referred.

The medical record assists the health-care team in generating a diagnosis for the patient and, subsequently, a treatment plan. Every member of the team is responsible for making sure all findings, treatments, owner communications, and so forth are written in the patient's medical record. For example, physical examination findings must be entered into the medical record. The veterinarian must document the diagnostic procedures and tests that have been ordered in the medical record, and health-care team members must confirm when these procedures are completed and their results. The veterinarian also documents the differential diagnoses that she/he is working to rule out. Another important item of the medical record is documentation of the patient response to treatment. This allows for treatment plans to be adjusted by the veterinarian.

In the event of staff turnover or the patient going to another hospital, the medical record allows for continuity of care. Medical records allow for the prior history of a patient to be reviewed and help health-care teams unfamiliar with a patient to gain a better understanding of the history and condition of the patient. Medical records also promote continuity of patient care, especially if more than one veterinarian or technician manages the patient over its lifetime.

As we know, communication with a client is integral to the treatment of a pet. The medical record should reflect all communications with the client regardless of which health-care team member has had the communication. There may be many team members assisting a single patient and communicating with the owner; for this reason every interaction must be documented and all instructions or communication sheets should be included in the medical record. This ensures all members of the team have a clear understanding of what was communicated to the client. Other important information in the medical record includes the names of other members in the household, other pets, and so on.

The medical record lists all services completed on the patient whatever the reason or length of stay. By listing all the services, the documentation also serves as a way to verify billing and the legal evidence that certain services were performed on the patient and received by the owner. Medical records also can be used by practice managers and owners to assess a variety of hospital functions:

- the workload of various health-care team members
- hospital budget
- business income
- inventory management
- development of marketing plans for the hospital
- compliance with standards of care.

Textbook for the Veterinary Assistant, Second Edition. Kara M. Burns and Lori Renda-Francis.
© 2022 John Wiley & Sons, Inc. Published 2022 by John Wiley & Sons, Inc.
Companion website: www.wiley.com/go/burns/textbookvetassistant2

The medical record is a legal document and may be used in a court of law. Medical records are invaluable should litigation ever occur. The medical record is the proof that procedures were or were not performed and treatments were administered. Specific dates and times should always be entered. The medical record must always be up-to-date and accurate. If it is not in the medical record, then legally it is viewed as not having been performed. The office or practice manager should make it a practice to pull out charts at random and check that all the information is complete and accurate. In a veterinary hospital, things move quickly, and the medical record gets passed around to the various team members. However, there are no shortcuts when it comes to medical records. All members of the team *must* document in the patient record when something has been performed, ordered, received, and so on, every time! After each entry, the team member must initial the record entry. See Figures 22.1, 22.2, and 22.3.

Regardless of whether the hospital at which you work uses computerized or paper medical records, there are certain criteria that must be followed.

- One medical record for every patient. Even in multipet households, each pet must have its own medical record.

- Medical records must be easily retrievable and readily available at all times.

- Medical records must be complete and accurate.

- Records should be written as legal, professional, and medical documents. They can be admissible in court if requested.

- Medical records must be legible and contain no misspellings. Illegible medical records are a risk to patient safety as calculations and dosages may be misread. Also, the owner and possibly a court of law will need to read these and be able to understand the words written on the record.

- Medical records should always be written in blue or black ink.

- If a mistake is made in the medical record entry mistake, simply cross out the error and initial it. White-out should never be used in a medial record.

Medical records must maintain consistency regardless of the pet, client, or (if computerized) the type of software. The majority of medical records are written with the most recent event listed first (reverse chronological order). Recent records should be placed on the top of the file. Laboratory results, consultations, and estimates should be placed after the written portion of the medical record.

The medical record most commonly used in veterinary hospitals today is known as the problem-oriented medical record (POMR). The POMR is used by the American Animal Hospital Association Standards of Accreditation and supports an organized approach to clinical veterinary medicine and promotes great communication, team-approached patient care, and quick retrieval of patient information.

All medical records must contain the following information in every patient record:

1. client and patient information
2. medical history
3. vaccination history
4. presenting complaint
5. physical examination
6. diagnosis/differential diagnosis
7. laboratory reports
8. treatment
9. prognosis
10. surgical report
11. estimates and fee information
12. consent forms.

Each hospital may have slightly different terms for the list above, but they still need to have the information listed in each medical record.

Client and patient information includes the name, address, and phone number of the client. Phone numbers to be listed should include cell phone, work phone, and home phone; contact numbers for other members of the household should also be listed. It is also important to ask the client which times are appropriate for the health-care team to call with updates or to gather information. Special attention should be given to the proper spelling of the client's name and address, as there may be multiple ways of spelling a name or a street address

The age, breed, gender, and species of the patient should be listed in this section. This is known as the patient's signalment. Owners do not appreciate their pet being referred to by the wrong gender or breed. All health-care team members should check the medical record to confirm gender, breed, and name of the patient prior to communicating with the client. Furthermore, the patient's date of birth (DOB) rather than age should be recorded. It is not wise to write "2 years old" on a chart because the patient will age through the years, but the health-care team will always look at the chart and see "2 years old." The patient's DOB should be documented during the initial visit, and during subsequent visits, the DOB can be subtracted from the current date to yield the patient's current age. Information should be confirmed for accuracy each time the client comes in to ensure that the information in the medical record is correct and up to date.

The medical history portion of the medical record should include all prior history of the patient, even if the patient visited a different veterinary hospital in the past. The vaccination history should be recorded as part of the patient history, including the area on the body where specific vaccinations were administered. Parasite control, dental health, nutritional history, prior body conditioning score (BCS), weight, the patient's typical temperament, any unusual behavior, environment where the pet resides, other pets in the household, indoor versus outdoor status, exposure to other animals, known allergies and reactions, and any prior medical conditions, trauma, or surgeries should be listed in this section.

The next part of the medical record should include the presenting complaint, or why the pet is at the hospital. Health-care team members must listen to the clients and what they are (and

DATE_____   PATIENT NUMBER_____

HAPPY TAILS VETERINARY HOSPITAL
CLIENT/PATIENT INFORMATION FORM

Owner Information – Please print in Ink

Owner's Name _____

Address _____

City, State, Zip Code _____

Phone Numbers:

Home_____ Work_____ Cell _____

Pet Information

Species (Dog, Cat, Other) _____ Breed _____

Pet's Name _____ Gender _____ Altered - Y or N

Birthdate_____ Color _____

Microchip – Y or N   Microchip ID Number _____

STATEMENT OF OWNERSHIP AND CONSENT

I am the owner of the animal described above, or have authorization from the above owner to consent to recommended treatment.

I hereby authorize the professional and medical services including, but not limited to: diagnostic, therapeutic, anesthetic, and surgical recommended as necessary for treatment.

I accept the financial responsibility for the professional veterinary services.

I have read the consent and have been educated as to why the recommended procedures are necessary. Additionally, I have been told of potential complications and alternatives to the procedures.

Signature (Owner/Agent) _____Date_____

Figure 22.1   Client/patient form.

HAPPY TAILS VETERINARY HOSPITAL
CLIENT/PATIENT ASSESSMENT FORM

Owner's Name _____Patient Number_____

Address _____

City, State, Zip Code _____

Phone Number: _____

Pet's Name _____ Gender _____ Altered - Y or N

Birthdate_____ Color _____

Date	
	History –
	Presenting Complaint –
	Physical Examination – Temperature: Pulse: Respiration: Pain Assessment: Nutritional Assessment:
	Differential Dx:
	Orders:
	Lab Results:
	Prognosis:

Figure 22.2   Client/patient assessment form.

HAPPY TAILS VETERINARY HOSPITAL
CLIENT/PATIENT ASSESSMENT FORM

Owner's Name _____ Patient Number_____

Address _____

City, State, Zip Code _____

Phone Number: _____

Pet's Name _____ Gender _____ Altered - Y or N

Birthdate_____ Color _____

Date	Notes

Figure 22.3   Client/patient notes form.

sometimes are not) communicating. This will help team members ask the proper questions regarding the pet's presenting problem.

A complete, head-to-tail physical examination must be performed and documented in the medical record. The vital assessments (temperature, pulse, respiration, pain level, and nutritional assessment) are the first to be observed in the physical exam. Weight, mucous membrane appearance and findings from auscultation of the chest, abdominal palpation, and examination of the lymph nodes and musculoskeletal system all must be documented. Health-care team members should be familiar with the abbreviations used in their hospital. The American Animal Hospital Associations abbreviation guide can also be referred to.

At this point, the veterinarian will have developed a differential diagnosis (possible diseases or conditions that may be causing the presenting complaint). This diagnosis (or, if more than one, these differential diagnoses) should be documented along with diagnostic tests ordered by the veterinarian. If the patient is found to have more than one diagnosis or disease condition, all must be documented at this time.

Laboratory results should be documented next. This includes all results, normal and abnormal. Results of all medical testing must be documented, including radiograph results, ultrasound testing and results, electrocardiogram results, and referral to another veterinarian or a board-certified veterinarian.

Treatment recommendations, orders, and medications prescribed by the veterinarian must all be documented. Along with this is the health-care team's follow-through and administration of the veterinarian's orders for treatment. Every time an animal is examined, treated, medicated, and so forth by a health-care team member, documentation must be made in the patient's medical record and initialed by the team member who administered the procedure.

A veterinarian makes a prognosis for each patient. This prognosis is communicated to the pet owner. The prognosis is the predicted outcome of the disease based on all the data the veterinarian and the health-care team have gathered. The prognosis itself and the client communication must both be documented in the patient's medical record.

If surgery is performed, or if a medical referral has been made, the full detailed report from the surgeon or the referral veterinarian must be added to the patient's medical record. Any forms that are used during any procedure must also be added to the record. For example, if surgery is to be performed, documentation sheets including anesthetic protocol, blood pressure readings during the surgical procedure, length of surgery, complications to watch for post surgery, and so on should be documented and added to the patient's medical record.

The health-care team should discuss cost estimates for care with the client and keep a copy for the client and a copy in the medical record. This discussion should happen prior to any services being performed. The client should sign the estimate to indicate that it was discussed. This form should be placed in the medical record. Also, if consent forms are required, signed consent forms must be placed in the medical record. Consent forms document the understanding among the veterinarian, client, and veterinary hospital of the specific conditions, risks, and responsibilities of each party. Completed and signed consent forms provide veterinary practices with legal evidence that the health-care team, on behalf of the veterinary hospital, informed the patient's owner of the important information regarding the procedure and that the owner consented to this recommended and planned course of action. Obtaining authorization or consent to perform surgery, *necropsy*, and euthanasia are a few examples of situations where written owner consent, in addition to verbal communication, is important.

Each entry into a POMR typically follows a specific format:

- the defined database
- the problem list
- the plan
- the progress section.

The database is the signalment, history, physical examination, and diagnostic tests combined. The problem list includes the patient's name, gender, species, breed, age, nutritional status, allergies, medications the pet is currently taking, and any vaccinations received. The plan contains the differential diagnosis, the diagnostic tests, medications prescribed, and treatment that has been ordered for the patient.

Within the progress section, the standard SOAP format is followed. The SOAP format is used by veterinary and human medical professionals when assessing patients' progress. The progress of a patient is followed by updating the Subjective information, Objective information, Assessment, and Plan. Subjective information is the reason the client and patient are at the hospital. It is inclusive of the office visit itself, observations from the owner, and the history of the patient. Objective information is the information that the team receives directly from the examination, diagnostic work-up, and interpretation of lab results. Assessment includes conclusions reached after the data are reviewed. Assessment also includes a differential diagnosis. Any tentative diagnoses should be listed here along with the documentation of rule-outs. In ruling out a disease, the health-care team is looking at the data gathered to see if all fit the diagnosis; if not, that particular disease/diagnosis can be ruled out by the veterinarian. A plan is subsequently developed from the assessment and includes treatment, surgery, medication, diagnostic tests, and client communication.

All health-care team members should be aware of the importance of the patient's medical record and should document all information and findings into the medical record. Medical records should be legible, so care should be taken when information is entered. Medical records are a major component of the veterinary hospital and are legal documents.

References

Bassert, J.M. 2018. Medical records. In: *McCurnin's Clinical Textbook for Veterinary Technicians*, 9th edition. Bassert, J.M., Beal, A.D., Samples, O.M. (eds). Elsevier Saunders, St Louis, MO, pp. 77–104.

Pattengale, P. 2005. *Tasks for the Veterinary Assistant*. Lippincott Williams & Wilkins, Philadelphia, PA, pp. 33–95.

Prendergast, H. 2020. Medical records management. In: *Front Office Management for the Veterinary Team*. Elsevier, St Louis, MO, pp. 292–308.

Sirois, M. (ed.). 2017. Practice management. In: *Principles and Practice of Veterinary Technology*, 4th edition. Elsevier, St Louis, MO.

www.wiley.com/go/burns/textbookvetassistant2

Please go to the companion website for assignments and a PowerPoint relating to the material in this chapter.

Chapter 23 Occupational Safety and Health Administration

Working with animals! That's what you've always wanted to do. As a veterinary assistant, you are finally realizing your dream of a career helping animals. Veterinary assistants are valued members of the veterinary team and will be utilized in many roles. There are so many things to learn: caring for animals, helping in the lab, assisting the licensed veterinary technician with nursing care, and much, much more. To work effectively in a veterinary hospital, one of the most important areas you must learn about is safety. This is crucial to your wellbeing as well as that of your fellow employees and even the animals you care for.

What is the Occupational Safety and Health Administration?

The Occupational Safety and Health Administration (OSHA) is part of the US Department of Labor. Created in 1970 by the US Congress, the OSHA's mission is to help employers and employees reduce on-the-job injuries and deaths. The OSHA assures safe and healthy working conditions for working people by setting and enforcing standards and providing training, outreach, education, and assistance. As a veterinary assistant, you will be protected by safety measures that your clinic has in place due to either federal OSHA regulations or an OSHA state-approved program. It is interesting to note that state programs must exceed federal OSHA standards for workplace safety and health.

The OSHA provides a wide selection of training courses and educational programs and materials that help employers train their employees. When you are hired as a veterinary assistant, your employer will have you spend some time learning the clinic's OSHA information.

Material safety data sheets

Material safety data sheets (MSDSs) provide information to help employees work with all products that are found in their workplace. MSDSs are produced by chemical manufacturers and must be provided by the company that sells the chemical or substance. The MSDS is updated each time the material changes. It is important to make sure your clinic has the updated MSDSs on file. The Hazard Communication Standard (HCS) requires employers to maintain an MSDS on file for each hazardous substance in use at their facility. MSDSs should be meticulously filed in a logical way. It is best to file them alphabetically by product name. The use of a designated three-ring binder is recommended and it should be inspection-ready at all times.

All MSDSs must be in English (they can be bilingual) and stored in an area that all staff have access to. Staff members must know how to find and use all MSDSs.

The MSDS must be for the exact product and must be from the manufacturer of the current items being used. Some practices will buy several different brands of a product, depending on availability or price. Always keep an MSDS for each brand in the MSDS binder, so that the correlating information per product is available.

OSHA labeling of secondary containers

All secondary containers in use in your clinic must be labeled with an OSHA label. These labels indicate specific hazards. The labels are divided into four sections by color and hazard: blue (health), red (flammability), yellow (reactivity), and white (personal protection). In each color bar, there is a white box in which the hazard rating

Textbook for the Veterinary Assistant, Second Edition. Kara M. Burns and Lori Renda-Francis.
© 2022 John Wiley & Sons, Inc. Published 2022 by John Wiley & Sons, Inc.
Companion website: www.wiley.com/go/burns/textbookvetassistant2

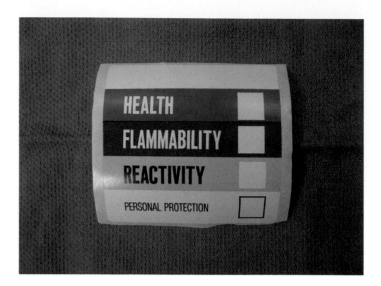

Figure 23.1 Secondary labeling. Source: Courtesy of Dr Lori Renda-Francis, LVT.

number must be written (Figure 23.1). One of your responsibilities as a veterinary assistant will be to accurately write in the correct hazard code for each product. This information is found on the MSDS that accompanies each product. Precise labeling is extremely important and will be checked during OSHA inspections.

OSHA inspections

OSHA inspections are usually unannounced. There are special conditions when OSHA may inform an employer of an imminent inspection, but notification will most likely be less than 24 hours. Any employer who receives advance notice must inform employees or employee representatives of the upcoming inspection. When the OSHA inspector, arrives he or she will show a valid official credential. Then the plan for the inspection overall will be explained. At this point, the OSHA representative and designated practice employee will walk through the clinic. The OSHA officer will look for safety and health hazards. It is important to know that the OSHA officer must consult with a reasonable number of employees regarding safety and health in the workplace. If you are a little worried about this potential interview, you should be aware that as an employee you are protected under the Act from discrimination by the employer for exercising your health and safety rights.

The official OSHA website describes standards for veterinary workplaces as follows.

> "Veterinary-specific standards enforced by OSHA cover the following health and safety issues; formaldehyde exposure, precautions for zoonotic disease prevention, anesthetic gas monitoring and safety, blood borne pathogens, laser safety, chemical hazard communications, monitoring exposure of ethylene oxide, glutaraldehyde exposure, ionizing radiation, means of egress, latex allergy, ergonomics control, walking-working surfaces, record-keeping requirements, an emergency action plan and electric/fire safety standards. OSHA inspections require evidence that the clinic is following these standards.

The inspection tour may cover all or just part of your clinic. The OSHA officer will inspect clinic records of deaths, injuries, and illnesses, which the employer is required to keep. The inspector will also check to see that the clinic has in place a written, comprehensive, communication program that includes container labeling, MSDSs, and an employee OSHA training program."

Prior to any inspection, all veterinary team members should prepare by becoming informed. As a veterinary assistant, you may be one of the employees consulted, so it is smart to be informed about various health and safety measures your clinic is taking. Another of your responsibilities is to make sure all of your clinic's secondary containers are properly labeled. Last but not least, know where the MSDS sheets are filed.

Common OSHA veterinary violations

- Labeling of secondary containers. These are containers used to hold chemical products other than the original; for instance, a spray bottle of disinfectant.
- An employee who doesn't know how to access the MSDS binder.
- Paperwork violations.
- Lack of practice-specific training records and safety manuals.
- Lack of displayed federal and state posters.

Fines

If the OSHA inspection finds your clinic is not in compliance with OSHA standards, a fine of $7000 per incident will be issued. An incident includes each instance of incorrect labeling, so if your clinic has two or three incorrectly labeled secondary containers, the fines will be $14000–21000. Even if you appeal your fine and it is reduced, you are still looking at a lot of money. Fines for incorrect paperwork start at $1000 per incident. What seems like a minor oversight can become a very serious financial issue. Obviously, it pays to be very diligent with OSHA compliance.

The OSHA's mission is ensuring that health and safety practices are in place for the protection of all. It is an important government agency that takes its responsibilities very seriously, and you should too. As a veterinary assistant and a valued employee, the OSHA sees to it that you are protected in your place of employment.

References

Prendergast, H. 2020. Safety in the veterinary practice. In: *Front Office Management for the Veterinary Team*, 3rd edition. Elsevier, St Louis, MO.

SafetyVet. Frequently asked OSHA questions. www.safetyvet.com/osha/OSHAdefault.html

Siebert, P. 2018. Occupational health and safety in veterinary hospitals. In: *McCurnin's Clinical Textbook for Veterinary Technicians*, 9th edition. Bassert, J.M., Beal, A.D., Samples, O.M. (eds). Elsevier Saunders, St Louis, MO, pp. 106–123.

Tiffany, L.M. 2012. "Surprise! The OSHA inspector is here!" *Veterinary Practice News*. www.veterinarypracticenews.com/surprise-the-osha-inspector-is-here/

www.wiley.com/go/burns/textbookvetassistant2

Please go to the companion website for assignments and a PowerPoint relating to the material in this chapter.

Chapter 24 Pet Health Insurance

Pet insurance has a fairly recent history in the United States. The very first pet insurance policy was actually written for a dog in Sweden in 1924. Not until 1982 was the first policy written in the United States. That policy was written to cover the television canine hero, Lassie.

Although the US pet population is increasing, access to veterinary care continues to be a concern. Affordability of veterinary services is a challenge for some pet owners. Pet health insurance is one tool that can help alleviate this burden. The North American Pet Health Insurance Association (NAPHIA) report shows that close to 3.45 million pets were insured in North America at the end of 2020 and that pet health insurance has been increasing at an average annual growth rate of 23.4% over the past 5 years. This supports the belief that pet parents do believe in the value of pet insurance. Pet insurance gives pet owners the comfort of knowing financial support is available should their pet family member need medical care.

Pets are now considered members of the family by many people. In the United States, there are an estimated 63.4 million households that own at least one dog, and 42.7 million households that own at least one cat. A recent survey reinforced this as 95% of dog owners and 94% of cat owners agreed (strongly or somewhat) that their pets are part of the family. This belief is even stronger in the millennial population. Consequently, if pets are considered family members and owners are willing to care for their pet's well-being, the need for pet health-care is obvious. We recognize that for pet owners, the economic risk associated with veterinary care is growing. However, it should be stated that a well-established tool that pet owners can use to manage financial risk in their lives does exist = insurance. Therefore, the prospect that pet owners will need and opt for pet health insurance is growing.

Pet health insurance helps pay for the costs of treatments that are difficult to foresee in the future, similar to human health insurance. Policy holders pay a small monthly premium to avoid future significant financial burden. Additionally, pet owners with pet health insurance have been reported to spend more towards the end of a pet's life, as is seen in humans with health insurance. Veterinarians and the veterinary health-care team play an important role in communicating the benefits of pet health insurance for the owner as an option for payment, as well as benefiting the veterinarian and practice as well.

From a regulatory perspective, pet insurance falls under the property/casualty area of insurance, as pets, even in 2021, are legally considered property. Pet health insurance functions like human health insurance, but is underwritten like property and casualty.

Many plans offered by insurance companies cover accident and illness. Also, some carriers have wellness plans that include things such as routine dental cleaning. And while most insurers only cover dogs and cats, the coverage is beginning to expand to other pets considered to be companion animals—birds, rabbits, snakes and other reptiles, pot-bellied pigs, etc. Also, one of the most frequently asked questions revolves around multipet households and although coverage of more than one pet in the same household varies by the provider, owners are able to get a multipet discount in many instances.

Other more nontraditional treatments are available and could be covered by insurance too, including behavioral treatment. Remember that animals can develop anxiety or posttraumatic stress disorder from trauma, similar to human beings. As pet health insurance grows, so does the coverage of alternative treatments, including acupuncture, therapeutic massage, and pain management.

Textbook for the Veterinary Assistant, Second Edition. Kara M. Burns and Lori Renda-Francis.
© 2022 John Wiley & Sons, Inc. Published 2022 by John Wiley & Sons, Inc.
Companion website: www.wiley.com/go/burns/textbookvetassistant2

Policies have no face value death benefit akin to human life insurance, although they can cover euthanasia.

The veterinary profession has struggled to improve compliance with veterinary recommendations for years. A primary benefit of health insurance is believed to be increased compliance with responsible pet care. It is thought that those owners who have pet insurance are more likely to treat an injured pet and use veterinarian services versus euthanizing a pet than those who do not.

The most common pet health insurance in the US is accident and illness insurance that typically insures against unforeseen health incidents, whether illness, disease, or injury. From that standpoint, the primary function is to make sure money is available to treat a sick or injured animal.

Veterinary medicine has made great advancements in the level of specialty care and these technological improvements will continue and mirror many of the developments in human medicine. Many procedures commonly performed on humans are now being performed on animals and these cutting-edge therapies are being made available to pet owners to aid their ill pet. However, these procedures can be very costly. Given that, along with the routine care of owning a pet, who would benefit most from a pet insurance policy?

The answer is threefold—the pet, obviously, the owner, and the veterinarian. Many animals are euthanized when an emergency occurs or a complex disease process is diagnosed. Owners who obtain pet insurance are much more likely to make the decision to treat instead of euthanize or settle for substandard care due to cost restrictions. The pet owners are the next to benefit from pet insurance. By budgeting for their pet's routine care and planning for the unexpected by purchasing a pet insurance policy, owners can have peace of mind. They know that their pet is receiving the best standard of care and they have taken the financial worry out of the picture. This allows owners to focus their attentions on their animal and the veterinarian's recommendations. The veterinarian will also benefit from clients who carry pet insurance for their animals. Many diagnostic tests that aid in an accurate diagnosis are not performed when they become cost-prohibitive. Clients who carry pet insurance will authorize their veterinarian to perform more of these necessary tests. Not only is the diagnosis more accurate when this occurs, but it also increases the profitability of the veterinary practice.

Pet insurance policies are similar to human medical insurance plans in that they are based upon annual premiums, deductibles, and different coverages. Policies are generally based upon species, pet's age, and presence of preexisting conditions. Lifestyle (indoor versus outdoor) may also play a role. Pet insurance generally has an annual deductible, just like human health plans, and runs an average of $50–$100 per month. Annual policy costs depend on individual annual deductibles and package selections. Insurance packages can be comprehensive, which means they cover annual check-ups, vaccines, and routine and preventive care such as spaying and neutering. A less expensive plan may have less coverage and only insure for accidents and illness. Many policies offer multipet discounts.

Table 24.1 Comparison of two pet insurance companies for a 6-month-old intact Labrador Retriever.

	Plan A	Plan B
Reimbursement percentage	90%	90%
Monthly price with exam fee coverage	$48.00	$67.00
Monthly transaction fee	$2.00	$2.00
Optional wellness plan cost/month	$16 or $26	$10 or $25
Total monthly premium	$66 or $76	$79 or $94
Deductible	$250 annual	$250 annual
Payout	Unlimited	$10,000

Table 24.1 is a comparison of two pet insurance companies. It is a good demonstration of monthly premiums, deductibles, and feature differences.

There are many specifics regarding pet insurance that differ by company. It is a good idea to comparison shop among insurance providers. There seem to be few companies that will insure for preexisting conditions, congenital disorders, and developmental defects, including cruciate ligament injuries occurring within the first 12 months of age.

Even with all the evidence pointing to the benefits of purchasing pet insurance, it has taken a long time for the concept to gain popularity. Why is this? The Brakke Veterinary Practice Management Group reports one of the reasons is that veterinary services have historically been priced at bargain levels. Historically, pet owners were less inclined to go to advanced levels to save their farm dogs or barn cats. And it was not very long ago (relatively speaking) that 24-hour emergency care and specialty hospitals were not available for pets. Pet insurance companies report that the pet owners most likely to purchase pet health insurance are those unfortunate families who have experienced high treatment expenses and emotional loss of a beloved pet. Veterinarians have been reluctant to promote pet health insurance in the past and without the veterinarian's recommendation, clients have not taken pet insurance seriously. In addition, in the last 20+ years there has been very limited marketing of pet health insurance other than brochures sitting on the counter of the veterinary hospital and, more recently, the internet. Thankfully, for all involved, especially the pet, this is changing.

Economic times have definitely changed through the years. For the many reasons mentioned earlier there is a huge benefit to pet insurance. The AVMA has some recommendations to make pet insurance work for most practices. Identify one team member to be the insurance coordinator for the practice. Choose two or three insurance companies to support and develop a deeper understanding of how they work. Train the entire veterinary team so all personnel are able to educate the clients. Educate the clients about pet insurance by informing all new and existing clients that your practice supports pet insurance. Keep insurance claim forms for the companies you support in the reception area so staff can help complete the necessary paperwork accurately and claims can be submitted promptly.

The bottom line is to become knowledgeable as a team member and a pet owner in the options of pet health insurance. There are many choices of companies and individual plans available. The demand for pet health insurance seems to be on the rise for many emotional, economical, and medical reasons. As veterinary professionals, it is important that we understand the changing needs of our clients and patients and continue to be informed and educate our clients.

References

Alt K. Pet Insurance Comparison Charts 2021: Compare Quotes, Plans, Coverage, and Waiting Periods. Canine Journal. www.caninejournal.com/pet-insurance-comparison/

Animal Sheltering. Pets by the Numbers. www.animalsheltering.org/page/pets-bythe-numbers

Carlson, D., Haeder, S., Jenkins-Smith, H., Ripberger, J., Silva, C., Weimer, D. 2019. Monetizing Bowser: a contingent valuation of the statistical value of dog life. *JBCA*, 11, 131–149.

Einav, L., Finkelstein, A., Gupta, A. 2017. Is American pet health care (also) uniquely inefficient? *American Economic* Review, 107, 491–495.

Malloy, M.G. 2018. A policy for Fluffy: pet insurance is a small industry—but it's poised for big growth in the U.S. *American Academy of Actuaries Contingencies*, Sep/Oct, 16–24.

NAPHIA. 2021. *State of the Industry (SOI) Report.* https://naphia.org/industry-data/

Packaged Facts. 2020. U.S. Pet Market Outlook, 2020–2021: The COVID-19 Impact. Packaged Facts, Rockville.

Veterinary Economics Division. 2018. *AVMA Pet Ownership and Demographic Sourcebook.* American Veterinary Medical Association, Schuamburg.

Williams, A., Williams, B., Hansen, C.R., Coble, K.H. 2020. The impact of pet health insurance on dog owners' spending for veterinary services. *Animals*, 10, 1162.

Resources

- www.avma.org/resources/pet-owners/petcare/do-you-need-pet-insurance
- www.caninejournal.com/pet-insurance-comparison/
- www.avma.org/resources-tools/avma-policies/pet-health-insurance

www.wiley.com/go/burns/textbookvetassistant2

Please go to the companion website for assignments and a PowerPoint relating to the material in this chapter.

Glossary

Acceptance Period the period of time in which the bitch is most likely to allow the act of reproduction to occur

Acetabulum the hip socket in which the head of the femur sits

Acidosis metabolic acidosis occurs when the accumulation of nonvolatile acids or loss of bicarbonate exceeds the body's buffering capability. A condition that occurs when there is an excessive level of acidity in the blood

Alkalosis a condition in which the body fluids have excess base (alkali). Alkalosis is excessive blood alkalinity caused by an overabundance of bicarbonate in the blood or a loss of acid from the blood

Allergen an antigen that elicits an allergic or hypersensitivity reaction

Alveolar Bone the thick ridge of bone which contains the tooth sockets. The alveolar bone is located on the jaw bones which hold the teeth

Amputate to surgically remove a limb

Anal Sac two small glands located under the skin on either side of the anus that produce and secrete material used by dogs and cats as a sexual pheromone, territory marker, or defense mechanism

Anal Sacculectomy surgical removal of the anal sacs

Analgesic medication to relieve pain

Anaphylaxis a serious hypersensitivity reaction, often characterized by profound hypotension, pulmonary edema, and collapse

Anatomical Position the normal standing position of an animal

Anatomy the study of the structure of the body and the relationship of its parts

Anesthetic Gas inhalation substance used to anesthetize patients usually by means of an anesthetic machine

Anisodactyl the shape of the foot in passerine species which manifests as three toes pointing forward and one toe pointing to the rear

Annual Deductible the fixed dollar amount an individual pays per calendar year for covered services

Annual Premium a method of measuring the comparison in price for purchasing a year's period of services if paid at once

Anterior Pituitary Gland the front portion of the pituitary gland which is located at the base of the brain and is responsible for the production and release of specific hormones

Anterior refers to the front of the body

Anticoagulant medication to help prevent blood clots

Antigen a substance capable of eliciting an immune response

Anus the opening at the end of the alimentary canal

Textbook for the Veterinary Assistant, Second Edition. Kara M. Burns and Lori Renda-Francis.
© 2022 John Wiley & Sons, Inc. Published 2022 by John Wiley & Sons, Inc.
Companion website: www.wiley.com/go/burns/textbookvetassistant2

Appendicular Skeleton is composed of the bones of the limbs, clavicle, scapula, humerus, radius, ulna, carpus, metacarpals, phalanges, pelvis, femur, patella, tibia, fibula, tarsus, metatarsals, and phalanges

Arrhythmia a condition in which the heart beats with an irregular or abnormal rhythm

Artery a blood vessel that carries oxygenated blood away from the heart and delivers it throughout the animal's body

Artificial Insemination the placing of semen in the vagina of an animal to achieve conception by means other than coitus

Asepsis the complete absence of infection

Aseptic Technique measurements taken to avoid the contamination of a surgical wound

Asocial not social; withdrawal, marked by indifference, from community

Atmospheric Nitrogen nitrogen is one of the primary nutrients critical for the survival of all living organisms. Although it is very abundant in the atmosphere, it is largely inaccessible in this form to most organisms. Only when nitrogen is converted from dinitrogen gas into ammonia (NH_3) does it become available to primary producers. Nitrogen exists in many different forms, including both inorganic (e.g., ammonia, nitrate) and organic (e.g., amino and nucleic acids) forms. Thus, nitrogen undergoes many different transformations in the ecosystem, changing from one form to another as organisms use it for growth and energy

Atom smallest unit into which matter can be divided without the release of electrically charged particles. It is also the smallest unit of matter that has the characteristic properties of a chemical element. As such, the atom is the basic building block of chemistry

Atraumatic causing minimal tissue injury

Atrophy to waste away, especially as a result of the degeneration of cells. The decrease in size of a body part, cell, organ, or other tissue

Aural Hematoma a collection of blood within the cartilage of the ear and the skin

Auscultation listening to sounds within the body, typically of the heart and lungs

Autoclave a mechanism used to sterilize items by the application of steam under pressure

Autoclave Tape specialized tape used to label surgical and indicate steam exposure on items that are sterilized by the autoclave

Autoimmunity a misdirected immune response that occurs when the immune system goes awry and attacks the body itself

Autotomy ability of the lizard to break away part of the tail at points of fracture planes of cartilage through the vertebral bodies

Axial Skeleton is composed of the bones of the skull, the hyoid bones, ribs, sternum, and vertebral column

Axilla an anatomical region under the shoulder joint where the arm connects to the shoulder

Back the area from the withers to the root of the tail

Belly the underside of the abdomen

Biceps the posterior muscle of the hind leg

Biological Vector an animal vector in whose body the pathogenic organism develops and multiplies before being transmitted to the next host

Biology the study of all forms of life

Bladder a small, balloon-shaped structure that serves as a receptacle for fluid waiting to be eliminated

Blood-Borne Pathogen a disease present in the blood or bodily fluids that is transmissible from animal to animal after ingestion or contact has occurred

Body Language a form of nonverbal communication whereby animals can express emotions and intentions through bodily movements

Borrowing the act of temporarily taking an item from another entity with intentions of bringing it back or replacing it

Brachycephalic short-muzzled dog with a flattened face. It is the result of a genetic mutation which alters the way that the bones in the skulls grow. As a result, the shape of the skull is wide and short

Bradycardia a slower than normal heart rate

Breeding the act of producing offspring

Brisket the front portion of the body located between the forelegs and below the chest

Bronchi any of the major air passages of the lungs which diverge from the windpipe

Buccopharyngeal relating to or near the cheek and the pharynx; the buccopharyngeal fascia of the buccinator

Budgeting a plan to utilize expenditures and future income to use as a guideline for saving and spending

Bullae fluid-filled sacs or lesions that appear when fluid is trapped under a thin layer of skin

Capillary any of the fine branching blood vessels that form a network between the arterioles and venules

Capillary Refill Time the time required for blood to refill capillaries after applying finger pressure and blanching the area

Carcinoma a type of cancer that starts in cells that make up the skin or the tissue lining organs, such as the liver or kidneys. Like other types of cancer, carcinomas are abnormal cells that divide without control. They are able to spread to other parts of the body, but do not always do so

Cardiac Sphincter a thin ring of muscle that helps to prevent stomach contents from going back up into the esophagus

Cardiovascular System includes the heart and blood vessels

Carotenoid pigments in plants, algae, and photosynthetic bacteria. These pigments produce the bright yellow, red, and orange colors in plants, vegetables, and fruits

Carpus consists of the joint and several carpal bones

Catabolism the breakdown of complex molecules in living organisms to form simpler ones, together with the release of energy; destructive metabolism

Caudal refers to the tail portion of the body

Cecal Dysbiosis the disruption of the delicate balance of organisms within the rabbit's digestive tract

Centrifugal Force an apparent force that is felt by an object moving in a curved path that acts outwardly away from the center of rotation

Cephalic Vein located on the anterior surface of the forearm

Cere the flesh-colored skin located at the base of the upper beak; found in many bird species

Cervical Vertebrae the vertebrae of the neck

Cesarean Section a surgical procedure used to deliver a baby through incisions in the abdomen and uterus

Chelonian the turtle and tortoise species

Choana found in the roof of the mouth of avian species; the V-shaped notch that allows for communication between the nasal cavity and the oropharynx

Chromosome a thread-like structure of nucleic acids and protein found in the nucleus of most living cells, carrying genetic information in the form of genes

Clavicle also known as the collarbone; a skinny bone that connects the sternum to the scapula

Cloaca the terminal end of the urinary, reproductive, and gastrointestinal tract in birds

Cluster Seizures seizures that start and stop, but occur in groups one after another

Coccygeal Vertebrae the vertebrae of the tail

Coelom body cavity found in birds and reptiles, consisting of the thoracic and abdominal cavities

Cold Sterilization the soaking of instruments in a disinfectant solution in an attempt to eliminate or inhibit growth of microorganisms on inanimate objects

Colic a term used to describe a symptom of abdominal (belly) pain, which in horses is usually caused by problems in the gastrointestinal tract

Colostrum the first form of milk produced by the mammary glands of mammals (including humans) immediately following delivery of the newborn

Combining Form when a root word is combined with a vowel, e.g., orthopedic

Complete Feeds a mixture of roughage and concentrate

Concentrates typically a cereal grain that may or may not have supplemented protein, minerals, and vitamins; high in energy

Conception the starting formation of a new organism after successful fertilization has occurred

Conformation an animal's structure, form, symmetrical disposition, and arrangement of body parts

Contact Dermatitis a condition that results in inflammation from contact with allergens or substances that damage or irritate the skin. It can affect animals of any age, though some breeds with genetic predispositions and those with weakened immune systems are more likely to show signs

Controlled Substance a substance placed in a given schedule of drugs created by the DEA based on whether it has a current accepted medical use for treatment in the United States; also refers to the drug's relative potential and likelihood of causing dependence

Coprophagic the eating of feces that is normal behavior among many animals

Copulation a scientific word to describe the sexual practices of both humans and animals

Cornified a process wherein a horny layer of epidermis is formed and acts as an epidermal barrier. It is characterized by the production of keratin

Cortical Bone the dense outer surface of bone that forms a protective layer around the internal cavity. This type of bone, also known as compact bone, makes up nearly 80% of skeletal mass and is vital to body structure and weight bearing because of its high resistance to bending and torsion

Costal Cartilage the cartilage at the end where the rib attaches to the sternum

Cranial refers to the head portion of the animal's body

Cranium the skull, especially the part enclosing the brain

Cremation the use of high-temperature burning, vaporization, and oxidation to reduce deceased bodies to basic chemical compounds

Crest the upper arched area of the neck

Cross-Training training all members of the health-care team to perform all the responsibilities of all positions in the hospital

Croup the area of the back from the root of the tail to the front of the pelvis

Cutaneous relating to or affecting the skin

Cystocentesis the insertion of a needle into the patient's bladder through the ventral abdominal wall

Cytotoxic cytotoxic drugs (sometimes known as antineoplastics) are a group of medicines that contain chemicals which are toxic to cells, preventing their replication or growth, and so are used to treat cancer

Database an organized collection of data, usually located on a computer

DEA License a license obtained by a veterinarian that allows the purchasing or dispensing of controlled substances to take place under their supervision

Deciduous Teeth the animal's first set of teeth, otherwise known as the baby teeth

Decubital Sores sores that develop from pressure exacerbated by recumbency, increased skin moisture, and irritation

Defective having flaws, imperfections, or faults

Depot Fat chiefly composed of the glycerides of various fatty acids and usually contain 75% of oleic acid, 20% of palmitic acid and 5% of stearic acid. They remain as mixed triglycerides; that is, one glycerol molecule is attached to three fatty acid molecules of either similar or dissimilar varieties

Dermatological relating to the skin

Dermatopathy any disease of the skin. Also known as dermopathy

Dermatophytes a group of fungal infections that can affect the skin, hair, and nails

Dewclaw the extra toe found on the inside of a dog's front leg. It is a completely normal digit with three bones, two joints and a nail

Diabetes Insipidus rare disorder that affects water metabolism, preventing the body from conserving water and releasing too much of it. This condition is characterized by increased urination, dilute urine (so-called insipid, or dull, urine), and increased thirst and drinking. This disease is not related to diabetes mellitus (insulin diabetes)

Diaphragm the muscle that divides the thoracic and abdominal cavities

Differential Diagnosis possible diseases or conditions that may be causing the presenting complaint as determined by the veterinarian

Digestive System includes the mouth, teeth, salivary glands, esophagus, stomach, intestines, pancreas, colon, liver, and gallbladder

Digits relate to human fingers

Direct Auscultation using the ear (no instrument) to listen to sounds produced by the body

Disaccharide the sugar formed when two monosaccharides are joined by glycosidic linkage

Distal describes a structure that is farther from the point of origin or away from the body

Distributor an entity that purchases noncompeting products, houses them, and then resells them to various retailers or businesses

Dorsal pertains to the back of the animal or toward the spine

Dorsal Plane an imaginary line that divides the body into dorsal and ventral portions

Dorsal Recumbency a position in which the animal is laying on its dorsum or back

Dose amount of a medication given at a single time

Drug Enforcement Agency US federal law enforcement agency that practices under the US Department of Justice and aids in the enforcement of the domestic Controlled Substance Act and governs the use of all controlled substances

Duodenum the first part of the small intestine immediately beyond the stomach, leading to the jejunum

Dystocia difficult birthing process

Ears located on or near the top of the head and can vary in size, placement, and shape depending on the breed

Ecdysis the process of shedding the old skin (in reptiles) or casting off the outer cuticle (in insects and other arthropods)

Echocardiography a test that uses sound waves to produce live images of the heart. The image is called an echocardiogram

Ectoparasites parasites that live and thrive on the outside surface of an animal's skin

Ectothermic a reptile that regulates its body temperature largely by exchanging heat with its surroundings; cold-blooded

Edema swelling that is caused by fluid trapped in the body's tissues

Egress the act of leaving or "going" from a given enclosure

Ejaculation the expelling of discharge containing semen from the male reproductive tract

Elbow the joint that connects the upper arm and the forearm

Electrocardiography measurement of electrical activity in the heart and the recording of such activity as a visual trace (on paper or on an oscilloscope screen), using electrodes placed on the skin of the limbs and chest

Electrolyte any substance that separates into ions when in solution

Electromagnetic Radiation a kind of radiation including visible light, radio waves, gamma rays, and x-rays, in which electric and magnetic fields vary simultaneously

Embryology the study of the origin and development of an individual organism, beginning after conception, or fertilization of the egg, and continuing through parturition, or birth

Empathy the feeling that you understand and share another person's experiences and emotions

Endocrine System includes the thyroid glands, adrenal glands, and parathyroid glands

Endogenous substances and processes that originate from within a system such as an organism, tissue, or cell

Enterotoxemia condition induced by the absorption of large volumes of toxins produced by bacteria such as *Clostridium perfringens* from the intestines

Epaxial situated on the dorsal side of an axis

Equal Opportunity Employment Act enables employees to avoid employer discrimination within the work environment by allowing employees to practice their given health and safety rights

Ergonomics the study of employees and their work environment

Ergosterol sterol found in cell membranes of fungi and protozoa, serving many of the same functions that cholesterol serves in animal cells

Esophagus the tube that connects the mouth to the stomach

Estrous Cycle also referred to as coming "into season"; the first day in which the bitch experiences bloody discharge expelled from the vulva

Ethylene Oxide a toxic colorless gas compound usually obtained by the oxidation of ethylene and commonly used for ethylene glycol synthesis

Eustachian Tube a structure located within the middle ear that aids in the equalization of pressure from the atmosphere

Euthanasia ending a patient's life utilizing humane measures

Euthanize the act of inducing a painless death

Expiration act or process of releasing air from the lungs through the nose or mouth

External refers to the outer surface of the body, which is more superficial

Exudate any fluid that filters from the circulatory system into lesions or areas of inflammation

Fecundity term often used to describe the rate of offspring production after one time step (often annual)

Feedstuff any dietary component that provides some essential nutrient or serves some other function

Femoral Vein extends from the groin on the medial aspect of the thigh

Femur the longest bone in the body, located just distal to the pelvis

Fertility the ability of an animal to produce offspring

Fibula the longer thinner bone of the lower hindlimb

Fight or Flight Principle all animals operate on this; when threatened, they will try to get away or they will stand their ground and fight (especially if the animal feels restrained)

Flea wingless insect that consumes blood from warm-blooded animals in order to survive

Flews the upper lips

Floating Ribs the ribs that are not attached to cartilage

Fomite object or material which is likely to carry infection, such as clothes, utensils, and furniture

Forage feeds made up using the majority of or the complete plant

Forearm the top area of the upper front leg

Forehead area just above the eyes and just before the stop

Foreign Body a foreign body (FB) is any object originating outside the body of an organism

Formaldehyde a pungent colorless gas made into a solution by oxidizing methanol; often used for the preservation of tissues

Forward Booking forward booking simply means scheduling all patients' next appointments before they leave the practice after their current visit

Fructosamine the fructosamine test is a blood test that measures average blood glucose levels over the 2–3 weeks prior to when the test is performed

Gait the manner in which an animal moves and walks

Gallbladder a pear-shaped structure lying between the lobes of the liver

Genetic Damage radiation may alter the DNA within any cell

Genetics the science governed by the laws and processes of plant and animal inheritance; the study of an animal or special organism's ancestry

Germinative capable of germinating, developing, or creating; of or pertaining to germination

Gingiva the gingiva surrounds the teeth and the marginal parts of the alveolar bone, forming a cuff around each tooth

Glutaraldehyde a nonflammable, toxic, and irritable liquid commonly used to fix slides to be viewed under an electron microscope

Hamstrings muscles in the back of the upper thigh

Hay forage that is cut and dried and then stored as bales

Hazard Rating Number a number code found on MSDS that correlates to the chemicals hazard written on all OSHA labels

Heart the main blood-pumping organ in the chest

Heart Rate the total number of heart beats consisting of two sounds, "lub-dub," counted during 1 minute

Heat Cycle the period of time in which the female is sexually receptive

Hematoma collection of blood outside blood vessels

Hemostat an instrument used to control bleeding

Hepatic Lipidosis characterized by the excess accumulation of fat in the liver and a common cause of potentially reversible liver failure in cats

Hepatotoxicity injury or damage to the liver caused by exposure to drugs; it is an adverse drug reaction that may be uncommon but serious

Herbivore animal that feeds on plants

Hereditary the passing of genes from one generation to the next through sperm and ova

Histology the microscopic study of the minute structure, composition, and function of normal cells and tissues

Homeostasis state of steady internal, physical, and chemical conditions maintained by living systems

Homogenous consisting of parts or elements that are all the same. Something that is homogenous is uniform in nature or character throughout

Hormone a chemical substance produced by various organs and carried by the bloodstream which aids in the activity and function of another organ

Human–Animal Bond the relationship between humans and animals that enhances quality of life for both, but especially humans

Humerus the long bone of the forelimb that extends from the shoulder to the elbow

Husbandry the management, housing, and upkeep of animals

Hyoid Apparatus the hyoid apparatus holds the larynx in place and supports the pharynx and tongue. It is made up of five different bones, which vary in length and size depending on the species

Hyoid Bone U-shaped structure located above the larynx and below the mandible and is suspended by ligaments

Hyperglycemia hyperglycemia (high blood glucose) means there is too much sugar in the blood because the body lacks enough insulin to deal with it

Hyperthermia condition of having a body temperature greatly above normal

Hypovolemic a decrease in the volume of blood in the body, which can be due to blood loss or loss of body fluids

Hypoxia deficiency in the amount of oxygen reaching the tissues

Hypsodont a pattern of dentition with high-crowned teeth and enamel extending past the gum line, providing extra material for wear and tear

Ileum the distal part of the small intestine

Ilium a part of the pelvis

IM Injection an intramuscular injection is used to deliver a medication deep into the muscles

Immunosuppression reduction of the activation or efficacy of the immune system

Impacted pressed firmly together

Inactivated Vaccine a vaccine that is made up of a noninfectious agent (e.g., whole killed pathogens or selected antigenic subunits) such that immunity is induced

Indicator Strip a strip of paper-like material used to indicate adequate sterilization has occurred

Indirect Auscultation using a stethoscope to magnify sounds within the body

Inflammatory Response occurs when tissues are injured by bacteria, trauma, toxins, heat, or any other cause

Inseminate to place semen in the vagina of an animal during coitus

Inspiration the act of breathing in

Insurance the transfer of risk and loss; occurs from one entity to another by means of exchange for payment

Integumentary System includes skin, hair, nails, sweat, and sebaceous glands. The skin is considered the largest organ in the body and has many functions

Intercostal Joint synovial joint between the tips of adjacent costal cartilages of ribs 6–10

Internal refers to deep inside the body

Intestinal Epithelial Brush Border the brush borders of the intestinal lining are the site of terminal carbohydrate digestion

Intramuscular (IM) Administration injecting a drug into a muscle mass

Intranasal located or occurring within the nose or taken through the nose

Intraosseous route of injection directly into the marrow of the bone

Intraperitoneal (IP) Injection injection into the abdominal cavity

Intravenous (IV) Injection injection into a vein

Inventory Counts keeping track of quantities of drugs and supplies used over a period of time along with the cost of each item

Inventory items a business has in stock or a recorded register of goods within a business

Ionizing Radiation any form of radiation (x-rays or alpha particles) that, upon passing through a medium, will produce ionization

Jejunum the part of the small intestine between the duodenum and ileum

Jugular Vein large superficial veins located on either side of the trachea on the neck

Keel the bony ridge along the sternum in avian species allowing for the attachment of flight muscles

Keratin the fibrous protein responsible for the formation of skin, hair, and nails

Kidneys bean-shaped structures designed to excrete urea, uric acid, and other wastes

Laceration wound that is produced by the tearing of soft body tissue. This type of wound is often irregular and jagged

Lagomorph small to medium-sized animal that in many ways resembles a large rodent

Laminar Flow a type of flow pattern of a fluid in which all the particles are flowing in parallel lines, as opposed to turbulent flow, where the particles flow in random and chaotic directions. A flow is either turbulent, laminar, or somewhere in between

Laminitis damage and inflammation of the tissue between the hoof and the underlying coffin bone (distal phalanx, P3)

Large Intestine connects the small intestine to the anus. The primary function is to absorb water from feces as needed in order to keep the animal hydrated

Lateral farther from the midline or median plane or toward the side of the body

Lateral Recumbency a position in which the animal is lying on its side

Lateral Saphenous Veins small superficial veins that run diagonally across the lateral surface of the distal part of the tibia

Latex finely divided rubber particles present in synthetic plastic or rubber

Legume plant in the family Fabaceae (or Leguminosae), or the fruit or seed of such a plant

Lending to give or allow the use of a given item temporarily under the circumstance that it will be returned or replaced with that of its equivalency

Lethargic a state of tiredness, weariness, fatigue, or lack of energy. It can be accompanied by depression, decreased motivation, or apathy

Lice parasites that feed off birds, humans, and other animal hosts by the action of biting or suction

Lingual the surface toward the tongue

Lipemia presence of a high concentration of lipids (or fats) in the blood

Liver reddish brown lobed organ that secretes bile

Loin the area on both sides of the vertebrae between the last few ribs and the hindquarters

Lumbar Vertebrae the vertebrae of the lower back

Lumbodorsal or Dorsal Lumbar located on either side of the midline

Lumen in biology, a lumen (plural lumina) is the inside space of a tubular structure, such as an artery or intestine

Lung the main respiratory organ composed of several lobes

Lysing to cause dissolution or destruction of cells

Mammary Tumors tumors present in the milk-producing glands of female animals

Mandible facial bone that forms the lower jaw

Manufacture the production of goods through various forms of labor that are created for use or sale within the economy

Mate the pairing of two animals of opposite sex for reproduction to take place

Material Safety Data Sheet (MSDS) informational sheet produced by manufacturers of various chemical products that must be provided with the chemical at the time of purchase; used as a reference tool in practice to appropriately clean up, avoid errors, and utilize different chemicals in a safe manner to avoid hazardous outcomes associated with the given chemical

Maturation the process of becoming mature; the emergence of individual and behavioral characteristics through growth processes over time

Maxilla facial bone that forms the upper jaw

Mayo Stand portable instrument stand with a tray on top used to hold surgical instruments and materials during operating room and in-office procedures. Mayo stands provide a convenient location which can be sterilized and positioned close to surgical sites without getting in the way

Medial nearer or toward the midline or median plane

Median Plane an imaginary line that extends directly down the middle of the body, dividing it into equal right and left portions

Medical Record a permanent written description of the medical services recommended and administered in the client–patient–health-care team relationship

Mentation the overall mental status of a patient

Mesonephric the mesonephric duct is a paired organ that forms during the embryonic development of humans and other mammals and gives rise to male reproductive organs

Metabolic Acidosis a serious electrolyte disorder characterized by an imbalance in the body's acid–base balance

Metacarpals long bones found just distal to the carpus

Metatarsals the long bones found just distal to the tarsus

Metritis inflammation of the uterus

Middle Nasal Meatus an air passage of the lateral nasal cavity located between the middle nasal concha and lateral nasal wall

Midsection the portion of an animal's body between the chest and pelvis

Mites arthropods, not insects; close cousins of spiders and ticks

Modified Live Vaccine a vaccine made from a weakened version of the pathogen, which will induce an immune response but is weakened enough so that it will not cause disease

Monetary Investment the way in which one spends or defers money

Mount the step taken by the male animal in preparation to mate by climbing on top of another animal or object; to copulate as a male

Mouth where digestion begins

Musculoskeletal System includes all the muscles, bones, and joints. It permits motion and movement of the body

Muzzle the area between the stop and the nose

Myocardium the muscular layer of the heart

Narcotics also called opioid pain relievers. They are only used for pain that is severe and is not helped by other types of painkillers

Nasolacrimal Gland the nasolacrimal duct (also called the tear duct) carries tears from the lacrimal sac of the eye into the nasal cavity. The duct begins in the eye socket between the maxillary and lacrimal bones, from where it passes downwards and backwards

Necropsy a surgical examination of a dead body, most commonly a dead animal, in order to learn why the animal died

Neoplasia new, uncontrolled growth of cells that is not under physiological control

Nephrotoxic toxicity in the kidneys. It is a poisonous effect of some substances, both toxic chemicals and medications, on kidney function

Nervous System includes the brain, spinal cord, and nerves

Neurotransmitter chemical messengers that transmit a signal from a neuron across the synapse to a target cell, which can be a different neuron, muscle cell, or gland cell

Nits nits are lice eggs and it is important to get rid of them so that the head lice don't just come back when all the new eggs hatch

Nociceptors neural processes of encoding and processing noxious stimuli

Nose located on the front of the face

Nosocomial Infection also called health-care-associated or hospital-acquired infection, is a subset of infectious diseases acquired in a health-care facility

Occluded closed up or blocked off

Occlusal Surface the surface of the tooth that is used for chewing or grinding

Occupational Safety and Health Administration a division of the US Department of Labor created in 1970 by the US Congress in order to assist employers and employees to reduce the occurrence of injury and/or death during work

Olfactory relating to the sense of smell

Oocyte the immature state of eggs or ova

Operculum the operculum is a hard, plate-like, bony flap that covers the gills of a bony fish (superclass: Osteichthyes). It protects the gills and also has a role in respiration

Ophthalmic relating to the eye and its diseases

Orbits the eye sockets in the skull

Order Quantity the quantity of a given product to be ordered by management or supervision personnel in charge of maintaining inventory

OSHA Label labels created according to OSHA standards used to indicate specific hazards of all chemicals used in secondary containers; OSHA labels are divided into four colored sections that correlate to different hazards: blue (health), red (flammability), yellow (reactivity), and white (personal protection)

Osteology the study of bones

Otitis general term to describe an infection and/or inflammation occurring within the ear

Ovaries produce ova and secrete hormones

Over-the-Counter (OTC) Medication medications that do not need a prescription

Ovulation the process of egg release after maturation has taken place

Palmar the caudal surface of the forelimb below the carpus

Palpebral Reflex the corneal reflex, also known as the blink reflex or eyelid reflex, is an involuntary blinking of the eyelids elicited by stimulation of the cornea (such as by touching or by a foreign body), though it could result from any peripheral stimulus

Pancreas an organ that secretes insulin

Papillae small projecting body parts similar to a nipple in form

Parasite an organism that lives inside or on the surface of another animal in order to survive

Patella a large flat bone located over the stifle joint

Pathogenic capable of causing disease

Pathogens agents capable of producing diseases, including viruses, bacteria, and other microorganisms

Pathology the study of the causes and effects of diseases or injury

Paws include the toes, feet, and paw pads of all four of the animal's legs

Pelvis large bony structure of the hindlimbs made up of three bones

Penetration the act of power used to permeate, enter, or pass into

Penis the male sex organ

Per Os by mouth

Perfusion the passage of oxygenated blood through body tissues; ability of blood to travel to the periphery of the animal

Peri- prefix that refers to around or the surrounding of a given area

Perianal situated in or affecting the area around the anus

Pericardial relating to or affecting the pericardium

Peripheral Edema edema is characterized by swelling due to an excessive accumulation of tissue fluid within the interstitium, which is a small space or gap in the substance of the body's tissues or organs

Peri-Rectal the area around the anus

Permanent Teeth the animal's second set of teeth, which replaces the deciduous teeth and remains throughout the duration of the animal's life

Phalanges the bones of the digit

Pharmaceutical relating to medicinal drugs, or their preparation, use, or sale

Pharynx a muscular tube that connects the oral and nasal cavity to the larynx and esophagus

Pheromone a chemical substance produced and released into the environment by an animal, especially a mammal or an insect, affecting the behavior or physiology of others of its species

Phlebitis inflammation of a vein

Photostimulable Phosphor the release of stored energy within a phosphor by stimulation with visible light, to produce a luminescent signal

Physiology the study of the normal functions and activities of organisms

Pinna the external or outside part of the ear

Plantar the caudal surface of the hindlimb below the tarsus

Plantigrade Stance in terrestrial animals, plantigrade locomotion means walking with the toes and metatarsals flat on the ground. It is one of three forms of locomotion adopted by terrestrial mammals

Plasma Proteins the collective term for the proteins present in the blood

Pleura membrane lining the thoracic cavity (parietal pleura) and covering the lungs (visceral pleura)

Pododermatitis inflammation of the skin of the paw

Point of the Shoulder consists of the front of the joint where the upper arm and shoulder blade come together

Polydipsia the term given to excessive thirst which is one of the initial symptoms of diabetes

Polyphagia polyphagia, also known as hyperphagia, is the medical term for excessive or extreme hunger

Polyuria production of abnormally large volumes of dilute urine

Portal Venous System the vessels involved in the drainage of the capillary beds of the GI tract and spleen into the capillary bed of the liver

Posterior refers to the rear end of the body

Posture a given position in which the animal's body is presented

Precocial precocial species are those in which the young are relatively mature and mobile from the moment of birth or hatching

Prefix the beginning of a word; consists of one or more syllables

Preoperative the preoperative phase is the time period between the decision to have surgery and the beginning of the surgical procedure

Prepuce the skin covering of the penis

Presenting Complaint the reason for the pet's visit to the hospital as communicated to the health-care team by the pet owner

Price Break a reduction given to purchasers in price per unit for a good if the order quantity exceeds a given amount determined by the seller

Primary Beam primary beam means the ionizing radiation coming directly from the radiation source through a beam port into the volume defined by the collimation system

Problem-Oriented Medical Record (POMR) the medical record format most commonly used by veterinary health-care teams, which follows a distinct format: the defined database, the problem list (also referred to as master list), the plan, and the progress

Proestrus the first week of a 3-week duration in which the bitch will expel bloody discharge

Prognosis the predicted outcome of the disease based on all the data the veterinarian and the health-care team have gathered

Prostaglandins a group of lipids made at sites of tissue damage or infection that are involved in dealing with injury and illness

Protocol a predetermined plan, rules, or series of guidelines within a business in the form of paper, electronic documents, or communication that individuals can refer to at any given time to minimize mistakes and carry out actions

Proximal describes a structure nearer to the point of origin or closer to the body

Pulmonic another term for pulmonary

Pyometra the presence of pus in the uterus

Quadriceps the muscle located anterior to the femur

Quick the area in which the nerve and blood supply are housed underneath the nail

Radius the cranial long bone of the forelimb that runs from the elbow to the carpus

Recombinant Vaccine a vaccine made from a live, nonpathogenic virus into which the gene for a pathogen-related antigen has been inserted

Rectum the lower part of the alimentary canal

Recumbent lying down

Renal relating to the kidneys

Reorder Point a system that records when a given product is running low or has run out and indicates to the personnel in charge of inventory maintenance to order more product

Reproductive Hormone a hormone produced by a gland, organ, or cell associated with the reproductive system which affects other parts of the body

Respiration Rate the total number of breaths taken by an animal for the duration of 1 minute

Respiratory System includes the mouth, nose, trachea, and lungs. It is responsible for absorbing oxygen and discharging carbon dioxide

Rhabdomyolysis a potentially life-threatening syndrome resulting from the breakdown of skeletal muscle fibers with leakage of muscle contents into the circulation

Rib one of the long curved bones occurring in 12 pairs in humans and extending from the spine to or toward the sternum

Rickettsiae the rickettsiae are rod-shaped or variably spherical, nonfilterable bacteria and most species are Gram negative. They are natural parasites of certain arthropods (notably lice, fleas, mites, and ticks) and can cause serious diseases – usually characterized by acute, self-limiting fevers – in humans and other animals

Root the central part of a word; the foundation or essential meaning of a word

Rostral pertaining to the nose end of the head

Ruff thick, dense hair located around the top of the neck

Sacral Vertebrae also known as the sacrum; consists of three fused vertebrae to which the pelvis is attached

Sagittal Plane an imaginary line that divides the body into right and left unequal parts

Saphenous Vein extends from the hock to the stifle on the medial aspect of the calf; becomes the femoral vein at the stifle

Scatter Radiation radiation that spreads out in different directions from a radiation beam when the beam interacts with a substance, such as body tissue

Schedule I a drug or substance that poses a high potential for abuse and has no currently accepted medical use for treatment in the United States; the drug or substance lacks accepted safety for use under medical supervision

Schedule II a drug or substance with a high potential for abuse and has currently been accepted for medical use in the United States or currently accepted medical use under severe restrictions; abuse of the drug or substance may lead to severe psychological or physical dependence

Schedule III a drug or substance with the potential for abuse less than the drugs or substances that fall under Schedules I and II; a drug or substance that has accepted medical use for treatment in the United States; the abuse of drugs or substances that may lead to moderate or low physical dependence or high psychological dependence

Schedule IV a drug or substance that has a low potential for abuse relative to the drugs or substances in Schedule III; a drug or substance that has been accepted for medical treatment in the United States; abuse of the drug or substance may lead to limited physical dependence or psychological dependence relative to drugs or substances in Schedule III

Schedule V a drug or substance that has a low potential for abuse relative to the drugs or substances in Schedule IV; a drug or substance that has a currently accepted medical use for treatment in the United States; the abuse of drugs or substances that may lead to limited physical dependence or psychological dependence relative to the drugs or substances in Schedule IV

Scrotum the sac-like formation of skin that houses the testes, located behind the penis

Seasonally Polyestrous those animals with estrous cycles occurring only during certain seasons of the year, due to the amount of daylight, are termed seasonally polyestrous

Seborrhea seborrheic dermatitis is a common skin disease that causes an itchy rash with flaky scales

Semimembranous/Semitendinous muscle group located in the rear leg; also known as the hamstring muscles

Sepsis a potentially life-threatening condition that occurs when the body's response to an infection damages its own tissues

Shoulder the muscular upper section of the upper arm

Signalment assists with proper identification of the patient, diagnosis, and predilections to traits and conditions as some conditions may be species, breed, gender, age, and color specific

Skeleton the jointed framework of the bones

Small Intestine composed of three parts: duodenum (attaches to the stomach), jejunum (middle and longest part), and ileum (last and smallest part, connects to the large intestine)

SOAP Format an acronym used by veterinary practices (Subjective, Objective, Assessment, and Plan)

Somatic Damage damage that is caused to the chromosomes in individual body tissue cells (such as skin cells or lung cells) by environmental factors (for example, UV light in the case of skin cells and tobacco smoke/air pollution or radiation from radon decay products in lung cells), which can accumulate over successive cell divisions and lead to cancer

Spay the surgical act of removing the uterus and ovaries from a female animal via the vulva

Standard Operating Procedures (SOP) guidelines set forth by the hospital management team. May or may not be professional standards, but will govern the procedures performed in the hospital

Standard Operating Procedures (SOP) Manual a handbook that lists all the written instructions for an organization's essential tasks. An SOP manual houses all an organization's individual SOPs in one place. The manual provides a comprehensive guide for overall operations

Standing Heat the period of time when the ova of a bitch have fully matured, thus making the bitch fertile from day 5 to 9 of the estrous cycle

Status Epilepticus a seizure that lasts longer than 5 minutes, or having more than one seizure within a 5-minute period, without returning to a normal level of consciousness between episodes

Sterile Field the area on and around the surgical table with which only personnel and sterile items may come in contact

Sternal Recumbency a position in which the animal is lying on its sternum or belly

Sternum also known as the breastbone; it forms the ventral midline of the rib cage

Stifle the joint located between the femur and the tibia

Stimulant a substance that raises levels of physiological or nervous activity in the body

Stock items available for distribution or sale from a business entity

Stomach a sac-like structure that stores large volumes of food

Stop indentation in the dog's forehead located just above the level of the eyes

Subcutaneous situated or applied under the skin

Subcutaneous (SQ or SC) Injection injection deep into (beneath) the skin, into the subcutis

Suffix the ending part of a word

Surgical Kick Bucket typically used as receptacles, stainless steel kick buckets are an essential part of any operating room

Suture the act of stitching; material used to close a wound or surgical incision by the act of suturing

Tachycardia a heart rate that is too fast

Tail part of the body just below the croup

Tarsus the joint that connects the crus (the lower leg) to the metatarsals, which are the beginning of the foot; the tarsus is distal to the tibia and fibula and consists of numerous, irregularly shaped bones arranged in several rows

Tease a technique used to stimulate an animal to accept coitus

Teeth used for chewing and grinding food

Temperament the mental, emotional, and physical traits of an animal in addition to its natural predisposition

Testicles two oval-shaped organs contained within the scrotum that are responsible for the production of sperm

Theriogenology a term used in veterinary medicine to relate to all aspects of reproduction

Thermoregulation a mechanism by which mammals maintain body temperature with tightly controlled self-regulation independent of external temperatures

Thigh the area of the hindquarters located between the hip and the stifle

Thoracic pertaining to the animal's chest

Thoracic Vertebrae the vertebrae of the chest

Thorax part of the body of a mammal between the neck and the abdomen, including the cavity enclosed by the ribs, breastbone, and dorsal vertebrae, and containing the chief organs of circulation and respiration; the chest

Thrombosis local coagulation or clotting of the blood in a part of the circulatory system

Tibia the larger of the two lower hindlimb bones, considered the more weight-bearing bone

Tick warm-blooded ectoparasite that attaches itself to warm-blooded animals to consume a blood meal

Tongue muscular structure located in the mouth

Toxicity the quality of being very harmful or unpleasant in a pervasive or insidious way

Trachea the tube that carries air to the lungs

Transducer a device that converts variations in a physical quantity, such as pressure or brightness, into an electrical signal, or vice versa

Transplacental passing through or occurring by way of the placenta

Transverse Plane an imaginary cross-section that divides the body into cranial and caudal parts

Triceps the muscle located caudal to the humerus

Truncal Alopecia hair loss on the trunk of the animal

Turnover Rate the time in which a given product is used and therefore should be replaced

Tympanic Membrane also referred to as the ear drum; aids in the transmission of sound and separates the external ear from the middle ear

Ulna the caudal long bone of the forelimb that runs from the elbow to the carpus

Ureters long tubes that funnel urine down into the bladder

Urethra the canal that carries the urine from the bladder

Urinary Catheterization in urinary catheterization, a catheter (hollow tube) is inserted into the bladder to drain or collect urine

Urogenital System includes the kidneys, urinary bladder, genitals, ureters, and urethra

Uterine Horns the uterus consists of two tubes or uterine horns that join with a short uterine body. This is the incubator that nourishes unborn puppies and kittens

Uterus houses the developing fetus; the dog uterus has two horns

Vaccine a biological product representative of a pathogenic organism responsible for stimulating immunity toward the pathogen

Vaginal Cytology the observation of vaginal discharge underneath a microscope to detect cells

Vasoconstriction narrowing or constriction of the blood vessels. It happens when smooth muscles in blood vessel walls tighten, which makes the blood vessel opening smaller. May also be called vasospasm

Vasodilation vasodilation, or the widening of blood vessels, happens naturally in the body when an increase in blood flow to tissues is needed. It is a normal process but it can also be part of health issues

Vein a blood vessel that carries deoxygenated blood toward the heart

Ventral pertaining to the belly or underside of the body

Vertebral Column also known as the backbone; it is made up of numerous vertebrae

Vibrissae whiskers, or vibrissae, are long, coarse hairs protruding from an animal's muzzle, jaw, and above its eyes

Viscosity the state of being thick, sticky, and semifluid in consistency, due to internal friction

Volatile Fatty Acids (VFAs) are linear short-chain aliphatic monocarboxylate compounds, such as acetic acid, propionic acid, and butyric acid, which are the building blocks of different organic compounds; VFAs have two (acetic acid) to six (caproic acid) carbon atoms

V-Trough a V-shaped device used to stabilize an animal placed in dorsal recumbency

Vulva the external opening to the vagina of female animals, characterized by a slit-like structure located below the anus

Withers the top of the shoulder blade and the highest point of the body; located just behind the neck

Wrist located lower on the front paw, also known as the carpus

Zoonotic a disease that is transmissible between animals and humans

Zygodactyl the shape of the feet in the psittacine species manifested as the second and third toes directed forward with the first and fourth toes directed backward

Index

Page locators in **bold** indicate tables. Page locators in *italics* indicate figures. This index uses letter-by-letter alphabetization.
